W9-BSA-209

MYOCARDIUM AT RISK AND VIABLE MYOCARDIUM

Developments in Cardiovascular Medicine

VOLUME 234

Myocardium at Risk and Viable Myocardium

Evaluation by SPET

edited by

JAUME CANDELL-RIERA

Department of Cardiology,
Hospital Universitari Vall d'Hebron, Barcelona, Spain

JOAN CASTELL-CONESA

Department of Nuclear Medicine,
Hospital Universitari Vall d'Hebron, Barcelona, Spain

and

SANTIAGO AGUADÉ-BRUIX

Department of Nuclear Medicine,
Hospital Universitari Vall d'Hebron, Barcelona, Spain

KLUWER ACADEMIC PUBLISHERS
DORDRECHT / BOSTON / LONDON

A C.I.P. Catalogue record for this book is available from the Library of Congress.

ISBN 0-7923-6724-3

Published by Kluwer Academic Publishers,
P.O. Box 17, 3300 AA Dordrecht, The Netherlands.

Sold and distributed in North, Central and South America
by Kluwer Academic Publishers,
101 Philip Drive, Norwell, MA 02061, U.S.A.

In all other countries, sold and distributed
by Kluwer Academic Publishers,
P.O. Box 322, 3300 AH Dordrecht, The Netherlands.

This book is an updated version of an edition originally publihed in Spanish as "Miocardio en riesgo y miocardio viable". Translated by Dr. Peter Turner; Translation revised by Dr. G. Permanyer-Miralda.

Printed on acid-free paper

All Rights Reserved
© 2001 Kluwer Academic Publishers
No part of the material protected by this copyright notice may be reproduced or
utilized in any form or by any means, electronic or mechanical,
including photocopying, recording or by any information storage and
retrieval system, without written permission from the copyright owner.

Printed in the Netherlands.

MYOCARDIUM AT RISK

AND VIABLE MYOCARDIUM

Evaluation by SPET

Edited by J. Candell-Riera, J. Castell-Conesa and S. Aguadé-Bruix

CONTENTS

Contents

LIST OF CONTRIBUTORS

Santiago Aguadé-Bruix
Department of Nuclear Medicine
Hospital Universitari Vall d'Hebron
Barcelona
Spain

Jaume Candell-Riera
Department of Cardiology
Hospital Universitari Vall d'Hebron
Barcelona
Spain

Joan Castell-Conesa
Department of Nuclear Medicine
Hospital Universitari Vall d'Hebron
Barcelona
Spain

Joan Cinca-Cuscullola
Department of Cardiology
Hospital Universitari Vall d'Hebron
Barcelona
Spain

Josefa Cortadellas-Angel
Department of Cardiology
Hospital Universitari Vall d'Hebron
Barcelona
Spain

Amparo García-Burillo
Department of Nuclear Medicine
Hospital Universitari Vall d'Hebron
Barcelona
Spain

David García-Dorado
Department of Cardiology
Hospital Universitari Vall d'Hebron
Barcelona
Spain

José Manuel González-González
Department of Nuclear Medicine
Hospital Universitari Vall d'Hebron
Barcelona
Spain

Domingo Ortega-Alcalde
Department of Nuclear Medicine
Hospital Universitari Vall d'Hebron
Barcelona
Spain

César Santana-Boado
Department of Cardiology
Hospital Universitari Vall d'Hebron
Barcelona
Spain

Jordi Soler-Soler
Department of Cardiology
Hospital Universitari Vall d'Hebron
Barcelona
Spain

FOREWORD

The clinical use of nuclear cardiology for the assessment of myocardial ischemia continues to grow at an unprecedented rate. Part of the reason for this growth is the technical advances in single photon emission computerized tomography (SPECT). SPECT has been shown to provide high contrast images superior to planar imaging techniques. An important and recent technical advancement in SPECT has been ECG-gated myocardial perfusion SPECT to generate simultaneous myocardial perfusion and function information from a single study. Automated, quantitative techniques have facilitated the widespread application of this breakthrough. Another recent advancement has been the use of attenuation correction techniques to help remove the effects of the physical phenomena that degrades the visual and quantitative accuracy of SPECT images. Another reason for the growth of the clinical use of nuclear cardiology is the large body of published evidence documenting the effectiveness of SPECT techniques for assessing myocardial ischemia, myocardium at risk, viable myocardium and stunned or hibernating myocardium. These assessments have been shown to be important not only in diagnosis but also in prognosis.

This book is divided into three major sections, each addressing the important topics that have led to the clinical success of nuclear cardiology. The first section is a description of the technical aspects of state-of-the-art myocardial perfusion SPECT imaging. This section deals with the radionuclides, instrumentation, image acquisition and analysis, interpretation and quantification techniques used in the most progressive nuclear cardiology clinics. The second section discusses different SPECT approaches for the assessment of myocardium at risk and compares them to other techniques. The third section addresses the assessment of viable myocardium with SPECT and includes discussions on the pathophysiology of stunned and hibernating myocardium, differential diagnosis of ischemia vs. necrosis and the clinical need for detecting viable myocardium.

This book is written by a team of cardiologists and nuclear medicine physicians who have been performing and interpreting nuclear cardiology procedures for about twenty years. For many years they have been contributing to the nuclear cardiology literature by reporting the results of their investigations and by providing state-of-the-art educational material. The content of the book reflects the practical understanding of the subject that comes from their day to day clinical experience. This book is beautifully illustrated and contains a wealth of references. It is yet another important contribution by this team of physicians that should be of value to the practitioners of nuclear cardiology procedures and referring physicians alike.

Ernest V. Garcia

Emory University

Atlanta

U.S.A.

PREFACE

In 1977 we performed the first cardiac scintigraphy with technetium-99m pyrophosphate in the Hospital General Universitari Vall d'Hebron. In 1980 we performed the first isotopic ventriculography, in 1982 the first planar myocardial scintigraphy with thallium-201 and, in 1988, with compounds labelled with technetium-99m. The technical skills that we acquired during these years and their clinical application were presented in the book *Cardiología Nuclear* that was first published in 1992 and which was subsequently translated into English under the title *Nuclear Cardiology in Everyday Practice*.

Over the last decade a fundamental shift in nuclear cardiology has occurred with the advent of the technique of tomography. From our point of view this represented a qualitative change in the evaluation and quantification of cardiac studies with radionuclides. New concepts in cardiology have emerged in parallel especially within the ambit of coronary artery disease: concepts such as "jeopardise myocardium", "culprit lesion", "open artery", "clandestine ischaemia", "reperfusion damage", "remodelled ventricle", "stunned myocardium" and "hibernating myocardium". These have represented a new stimulus for the development of nuclear cardiology techniques.

We feel that it is now time to publish our experience gained over these past few years in single photon emission tomography in the diagnosis of the jeopardised myocardium and the viable myocardium and the quantification of both. Parts of this material contained in the text have been derived from various publications. However, we think that it is convenient to group our results and to contrast them with those that have been published in the literature with the objective that Spanish speaking cardiologists and clinicians in nuclear medicine would have, in one text, a reference starting point.

This book is the fruition of work and experience from two clinical services that coincided in a hospital that favoured close collaboration. As such, we wish to thank not only the authors who have collaborated in putting-together the different chapters but also those who, over the years, have helped us to put these techniques into practice and to generate and to interpret the data on which this book is based. We are also grateful to Dr. Peter Turner, who translated the book, to Dr. G. Permanyer-Miralda, who revised the manuscript, and to Drs. G. Oller, O. Pereztol and G. Romero, for their collaboration in the editorial task.

Jaume Candell-Riera

Joan Castell-Conesa

Santiago Aguadé-Bruix

Hospital Universitari Vall d'Hebron

Barcelona

Spain

1. RADIONUCLIDES, INSTRUMENTATION AND PROCEDURES

DOMINGO ORTEGA-ALCALDE and SANTIAGO AGUADÉ-BRUIX

1. Radionuclides and Radiopharmaceuticals

The study of myocardial perfusion using radionuclides requires the use of a tracer that has a great avidity for the myocardium, a good uptake and distribution in the myocardium that is proportional to the regional blood flow.

To-date, the most widely used tracers are Thallium-201 and Technetium-99m-labelled compounds. All require a similar methodology with respect to timing of stress, injection, detection and processing. However, technetium-labelled tracers are less attenuated by anatomical structures compared to Thallium and its energy is more suited to the characteristics of the detectors that are normally used in Nuclear Medicine and, with which, images of better quality and better performance of the SPET (Single Photon Emission Tomography) are obtained.

1.1. THALLIUM-201

Thallium-201 is a cyclotron produced radionuclide with some chemical properties of a monovalent cation, analogous to potassium [1,2] and with a similar biological behaviour as an intracellular ion [3]. Its half-life (T1/2) is 73.5 hours. In its transition by electron capture to ^{201}Hg, it emits a small quantity of gamma photons (2.6% at 135 keV and 10% at 166 keV). The principal photon emission (87.4%) are as X-rays of low intensity (69-83 keV) from the ^{201}Hg. These physical characteristics limit the maximum activity of ^{201}Tl that can be administered to the patient [4].

Following its intravenous administration in the form of thallium chloride, it distributes itself in the organism in proportion to the regional blood flow [5]. It is incorporated in the cardiac myocyte membrane as a function of the existing coronary flow and of the uptake capacity of the membrane and, in the myocardium, reaches about 4% of the total administered dose. The rest distributes between the liver, spleen, skeletal musculature, brain and kidneys [6]. Incorporation into the membrane is in two ways: one is an active route via the Na^+-K^+-ATPase pump that requires cellular integrity for its action and which is proportional to the level of cellular metabolic activity; the other, a passive route which, given the small size of the hydrated ion of ^{201}Tl (1.44 Å)[3], is purely by diffusion.

The uptake of Thallium from the blood is rapid with a myocardium capture of up to 85% in the first pass [7], the relationship between the degree of capture and coronary blood flow remains linear over a wide range of coronary flows.

J. Candell-Riera et al. (eds.), Myocardium at Risk and Viable Myocardium, 1–25.
© 2001 *Kluwer Academic Publishers. Printed in the Netherlands.*

Following the incorporation into the myocardial cells and within a maximum of about 20 minutes, a tendency towards equilibrium between intra- and extra-cellular concentrations of Thallium begins (the washout effect) and in which the myocyte concentrations equilibrate with that of the bloodstream; a phenomenon known as redistribution [8]. This redistribution is much more rapid when the regional blood flow is high and, in general, is considered complete after 3-4 hours. In zones with poor blood flow this could be delayed up to 24 hours[6]. The final elimination of Thallium from the organism is very slow and is via, predominantly, the kidneys.

1.2. TECHNETIUM-LABELLED COMPOUNDS

Myocardium perfusion tracers labelled with ^{99m}Tc have a major role for the future essentially because of the better physical characteristics of ^{99m}Tc. The higher energy of its gamma radiation (140 keV) reduces signal attenuation that can be caused by the interposition of other organs (breast, diaphragm) during the detection and is more suited to the detector systems (crystal thickness, collimators etc..)[6]. Further, its short half-life (6 hours) allows a higher dose to be administered to the patient and with lower dosimetry than ^{201}Tl and, with the higher photon flow, the quality of the image is improved together with the possibility of reducing the time of image acquisition [9].

Also, using ^{99m}Tc as the radionuclide, it is possible to perform a first pass ventriculography simultaneously with the administration of the dose in the moment of maximum exercise or during the administration of the dose at rest [10,11].

1.2.1. ^{99m}Tc-Isonitrile:

Of the many compounds of isonitriles labelled with ^{99m}Tc that have been studied [12], methoxy-isobutyl-isonitrile (MIBI) has the best biological properties for clinical use.

It is a lipophyllic compound with great myocardial affinity. Its cellular uptake is by diffusion across the transmembrane negative potential and is independent of the extracellular pH and of the Na^+-K^+-ATPase pump. Its distribution is proportional to the regional coronary flow [13]. More than 90% binds to the mitochondria within the cytosol and is in proportion to the level of mitochondrial metabolic activity [14]. The rate of myocardial uptake of MIBI is between 1.5 and 2% of the administered dose and, of which, 60% is bound during the first pass [15]. The rest of the activity distributes, in proportion to the flow, in the liver, spleen, kidneys and skeletal musculature. Active excretion of the tracer is via the hepato-biliary route [13]. The rate of uptake of MIBI allows for a good level of activity contrast between the heart and the lungs starting from around 60-90 minutes at which time the detection needs to be done [16].

The phenomenon of redistribution is practically nil since it is retained within the cell without returning to the bloodstream. Hence, one dose of the radiolabelled agent needs to be administered in the stress test and another dose at rest [17].

1.2.2. ^{99m}Tc-Tetrofosmin:

A phosphated compound labelled with ^{99m}Tc [18,19] and which acts as a lipophyllic cation. The mechanism of action is related to the cellular transmembrane potential difference and with uptake in the cytosol proportional to the cellular metabolic gradient. Its bio-distribution parallels regional blood flow to each organ while, in the heart, there is a tendency to saturation at high coronary flows [20] similar to that observed for MIBI. The rest of the distribution is mainly in liver, spleen, skeletal musculature and kidneys. It has a good and rapid myocardial uptake (1.2-1.4% of administered dose) and with a lung and blood clearance that is considerable faster than MIBI and, as such, provides an optimum heart-lung contrast after 10 minutes [21]. Elimination is essentially via the hepato-biliary route. It does not exhibit the phenomenon of redistribution and so it is necessary to administer a different dose of the radiolabel for the evaluation of the myocardium at rest [22].

1.2.3 ^{99m}Tc-Teboroxime:

This is a ^{99m}Tc compound derived form boronic acid [23,24], ionically neutral, with high molecular weight, highly lipophyllic and which has a great affinity, though reversible [25], for the cell membrane proteins to which it binds without entering the cytosol. The rate of binding is independent of the grade of cellular metabolism. The compound has a level of myocardial uptake superior to that of ^{201}Tl (around 90%) and its uptake is proportional to the coronary blood flow, including at very high flow rates [26]. It has a low pulmonary capture and its principal route of elimination is hepato-biliary.

Following the incorporation into the myocardium, the tracer is cleared rapidly from the heart because of the reversibility of its binding to the proteins. The clearance dynamics are biphasic; a rapid phase (68%) having a period of 2-3 minutes in stress and 5-6 minutes at rest, and a slow phase of 78 minutes (32%) [27]. This rapid clearance makes it difficult to obtain images since they must be acquired very rapidly post-administration (less than 2 minutes) and over a short time interval so as to avoid differences between the first and the last SPET images acquired.

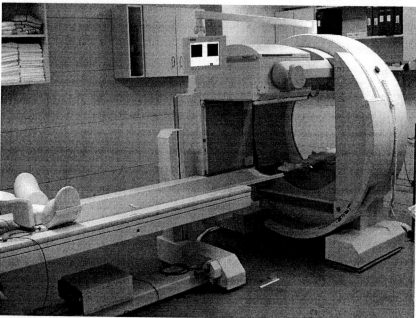

FIGURE 1: Dual head, adjacent (90º) gammacamera .

The clearance from the blood is very rapid and only 9.5% of the dose remains in the circulation at 15 minutes after the injection [28]. This facilitates the administration of the resting dose with a few minutes after the performance of the stress test.

At present its use is limited because of the speed with which the detection needs to be conducted and the need for multiheaded detectors (even up to three heads)[29].

2. Instrumentation

2.1. GAMMACAMERA

The gammacamera is the fundamental equipment of detection in Nuclear Medicine (Figure 1). It is composed of an Anger type detector head (single or multiple), fixed to a revolving support capable of orbiting in any plane and connected to a computer for the storage and processing of images.

2.1.1. *Detector head:*
The scintillation detector is a transducer that converts the radiation energy into electronic impulses and consists of: collimator, detector crystal, photomultiplier tubes, lead shielding and associated electronics.

The detector crystal is of sodium iodide with small traces of thallium and which has the property of fluorescing in response to the interaction of gamma-radiation; the quantity of light emitted being proportional to the energy of the incident radiation striking the crystal. Using a series of cathodes and photomultiplier tubes, the light emitted by the crystal is converted into electric impulses of a voltage proportional to the energy of the

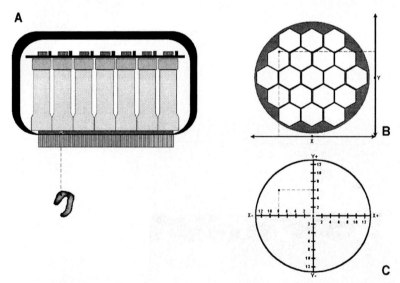

Figure 2: A) Scheme of an Anger type gammacamera (collimator, scintillation crystal, photomultipliers and associated electronics). B) Cover of the scintillation crystal surface with hexagonal cathodes. C) Spatial relationship of a gamma-photon detected.

radiation and which can be analysed using electronic slides [30].

The Anger type gammacamera [31] (Figure 2) is composed of a variable number of photomultiplier tubes that are distributed in the detector crystal in a hexagonal geometry within the cathode and which precludes any area of the crystal not being covered. Each radiation detected is codified by four parameters: its position in the X and Y axes of a system of co-ordinates centred in the detector field, the voltage of the impulse derived from its energy detection and the time at which the detection is made [32].

This information is transformed into digital impulses at the output end of the pre-amplifier of each photomultiplier and, subsequently, transferred to the computer. The information is used to spatially locate, relative to the X and Y axes, the point of interaction of the radiation with the detector for each time interval and for one or other energies of the specific emitters. The image is built-up with the integrated data.

The whole of the detector head is shielded with lead so as to preclude any radiation, other than that proceeding from the holes of the collimator, from striking on the scintillation crystal.

2.1.2   Collimator:

Before interacting with the detector crystal the radiation needs to be focussed. This is the function of the collimator. It consists of a grid of orifices over a matrix of lead and the characteristics of each collimator [33] are derived from the diameter of the orifices (wider at the septum and narrower at the lead matrix). For example, the greater the diameter of the orifice the greater the sensitivity and less the resolution; the greater the thickness of

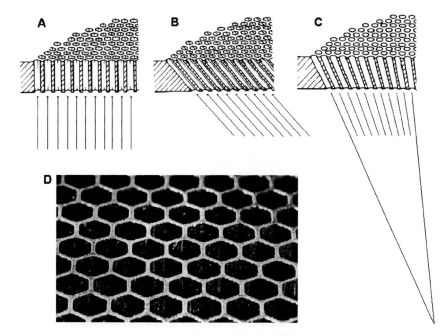

Figure 3:   A) Scheme of collimator with parallel holes perpendicular to the lead matrix.   B) Scheme of collimator with parallel holes inclined with respect to the lead matrix. C) Scheme of collimator with focalised asymmetric holes. D) Detail of the surface of a collimator with honeycomb orifices and lead partition .

the septum, the greater the energy of detection and less the sensitivity; the smaller the diameter of the orifice, the greater the resolution and the lower the sensitivity (Figure 3) [34].

Another characteristic of a collimator refers to the orientation of the holes: parallel, inclined, symmetrically focussed and asymmetrically focussed (Figure 3,C).

Usually a collimator of low energy, medium resolution and high sensitivity is used for the detection of ^{201}Tl and a collimator of high energy, high resolution and medium sensitivity for [99m]Tc.

2.1.3.   *Gantry support:*

This is a mechanical system for support of the detector and which allows a stable rotatory movement of the detector head. Its construction needs to be strong since the weight of the detector head can easily reach 300 kg.

It is possible to mount more than one detector head on the support. Dual headed detectors can be mounted in opposition at 180° or adjacent at 90° while triple headed detectors can be mounted in an equilateral triangle with an angle of 60° between each of them (Figure 4).

The conduct of a tomographic study implies the acquisition of multiple images each of which is a distinct projection taken while the detector rotates around the patient. The computer subsequently processes the data of each image to obtain three-dimensional information and which constitutes the basis of SPET [30].

The heart being situated asymmetrically in the thorax, it is not necessary for myocardial perfusion scintigraphy that the information from the tomography detection be acquired from a complete orbit of 360°. An arc of 180° (that includes the cardiac region) starting

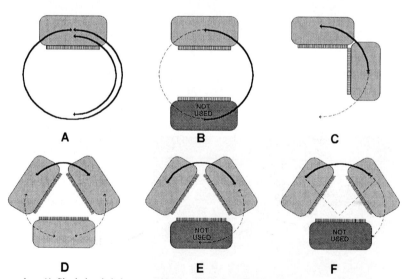

Figure 4:   A) Single-headed detector with circular and semi-circular orbit. B) Dual-headed detector in opposition and semi-circular orbit. C) Dual-headed detector in adjacent position and orbit of 90°. D) Triple-headed detector in adjacent position and orbit of 60°. E) Triple-headed detector in adjacent position and orbit of 120° (lower head not used). F) Triple-headed detector in adjacent position, collimators parallel and inclined at 15°, and orbit of 90° (lower head not used).

from the right anterior oblique (RAO) and ending in the left posterior oblique projection (LPO), is sufficient to obtain the images. The trajectory can be circular with a fixed radius, or elliptical. The latter fits better with the morphology of the thorax (Figure 5). The 180° arc allows for a reduction in the radius and a greater proximity of the detector to the patient compared to complete orbits (whether circular or elliptical) and, further, produces a variation at the centre of rotation which, in the circular orbit, is_shifted downwards (Figure 5). Some equipment offer the facility of detection at a distance and which adapts the radius of the elliptical orbit (contoured orbit) so as to disturb the patient less.

As a function of the number and geometry of the detector heads, the arc through which the support passes varies from 180° for the single detector to 90° for the double adjacent detectors and to 60° for the triple head. This reduction of the arc implies that, while maintaining the same rate of image acquisition, an arc of 90° reduces the total time by half and if the arc is 60° the reduction in time is to one third of that of only one detector head. (Figure 4).

The sequence of movement can be in two ways: continuous and stepwise (step and shoot). In the continuous detection mode the detector revolves without interruption, the velocity of rotation is fixed and so is the interval of angle for the acquisition of the image (every 2°, 3° or 6°). In the stepwise mode, the interval of angle and time for image acquisition is defined and the detector only registers the image when it is stopped at a pre-determined angle but not while turning to the next angular position. A mixed system within the stepwise mode of detection is one in which there is no stopping the image acquisition in the course of the detector rotation [35] and which increases the quality of the ultra-fast tomographic studies (2 to 5 minutes duration).

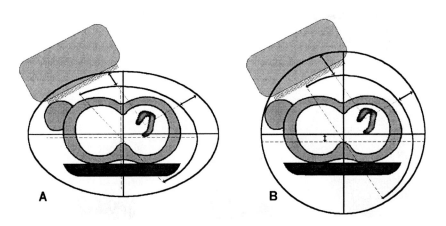

Figure 5: A) Elliptical orbits of 360° and 180°. Note the decrease in the major and minor radii of the ellipse in the 180° detection. B) Circular orbits of 360° and 180°. Note the considerable decrease in the radius and of the detector-subject distance in the 180° detection due to the descent of the centre of rotation .

2.1.4.   *Transmission image:*

Newer machines that incorporate the possibility for attenuation correction have an additional system to obtain a transmission image simultaneous to the detection of the scintigraphic image. This facilitates an individualised attenuation correction in each point of the image caused by the interpositioning of anatomical structures [36].

For this the manufacturers are incorporating in their gammacameras some external emitter sources such as gadolinium (^{153}Gd), gold (^{195}Au) or americium (^{241}Am) to be used in conjunction with ^{99m}Tc and cobalt (^{67}Co) for ^{201}Tl or ^{99m}Tc refills [37,38,39]. Independent of the radionucleide used, with multidetector gammacameras there are two types of transmission acquisition: the fixed linear source and the mobile source with electronic collimation.

In the dual-headed detector, the fixed linear source is for the emission image (scintigraphy) and the other for the transmission image (attenuation) and which has an asymmetrically focussed collimator. In the triple-headed equipment, two are used for the emission images and the third, with a symmetrically focussed collimator, for the transmission image. In these cases, the dedication of one head to the transmission image implies that the orbit to be described increases for the head that performs the emission image acquisition [39] (Figure 6; A, B and C).

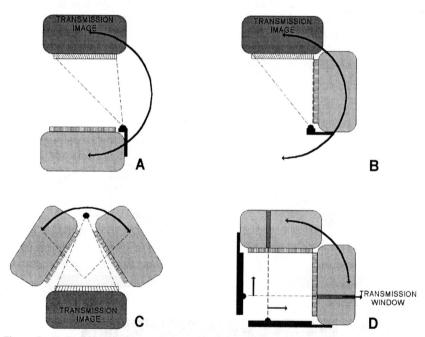

Figure 6: A) Dual-headed detector in opposition and semi-circular orbit. The opposed detector, with asymmetrically focussed collimator, acquires the transmission image proceeding from a fixed linear source. B) Dual-headed detector in adjacent position and semicircular orbit. One of the detectors with an asymmetrically focussed collimator acquires the transmission image proceeding from a fixed linear source. C) Triple-headed detectors in adjacent position, parallel collimators inclined at 15° and orbit of 90°. The lower with a symmetrical focussed collimator acquires the transmission from a fixed linear source. D) Dual-headed detector in adjacent position and orbit of 90° with a system of a double mobile source that sweeps lengthways for each image.

The mobile linear source and electronic collimator are installed above the adjacent double heads which simultaneously acquire emission and transmission images. A small strip of the detector situated across from the linear source acquires the transmission image while the rest of the detector acquires the transmission image (Figure 6; D). The source moves with constant velocity and is tracked by the electronic collimator so that for each transmission image the linear source performs a sweep. This system does not alter the orbit but the time of image acquisition needs to be increased as a function of the relationship between the width of the band of the electronic collimation and the dimension of the head.

The transmission images need to be processed so as to obtain the corresponding tomography slices that are then used to reconstruct the SPET and to correct for the attenuation caused by the structures of the thorax.

2.1.5. *Synchronised detection:*

For this type of detection it is required that, in addition to the signals of the gammacamera, the computer receives the R wave data (R-R interval in milliseconds) from the ECG, activated by the shutter release or trigger. This is taken as the duration of cardiac cycle and is divided into an equal number of time intervals, usually between 8 and 16. In a cyclic manner, and starting from each R wave, the information proceeding from the gammacamera undergoes the same fractionation as a function of time. Finally, a series of sequential summed images, corresponding to equal moments of consecutive cycles, are obtained and which constitute an averaged cardiac cycle (Figure 7).

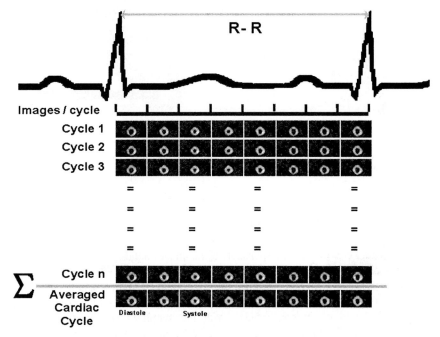

Figure 7: Scheme for synchronised detection. Division of the acquisition in fixed fractions of the R-R interval with summation of the cycles acquired during the projection.

As such, each of the multiple projections of the tomographic detection is formed, in essence, by a series of fractionated images of the cardiac cycle seen from this angle. Once the detection is completed and the images processed, a tomographic reconstruction (Gated SPET)[40] of each of the fractions of the cardiac cycles is obtained (Figure 8). The information so acquired contributes, in addition to the myocardial perfusion data, to the possibility of evaluating ventricular function [41,42], wall motion [43], systolic thickening [44] and myocardial mass [45].

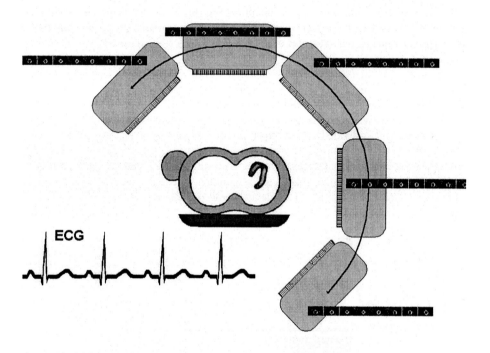

Figure 8: Synchronised SPET acquisition (Gated-SPET); a complete tomographic study being obtained for each fraction of the cardiac cycle acquired.

2.2. EQUIPMENT QUALITY CONTROL

The regular quality controls are indispensable if the images obtained are to be assessable in a viable manner. Normally, this is in two phases. The initial phase is the overall assessment of the equipment once installed [46] (requirement of the manufacturer). This includes verification of the head, the tomographic status and the collimators [47] and whose results should be in concordance with the supplier's specifications for the equipment (NEMA)[48] and which will serve as reference for subsequent actions. The second phase, or routine monitoring, is performed with variable periodicity based on the history of the equipment and preventive repair indications [49].

Monitoring includes the regular assessment for all gammacameras with respect to their uniformity of detection (uniformity map). This should indicate that the same activity is registered with the same signal whatever the position of the detector; its linearity (linearity map) which is the equivalent to astigmatism in classical optics; its sensitivity (electronic adjustment)[50] or the efficiency in the detection of minimum activities; its spatial resolution or the capacity to differentiate as being separate two points of close activity; its temporal resolution, or the capacity to distinguish two detections in temporal proximity; and its energy resolution or the capacity to discriminate the emissions of different radionuclides [51] (Table 1).

The spatial, temporal and energy resolution requirements are linked to the design of the detector (thickness of the crystal, geometry and number of photomultipliers together with their size and time-lag, collimator, etc.)[47,52] and which vary very slowly in parallel with the ageing of the equipment.

TABLE 1. Periodicity of quality control tests

TEST	PERIODICITY
Verification of uniformity	Daily/weekly
Verification of linearity/resolution	Weekly/monthly
Calibration of the matrix for correction of uniformity	Weekly/monthly
Correction of the centre of rotation	Weekly/monthly
Verification of pixel size	Weekly/monthly

Many of these measures, including those carried-out during image acquisition, are performed automatically (autocalibration) and are apparent to frequent users of such equipment [53].

What needs to be taken into account is the greater degree of uniformity required for SPET (<2% variation) than for planar scintigraphy (<5%). Each projection is a statistical assessment of counts detected and, in tomography, the activity detected at each point of the rotation is much less and small variations in the uniformity of the field can alter the quality of the images [54]. Hence, the manufacturers usually recommend correcting original tomographic images against a specific map for each type of acquisition (based on collimator, tracer, acquisition matrix, zoom, etc). This needs to be done periodically since conditions of gain on the photomulitpliers and the responses of the electronic systems vary with the weather [55].

Equipment that includes the correction facilities for attenuation needs to have the condition of the emission source checked, correction maps generated for each type of source that may be used and pixel size (unit of measurement of the acquisition matrix) calibrated. This is so that the superimposition of emission and transmission images may be performed with precision [53].

Other important aspects that need to be controlled are those related to the rotation of the head, such as the velocity and the center of rotation [56]. Also, the uniformity of the rotatory movement of the camera head needs to be evaluated regularly. The loss of mechanical stability can produce an excess of wobble or the de-alignment of the patient's couch/stretcher support with respect to the detector which can generate artefacts in the reconstruction and which are generally detectable as linear defects in the reconstruction sinograms.

3. Procedures

3.1. SPET DETECTION PROCEDURES

The specific procedure for tomographic detection is designed as a function of the tracer. For example, due to the rapid myocardial clearance of teboroxime, a maximum time for the acquisition of the image is about 6 minutes and tree-head camera are ideal since the tomography can be completed in 4 minutes [29], or 5 minutes for Gated-SPET using focussing collimators and tree-head camera detection [57].

Nowadays, the majority of authors [35,36,58] propose a circular arc of 180° (RAO-LPO) in step-and-shoot mode but this depends on the design of the gammacameras since there are machines that are designed to perform fixed elliptical orbits.

Generally, the position of the patient for the detection is in supine decubitus with the left arm or both arms placed above the head. Some reports recommend, especially in male patients, the prone decubitus position since this reduces the interference of the diaphragm on the inferior face of the left ventricle [59].

Once the patient is positioned, the height of the couch/stretcher and the radius of the rotation need to be adjusted so as to place the patient as close to the detector without making contact.

The differences in the acquisition between ^{201}Tl and the technetium-labelled compounds derive from their pharmacokinetic properties and their type of radioactive emission[60,61]. For example, ^{201}Tl has an energy and photon flow lower than that of ^{99m}Tc and requires a collimator of low energy and medium resolution (Low Energy Medium Resolution = LEMR) to obtain a sufficient level of counts for the image, but at the expense of a lower spatial resolution. Further, the time required to obtain a sufficient level of counts in each image is high (20-25 seconds). As a result, the total time of the study is prolonged and the last images detected show the signs of redistribution. As such, it becomes necessary to reduce the total number of images (30/60) when using Thallium-201 (Table 2)[4,62]. Finally, it is important to emphasise that, in case of problems, it is impossible to repeat the tomography detection since the Thallium redistribution phase will have already begun. The acquisition needs to be normalised, as previously, by the processor and the adjustment is with the energy map.

Technetium-labelled tracers have a better adaptation to the detector system. The greater energy and high photon flows (for medium and high doses of ^{99m}Tc) allow for the use of a collimator of low energy and high resolution (Low Energy High Resolution = LEHR) with good spatial resolution (Table 2)[4] and a relatively short (10-18 seconds) detection time; albeit these times varying as a function of the a function of the dose of ^{99m}Tc administered (Table 3)[61].

These studies require normalisation using an energy map but, also, because of the short half-life of ^{99m}Tc, a correction needs to be done for the decay of technetium i.e. the theoretical activity present in the first image acquired needs to be identical to that of the last image. In some equipment a summed normalisation factor is introduced which combines the factors of the different variables such as type of tracer (physical and biological half-lives) and the myocardial clearance of the tracer etc. As such, the normalisation factor needs to be determined in each nuclear cardiology unit based on individual experience.

TABLE 2. Characteristics of SPET acquisition

	SPET		Gated-SPET	
	^{201}Tl	^{99m}Tc	^{201}Tl	^{99m}Tc
Collimator	LEMR	LEHR	LEMR	LEHR
Matrix	64^2	$64^2/128^2$	64^2	$64^2/128^2$
Number of images	30/60	60/120	30*8	60*8/60*16
Detection range	180°	180°	180°	180°
Aperture	6°/3°	3°/1.5°	6°	3°
Images/cycle	-	-	8	8/16
Acquisition normalisation	Energy	Decay and energy	Decay	Decay and energy

LEMR = Low Energy Medium Resolution; LEHR = Low Energy High Resolution

TABLE 3. Overall estimated time (in minutes) of detection

Detector type	^{201}Tl	SPET ^{99m}Tc Dose			^{201}Tl	Gated-SPET ^{99m}Tc Dose	
		Low	Medium	High		Medium	High
1 head	22	22	15	12	45	45	30
2 heads	11	11	8	6	22	22	15
3 heads	7	7	5	4	15	15	10

3.2.   GATED-SPET (GSPET) DETECTION PROCEDURES

In addition to the characteristics for SPET (Table 2), those specific to the synchronisation with the R wave from the ECG need to be defined. GSPET detection supersedes normal SPET detection in clinical protocols and the data acquired in Gated-SPET (summation of the images of all of the cycle) constitutes a typical SPET study [40].

The number of images per cycle indicates the number of fractions into which each of the cycles is divided during the image acquisition. In general, 8 images per cycle are taken but with technetium-labelled tracers and high doses it is possible to acquire 16 images per cycle and which generates a better temporal resolution.

A very important aspect is that of frequency tolerance. In the studies of ventricular function (with radionuclide equilibrium ventriculography), the filtration criterion is important (10-15% of tolerance) so that evaluation is only on very similar cycles that have been widely averaged over 300 to 800 cycles [63]. In GSPET, on the other hand, the total number of cycles per projection is low (20 to 30; depending on the cardiac frequency of the patient) and, should the filtration criteria not be well controlled, very few (or none) of the cycles would be acceptable. The myocardial perfusion information would be lost in this projection and no image obtained.

So as to preclude this loss of information, the criterion of tolerance for cardiac frequency of the patient that is used in GSPET is based on a high (or very high) level of acceptance with tolerances greater than 75% or even 90% [42]. In contrast, the generation of each projection of an average cycle can give rise to the overall duration of the cycle varying in the long term of the study (up to 30 minutes) such that the temporal location of the systolic image can become altered.

3.3.   PROCEDURES: CLINICAL PROTOCOLS

In the design of the protocols for clinical use the most important factor to be taken into account is the bio-kinetics of the tracer [58,60] and, by implication, the time intervals between injection and detection, the possibility of repeating the detection, the requirement of a second dose of the tracer (Table 4) or the capability to perform delayed detections. Figure 9 schematically depicts comparisons of some of the procedures of myocardial perfusion studies.

TABLE 4. Dosimetry of myocardial perfusion studies

Tracer	Protocol	Activity (MBq)	Dosimetry (mSv)
^{201}Tl	Single dose	111-148 MBq	34-46 mSv
^{99m}Tc	Short	370 MBq + 1110 MBq	12.2 mSv
	Long	740 MBq + 740 MBq	12.2 mSv

Figure 10 shows the different protocols for the evaluation of the viable myocardium. In all of them the injection of the tracer is performed at rest with or without the administration of nitrates. The technetium-labelled tracers (MIBI and tetrofosmin) have all identical procedures, but the procedures for thallium have greater variations [64,65].

Inevitably, the design of the protocol would need to be adapted to the type of gammacamera available (number of heads, attenuation correction, etc).

3.3.1.   Thallium-201:

Stress/Redistribution protocol: Myocardial perfusion studies with ^{201}Tl begin with the conduct of a stress test with the injection of the radiotracer (148 MBq) at the point of maximum stress. The detection of the post-exercise images should be as early as possible and without a delay of more than 15 minutes. The detection of the redistribution images requires a wait of some 3 to 4 hours and it is recommended that the patient does not ingest anything between the two detections. This is the classical ^{201}Tl protocol [66].

Stress/Redistribution/Reinjection protocol: Similar to the preceding protocol but with a new dose of ^{201}Tl (37 MBq) administered at rest (reinjection)[67] so as to increase the level of circulating thallium and to obtain better resting images.

Stress/Redistribution/Delayed image protocol: This is the classical protocol in which the detection may be prolonged up to 24 hours and, due to the long half-life of ^{201}Tl, there is no loss in the quality of image while, at the same time, allow zones with low blood flow to reach equilibrium [68].

3.3.2.   *Technetium-labelled:*

Stress/Rest, Rest/Stress: Long protocol: This is the method that is, technically, most correct since it precludes interferences between the dose at stress and that administered at rest. However, the difficulty of repositioning the patient identically on two different days needs to be taken into account. The doses administered are the same in stress and at rest (740 MBq) and with which similar levels of counts are obtained in both sets of images.

When using MIBI, the detection needs to be conducted between 60 and 90 minutes of the administration of the doses. This is reduced to 20-30 minutes if tetrofosmin is used. A light food intake is recommended since this favours hepatobiliary elimination of the technetium tracer and which minimises interference in the images [16,61,69].

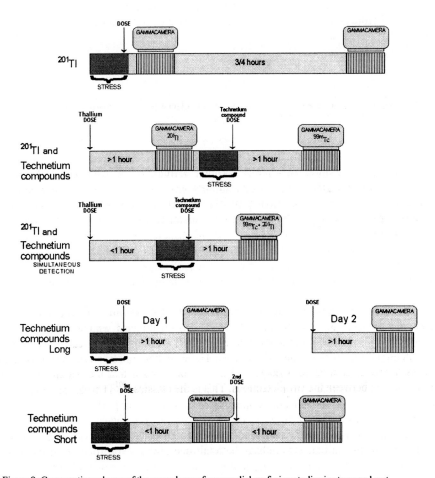

Figure 9: Comparative scheme of the procedures of myocardial perfusion studies in stress and rest

D. Ortega-Alcalde and S. Aguadé-Bruix

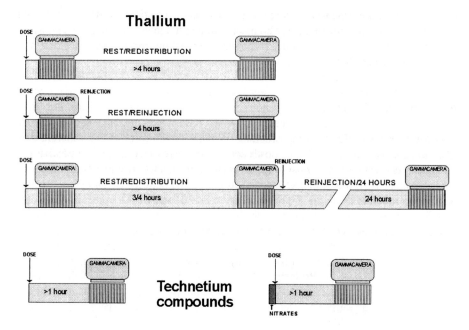

Figure 10: Comparative scheme of the procedures of the myocardial perfusion studies for the assessment of viability

Stress/Rest, Rest/Stress: Short protocol: The one-day, short protocol has a drawback that the second detection encounters residual activity of the first dose. So as to mitigate against this effect, the activity administered in the second dose needs to be three times higher than the first [70]. This difference in activities generates a discrepancy between the quality of the images obtained with the first and those of the second dose [71,72].

In our experience, the difference in the levels of counts produced by one or the other of the doses needs to be corrected for the time of acquisition of each of the doses injected such as, for example, 20-24 seconds per image for the lower dose and 8-10 seconds for the higher [71,73].

For the first detection and without food intake, the waiting time between dose administration and detection is reduced slightly to 60 minutes with MIBI and to 15 minutes with tetrofosmin. Following the administration of the second dose, the delay is 60 to 90 minutes for both tracers (albeit with tetrofosmin this can be shorter) and so gives the patient time for a light meal [74].

In reality, it is possible with tetrofosmin to perform a complete myocardial perfusion study, including stress and detections, in approximately one hour [75].

3.3.3. *Combined protocols of Thallium and Technetium:*
These are protocols designed to reduce the total time of the myocardial perfusion study by exploiting the bio-kinetic differences of the tracers. However, new difficulties such as

separating the simultaneously acquired images of ^{99m}Tc from those of ^{201}Tl are introduced. Also, the diffuse radiation emanating from the ^{99m}Tc image needs to be eliminated from the detector of the ^{201}Tl image so that no artefacts are generated and good quality images for both isotopes are obtained.

The limitations result from the characteristics of detection that apply to ^{201}Tl (low resolution collimator, long acquisition times) and, as such, the overall quality of the study with technetium is less [61].

Technetium Rest/Thallium Stress: This is a very short protocol. Following the administration and detection of the technetium, the stress test is performed and the detection with ^{201}Tl is immediate. On the other hand, the dose of technetium must not be very high so as to preclude, as much as possible, the diffuse radiation from the ^{99m}Tc on the ^{201}Tl detector.

Thallium Rest/Technetium Stress: This is a short protocol with an interval of more than one hour for the ^{201}Tl detection at rest followed by the stress and the injection of the technetium. The second detection has a delay of between 60 and 90 minutes for MIBI and of 30 to 60 minutes for tetrofosmin. This protocol allows for the correct detection of the ^{201}Tl with its appropriate characteristics of detection and followed by the detection of the ^{99m}Tc. Here the problem resides in comparing the images thallium and technetium obtained with different characteristics [76,77].

Thallium Rest/ Technetium Stress with simultaneous detection: This protocol is the shortest since, subsequent to the waiting interval of technetium, the stress is started and

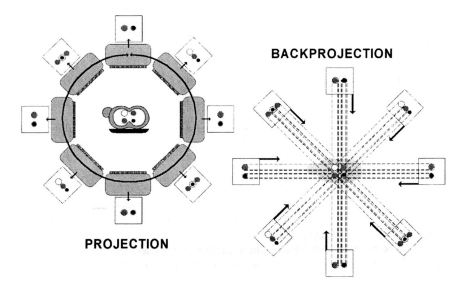

Figure 11: Projection) Scheme for the acquisition of tomographic images of a theoretical object as a function of the angle of detection. Backprojection) Backprojection diagram of the tomographic images. The virtual image of the theoretical object is by sketching-in the zone of superimposition of the projection lines.

D. Ortega-Alcalde and S. Aguadé-Bruix

detection of the ^{201}Tl and of the ^{99m}Tc is immediate and simultaneous. Detection is performed only once (^{201}Tl and ^{99m}Tc dual-isotope study) but with the characteristics of collimation, time and orbits appropriate for thallium [78].

3.4.   PROCESS

3.4.1   *Reconstruction*

Once the acquisition is completed and normalisation of the images performed by correcting with the appropriate energy map and, in the studies with technetium, correcting for isotope decay, the processing of the acquired tomographic studies begins [74]. Normally one begins with the emission tomography but with associated transmission tomographic study at one's disposal, as well.

The system of reconstruction that modern equipment use is that of filtered back projection (FBP) that is based on a linear back-projection superimposed on all the images obtained. This method is rapid, requires a moderate computation capacity but has the limitation of a loss of spatial resolution and of definition of the resulting image. The characteristic image contains artefactual spurious accumulated information on the edges of the object in the form of stars. (Figure 11)[79].

Filtration of the retroprojection minimises these drawbacks. The filters are

TABLE 5. Formulae for most frequently-used reconstruction filters

FILTER	FORMULAE
Ramp	$RM(w) = 1.0$
Butterworth	$BT(w) = \dfrac{(1.0 + Axw)}{\sqrt{1.0 + \dfrac{w}{(BxNq)^{(2xC)}}}}$
Hanning	$HN(w) = \dfrac{(1.0 + Axw)}{(0.5 + 0.5xcos[\pi + (\frac{w}{Nq})^{B}]^{C})}$
Metz	$MZ(w) = \dfrac{[1.0 - (1.0 - MTF^{2})^{P}}{MTF}$; $MTF = MTF(FWHM)$
Shepp-Logan	$SL(w) = sin[0.5x\pi x(\frac{w}{Nq})]$
Hamming	$HM(w) = 0.54 + 0.46\,xcos[\pi\,x(\frac{w}{Nq})]$

mathematical functions applied to each one of the back-projections so as to increase the difference between the signal-of-interest and the background signal (signal-to-noise ratio) so as to increase the contrast of the image. To apply the filters it is necessary to convert each projection into a mathematical function, applying the Fourier transformation (frequency domain). The resultant function, or Fourier transformation, is modified by the appropriate filter and is then reconverted to the "spatial domain" using the inverse transformation of Fourier (Table 5)[80].

The ramp filter is linearly proportional to the frequency and, as such, to the mean frequency potential where not only the information of interest resides but also the high noise. To eliminate the latter, the ramp filter is modified using a function (termed low-pass function) that introduces a higher cutoff level (Hanning, Butterworth, etc). The high cutoff levels produce images of better spatial resolution but with more noise. This may be usable when there is an abundance of counts; typical of the technetium-labelled compounds [81]. Low cutoff levels generate smoother images but with less spatial resolution. Low cutoff levels are employed, typically, for Thallium.

In practice, an ideal filter does not exist and each type of exploration requires adjustment for the best filter possible [82]. As such, the filter for Thallium will be different from that for technetium and the filter for studies with low dose technetium could be different from that used for the high doses. Hence, each centre needs to perform its own tests and to decide which type of filter is the most appropriate for each of the types of tomography (Table 6).

TABLE 6. Parameter values of most frequently-used filters

		FILTER	Gain (A)	Cut level (B)	Power (C)
^{201}Tl		Butterworth	0	0.35	5.0
		Hanning	0	1.00	1.0
^{99m}Tc	Low dose	Butterworth	0	0.35	5.0
	Medium dose	Butterworth	0	0.40	5.0
	High dose	Butterworth	0	0.50	5.0

For the studies reconstructed by filtered retroprojection, it is possible to perform a correction for linear attenuation using the method of Chang [83] which takes, as a weighting factor, the linear attenuation of water. This method is only effective for dense organs such as the head but is not applicable to cardiac studies due to the great differences in attenuation that exist between the different structures of the thorax (musculature, bone, lung, breast etc).

Other systems of tomographic reconstruction exist which are based on iterative processes [84] using variable weighting factors to facilitate convergence of results. These include weighted least-squares means (WLS)[85], the maximum-likelihood expectation maximisation (ML-EM)[86,87] and algebraic reconstruction techniques (ART)[88]. These systems incorporate as weightings, in the iteration process, the data derived from the transmission tomography so as to correct for attenuation once the tomographic reconstruction of the emission images is performed [89,90]. The final images corrected for attenuation show a better contrast and better definition than the non-corrected images.

The results obtained with iterative systems are invariably better than the classical filtered retroprojection but the enormous computational requirements and the time required for accurate iteration confine the systems to high-capacity computer work-stations [91].

3.4.2.   Creation and presentation of tomographic slices:

The reconstruction generates transaxial sclices of the thorax of the patient. For the best evaluation, the image of the cardiac area is amplified (zoom factor) and the image re-orientated such that the ventricular long axis is with the apex at the top, the lateral wall to the right of the observer and the right ventricle to the left. On these re-orientated slices, the images of the horizontal long axis (HLA) are generated and which cut the ventricle horizontally following the apex-base and presents views from the inferior wall towards the anterior (Figure 12). Perpendicular to these are coronal slices that are re-orientated as the short axis (SA) and which present views from the point and, progressively, from the apex to the base with the left ventricle to the right of the observer and the right ventricle to the left. Finally, the slices of the long vertical axis (LVA) are selected and are presented consecutively from the septum to the lateral wall of the left ventricle, seen from the septum, with the apex to the right of the observer. The presentation is according to the recommendations of the Society of Nuclear Medicine, American College of Cardiology and American Society of Nuclear Cardiology [92].

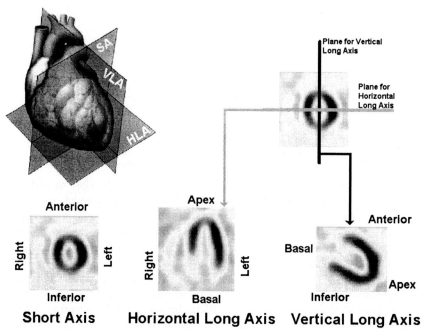

Figure 12: Scheme of the spatial re-orientation of the heart axes by the reconstruction according to the presentation format recommended by the Society of Nuclear Medicine, American College of Cardiology and American Society of Nuclear Cardiology [92].

It is very important that all the processes of reconstruction be repeated exactly the same way for the images of stress as for those of rest. Hence, programs that simultaneous process images of stress and of rest are recommended or, alternatively, programs that save the characteristics of the first study to be processed and then applies them, by default, to the second.

3.4.3. Gated-SPET processing:

At the start, the processing is practically identical to that of SPET but with some modifications. For example, for each of the fractions of the cycle (8 or 16) the filters need to be smoother since for each image of the cycle there would be 8 or 16 times less counts than the same image in SPET

The computing requirements for GSPET are very high since the memory space that these studies occupy is much greater than conventional SPET. For example, if the cardiac cycle is divided into 8 (the most usual) or 16 fractions, this means that 8 or 16 series would need to be generated for each one of the tomographic slices. Alongside this is the requirement for a processor with sufficient speed such that the reconstruction is not excessively slowed.

The final presentation of the images follow the same recommendations as that for SPET except that the data are viewed as a movie on the screen with the sequential images linked to the cardiac cycle. Myocardial contraction in the slices can be visualised and the activity of the ventricular walls during the cardiac cycle can be evaluated [93]. This facilitates evaluation of ventricular wall movement, myocardial activity increment during systole [94] (due to the systolic thickening of the wall) and, using programs based on the automatic delineation of the ventricular contours (endocardiac and epicardiac), a geometric estimation of cavity volume [95,96]. Also, it is possible to determine the principal haemodynamic parameters of left ventricular function: ejection fraction together with systolic and diastolic volumes [97,98,99].

References

1. Lebowitz E, MW Greene, R Fairchild et al. Thallium-201 for medical use I. J Nucl Med 1975; 16: 151-155.
2. Bradley-Moore PR, Lebowitz E, Green MW et al. Thallium-201 for medical use II: Biologic behavior. J Nucl Med 1975; 16: 156-160.
3. L'Abbate A, Biagnini A, Michelassi C et al. Myocardial kinetics of thallium and potassium in man. Circulation 1979; 60: 776-785.
4. Candell Riera J, Aguadé Bruix S, Castell Conesa J, Cortadellas Ángel J. Isonitrilos marcados con tecnecio-99m frente al talio-201 en la enfermedad coronaria. Rev Esp Cardiol 1994; 47 (Suppl 4): 101-115.
5. Strauss HW, Harrison K, Langan JK et al. Thallium-201 for myocardial imaging. Relation of thallium-201 to regional myocardial perfusion. Circulation 1975; 51: 641-645.
6. Beller GA (1995) Radiopharmaceuticals in nuclear cardiology, in Beller GA (ed.), Clinical Nuclear Cardiology, W.B. Saunders Company, Philadelphia, pp. 37-81.
7. Picard M, Dupras G, Taillefer R et al. Myocardial perfusion agents: compared biodistribution of 201-thallium, Tc-99m-tertiary-butyl-isonitrile (TBI) and Tc-99m-methoxy-isobutyl-isonitrile (MIBI). J Nucl Med 1987; 28 (Suppl.): 654-655.
8. Pohost GM, Alpert NM, Ingwall JS et al. Thallium redistribution: Mechanisms and clinical utility. Semin Nucl Med 1980; 10: 70-93.

9.   Beller GA, Watson DD. Physiological of myocardial perfusion imaging with technetium 99m agents. Semin Nucl Med 1991; 21: 173-181.

10.   Iskandrian AS, Heo J, Kong B et al. Use of 99mTc isonitrile (RP-30A) in assesing left ventricular perfusion and function at rest and during exercise in coronary artery disease, and comparison with coronary arteriography and exercise 201-Tl SPECT imaging. Am J Cardiol 1989; 64: 270-275.

11.   Maddahi J, Rodrigues E, Berman DS, Kiat H. State-of-the-art myocardial perfusion imaging. Cardiol Clin 1994; 12: 199-222.

12.   Jones AG, Agrams MJ, Davíson A et al. Biological studies of a new class of technetium complexes: The hexakis (alkylisonitrile) technetium (I) cations. J. Nucl Med Biol 1984; 11: 225-234.

13.   Wackers FJ, Berman DS, Maddahi J et al. Technetium-99m hexakis 2 methoxyisobutil isonitrile (hexamibi): Human biodistribution, dosimetry, safety, and preliminary comparison to thallium-201 for myocardial perfusion imaging. J Nucl Med 1989; 30: 301-311.

14.   Crane P, Laliberté R, Heminway S, Thoolen M, Orlandi C. Effect of mitochondrial viability and metabolism on technetium-99-sestamibi myocardial retention. Eur J Nucl Med 1993; 20: 20-25.

15.   Berman DS, Kiat H, Germano G et al. (1995) ^{99m}Tc-Sestamibi SPECT in cardiac SPECT imaging. De Puey EG, Berman DS, Garcia EV(eds.), Cardiac SPECT Imaging, Raven Press, New York, pp. 121-146.

16.   Taillefer R, Lafiamme L, Dupras G, Picard M, Phaneuf DC, Léveillé J. Myocardial perfusion imaging with 99mTc-methoxy-isobutil-isonitrile (MIBI): Comparison of short and long time intervais between rest and stress injections. Eur J Med 1988; 13: 515-522.

17.   Verzijlbergen JF, Oudheusden van D, Cramer MJ. Quantitative analysis of planar 99mTc-sestamibi myocardial perfusion images. Eur Heart J 1994; 15: 1217-1226.

18.   Higley B, Smith FW, Smith T et al. Technetium-99m-1,2-bis[bis(2-ethoxyethyl)phosphino]ethane: Human biodistribution, dosimetry and sefety of a new myocardial perfusion imaging agent. J Nucl Med 1993; 34: 30-38.

19.   Jain D, Wakers FJTh, Mattera J, McMahon M, Sinusas AJ, Zaret BL. Biokinetics of technetium-99m-tetrofosmin: myocardial perfusion imaging agent: implications for one-day imaging protocol. J Nucl Med 1993; 34: 1254-1259.

20.   Sinusas AJ, Shi Q, Saltzberg MT et al. Technetium-99m-tetrofosmin to assess myocardial blood flow: experimental validation in an intact canine model of ischemia. J Nucl Med 1994; 35: 664-671.

21.   Zaret BL, Rigo P, Wackers FJTh et al. Myocardial perfusion imaging with ^{99m}Tc tetrofosmin. Comparison to ^{201}Tl imaging and coronary angiography in a phase III multicenter trial. Circulation 1995; 91: 313-319.

22.   Kelly JD, Foster AM, Higley B et al. Tecnetium-99m-Tetrofosmin as a new radiopharmaceutical for myocardial perfusion imaging. J Nucl Med 1993; 34: 222-227.

23.   Narra RK, Nunn AD, Kuczynski BL et al. A neutral technetium-99m complex for myocardial imaging. J Nucl Med 1989; 30: 1830-1837.

24.   Leppo JA, Meerdink DJ. Comparative myocardial extraction of two technetium-labeled BATO derivatives (SQ30217), (SQ30014) and thallium. J Nucl Med 1990; 31: 67-74.

25.   Gewirtz H. Differential myocardium washout of technetium-99m-teboroxime: Mechanism and significance. J Nucl Med 1991; 32: 2009-2011.

26.   Rumsey WL, Rosenspire KC, Nunn AD. Myocardial extraction of teboroxime: Effects of teboroxime interaction with blood. J Nucl Med 1992; 33: 94-101.

27.   Henzlova MJ, Machac J. Clinical utility of technetium-99m-teboroxime myocardial washout imaging. J Nucl Med 1994; 35: 575-579.

28.   Johnson LL. Myocardial perfusion imaging with technetium-99m-teboroxime. J Nucl Med 1994; 35: 689-692.

29.   Chua T, Kiat H, Germano G et al. Rapid back-to-back adenosine stress/rest technetium-99m-teboroxime myocardial perfusion SPECT using a triple-detector camera. J Nucl Med 1993; 34: 1485-1493.

30.   Galofré-Mora P (1994) Physicochemical and technical fundamentals. in Candell-Riera J and Ortega-Alcalde D, (eds.), Nuclear Cardiology in everyday practice, Kluwer Academic Publishers, Dordrecht, pp. 1-28.

31.   Anger HO (1957) A new instrument for mapping gamma-ray emitters. Biology and medicine quarterly report UCRL-3653. Washington.

32.   Sorenson JA, Phelps ME. (1987) The Anger camera: Performance characteristics, in Sorenson JA and Phelps ME (eds.), Physics in nuclear medicine, Saunders, Philadelphia, pp. 318-345.

33. Moore SC, Kouris K, Cullum I. Collimator design for single photon emission-computed tomography. Eur J Nucl Med 1992; 19: 138-150.
34. Kircos LT, Leonard PF, Keyes Jr JW. An optimized collimator for single-photon computed tomography with a scintillation camera. J Nucl Med 1978; 19: 322-323.
35. Cao Z, Maunoury C, Chen CC, Holder LE. Comparison of continuous step-and-shoot versus step-and-shoot acquisition SPECT. J Nucl Med 1996; 37: 2037-2040.
36. Iskandrian AE, Maddahi J. Nuclear cardiology: new developments and future directions. J Nucl Cardiol 1997; 4: 189-192.
37. He ZX, Scarlett MD, Mahmarian JJ, Verani MS. Enhanced accuracy of defect detection by myocardial single-photon emission computed tomography with attenuation correction with gadolinium-153 line sources: evaluation with a cardiac phantom. J Nucl Cardiol 1997; 4: 202-210.
38. Ficaro EP, Fessler JA, Rogers L, Schwaiger M. Comparison of americium-241 and technetium-99m as transmission sources for attenuation correction of thallium-201 SPECT imaging of the heart. J Nucl Med 1994; 35: 652-663.
39. Ficaro EP, Fessler JA, Ackermann RJ et al. Simultaneous transmission-emission thallium-201 cardiac SPECT: effect of attenuation correction on myocardial tracer distribution. J Nucl Med 1995; 36: 921-931.
40. Cerqueira MD, Harp GD, Ritchie JL. Evaluation of myocardial perfusion and function by single photon emission computed tomography. Semin Nucl Med 1989; 17: 200-213.
41. Mazzanti M, Germano G, Kiat H, Friedman J, Berman DS. Fast technetium-99m labeled sestamibi gated single-photon emission computed tomography for evaluation of myocardial function. J Nucl Cardiol 1996; 3: 143-149.
42. Nichols K, DePuey EG, Rozanski A. Automation of gated tomographic left ventricular ejection fraction. J Nucl Cardiol 1996; 3: 475-482.
43. Hambye AS, Dobbeleir A, Derveaux M, Vandevivere J, van den Heuvel P. Determination of systolic thickening index with gated Tc-99m sestamibi SPECT. A new parameter of myocardial viability?. Clin Nucl Med 1997; 22: 172-175.
44. Fukuchi K, Uehara T, Morozumi T et al. Quantification of systolic count increase in technetium-99m-MIBI gated myocardial SPECT. J Nucl Med 1997; 38: 1067-1073.
45. Williams KA, Lang RM, Reba RC, Taillon LA. Comparison of technetium-99m sestamibi-gated tomographic perfusion imaging with echocardiography and electrocardiography for determination of left ventricular mass. Am J Cardiol 1996; 77: 750-755.
46. Kouris K, Clarke GA, Jarrit PH et al. Physical performance evaluation of the Toshiva GCA-9300A triple-head system. J Nucl Med 1993; 34: 1778-1789.
47. Graham LS. Quality control for SPECT systems. Radiographics 1995; 15: 1471-1481.
48. NEMA standards publication NU 1-1986. Performance measurements of scintillation cameras. NEMA sales office, Washington D.C..
49. Puchal R. Control de calidad de la tomogammacámaras. Rev Esp Med Nuclear 1995; 14: 257-260.
50. Fahey FH, Harkness BA, Keyes Jr JW et al. Sensitivity, resolution and image quality with a multi-head SPECT camera. J Nucl Med 1992; 33: 1859-1863.
51. Murphy PH. Acceptance testing and quality control of gamma cameras, including SPECT. J Nucl Med 1987; 28: 1221-1227.
52. Heller SL, Goodwin PN. SPECT instrumentation: performance, lesion detection and recent innovations. Semin Nucl Med 1987; 17: 184-199.
53. Baron JM, Chouraqui P. Myocardial single-photon emission computed tomographic quality assurance. J Nucl Cardiol 1996; 3: 157-166.
54. English RJ, Brown SE. (1986) Quality control requirements. In English RJ, Brown SE (eds.), SPECT, single-photon emission computed tomography: a primer, The Society of Nuclear Medicine, New York, pp. 25-46.
55. Kuikka JT, Tenhunen-Eskelinen M, Jurvelin J, Kiilianen H. Physical performance of the Siemens MultiSPECT 3 gamma camera. Nucl Med Commun 1993; 14: 490-497.
56. Graham LS, Fahey FH, Madsen MT, van Aswegen A, Yester MV. Quantitation of SPECT performance: Report of Task Group 4, Nuclear Medicine Committee. Med Phys 1995; 22: 401-409.
57. Everaert H, Vanhove C, Franken PR. Gated-SPET myocardial perfusion acquisition within 5 minutes usinf focussing collimators and tree-head gamma camera. Eur J Nucl Med 1998; 25:587-593.

58. Hicks R. (1994) Myocardial perfusion scintigraphy techniques using single photon radiotracers. in Nuclear medicine, Murray IPC, Ell PJ, Strauss HW (eds.), Churchil Livingstone, New York, pp. 1083-1098.

59. O'Connor MK, Bothun ED. Effects of tomographic table attenuation on prone and supine cardiac imaging. J Nucl Med 1995; 36: 1102-1106.

60. Dahlberg ST, Leppo JA. Myocardial kinetics of radiolabeled perfusion agents: Basis for perfusion imaging. J Nucl Cardiol 1994; 35:189-197.

61. Berman DS, Kiat HS, Van Train KF et al. Myocardial perfusion imaging with technetium-99m-Sestamibi: Comparative analysis of available imaging protocols. J Nucl Med 1994; 35: 681-688.

62. Van Train K, Maddahi J, Berman DS et al. Quantitative analysis of tomographic stress thallium-201 myocardial scintigrams: a multicenter trial. J Nucl Med 1990; 31: 1168-1179.

63. Ortega-Alcalde D. (1994) Gated blood-pool radionuclide ventriculography, in Candell-Riera J and Ortega-Alcalde D, (eds.), Nuclear Cardiology in everyday practice. Kluwer Academic Publishers, Dordrecht, pp. 145-157.

64. Mori T, Minamiji K, Kurongane H et al. Rest-reinjected thallium-201 imaging for assessing viability of severe asynergic regions. J Nucl Med 1991; 23: 1718-1724.

65. Maddahi J, Schelbert H, Brunken R, Di Carli M. Role of thallium-201 and PET imaging in evaluation of myocardial viability and management of patients with coronary artery disease and left ventricular dysfunction. J Nucl Med 1994; 35: 707-715.

66. Kiat H, Maddahi J, Roy LT et al. Comparison of technetium 99m methoxy isobutyl isonitrile and thallium 201 for evaluation of coronary artery disease by planar and tomographic methods. Am Heart J 1989; 117: 1-11.

67. Dilsizian V, Rocco TP, Freedman NTM, Leon Mb, Bonow RO. Enhanced detection of ischemic but viable myocardium by the reinjection of thallium after stress-redistribution imaging. N Engl J Med 1990; 323: 141-146.

68. Kiat H, Berman DS, Maddahi J et al. Late reversibility of tomographic myocardial thallium-201 defects: an accurate marker of myocardial viability. J Am Coll Cardiol 1988; 12: 1456-1463.

69. Maddahi J, Kiat H, Van Train KF et al. Myocardial perfusion imaging with technetium-99m sestamibi SPECT in evaluation of coronary artery disease. Am J Cardiol 1990; 66: 55E-62E.

70. Van Train KF, Areeda J, Garcia EV et al. Quantitative of same day Tc-99m-Sestamibi myocardial SPECT: Multicenter trial validation. J Nucl Med 1992; 33: 876 (Abstr).

71. Van Train KF, Areeda J, Garcia EV et al. Quantitative same day rest-stress technetium-99m-Sestamibi SPECT: Definition and validation of stress normal limits and criteria for abnormality. J Nucl Med 1993; 34: 1494-1502.

72. Sridhara B, Sochor H, Rigo P et al. Myocardial single-photon emission computed tomographic imaging with technetium 99m tetrofosmin: Stess-rest imaging with same-day and separate-day rest imaging. J Nucl Cardiol 1994; 1: 138-143.

73. Montz R, Perez-Castejon MJ, Jurado JA et al. Technetium-99m tetrofosmin rest/stress myocardial SPET with a same-day 2-hour protocol: comparison with coronary angiography. Eur J Nucl Med 1996; 23: 639-647.

74. Van Train KF, García EV, Maddahi J et al. Multicenter trial validation for quantitative analysis of same-day rest-stress technetium-99m-sestamibi myocardial tomograms. J Nucl Med 1994; 35: 609-618.

75. Santana Boado C, García Burillo A, Candell Riera J et al. SPET 99mTc-Tetrofosmin one day protocol in the diagnosis of CAD. J Nucl Med 1997; 41: 227 (Abstr).

76. Berman DS, Kiat H, Friedman JD et al. Separate acquisition rest thallium-201/stress Tc-99m sestamibi dual isotope myocardial perfusion SPECT: a clinical validation study. J Am Coll Cardiol 1993; 22; 1455-1464.

77. Heo J, Wolmer I, Kegel J, Iskandrian AS. Sequential dual-isotope SPECT imaging with thallium-201 and technetium-99m-sestamibi. J Nucl Med 1994; 35: 549-553.

78. Kiat H, Germano G, Friedman JD et al. Comparative feasibility of separate or simultaneous rest thallium-201/stress technetium-99m sestamibi dual isotope myocardial perfusion SPECT. J Nucl Med 1994; 35: 542-548.

79. English RJ, Brown SE (1986) Image Reconstruction, in English RJ and Brown SE (eds.), SPECT, single-photon emission computed tomography: a primer. The Society of Nuclear Medicine, New York, pp. 9-24.

80. Rosenthal MS, Cullom J, Hawkins W, Moore SC, Tsui BM, Yester M. Quantitative SPECT imaging: a review and recommendations by the Focus Committee of the Society of Nuclear Medicine Computer and Instrumentation Council. J Nucl Med 1995; 36: 1489-1513.

81. Garcia E, Cooke CD, Van Train KF et al. Technical aspects of myocardial SPECT imaging with technetium-99m-sestamibi. Am J Cardiol 1990; 66: 23E-33E.

82. Gilland DR, Tsui BMW, McCarTney WH, Perry JR, Berg J. Determination of the optimum filter function for SPECT imaging. J Nucl Med 1988; 29: 643-650.

83. Chang LT. A method for attenuation correction in radionuclide computed tomography. IEEE Trans Nucl Sci 1978; NS-25: 638-643.

84. King MA, Tsui BMW, Pan TS, Glick SJ, Soares EJ. Attenuation compensation for cardiac single-photon emission computed tomographic imaging: Part 2. Attenuation compensation algorithms. J Nucl Cardiol 1996; 3: 55-63.

85. Lalush DS, Tsui BM. A fast and stable maximum a posteriori conjugate gradient reconstruction algorithm. Med Phys 1995; 22: 1273-1284.

86. Walrand SH, van Elmbt LR, Pauwels S. A non-negative fast multiplicative algorithm in 3D scatter-compensated SPET reconstruction. Eur J Nucl Med 1996; 23: 1521-1526.

87. Knesaurek K, Machac J. Non-uniform attenuation correction in SPET using a modified conjugate gradient reconstruction method. Nucl Med Commun 1997; 18: 431-436.

88. Ros D, Falcon C, Juvells I, Pavia J. The influence of a relaxation parameter on SPECT iterative reconstruction algorithms. Phys Med Biol 1996; 41: 925-937.

89. King MA, Tsui BMW, Pan TS. Attenuation compensation for cardiac single-photon emission computed tomographic imaging: Part 1. Impact of attenuation and methods of estimating attenuation maps. J Nucl Cardiol 1995; 2: 513-524.

90. Lalush DS, Tsui BM, Performance of ordered-subset reconstruction algorithms under conditions of extreme attenuation and truncation in myocardial SPECT. J Nucl Med 2000; 41:737-744.

91. Passeri A, Formiconi AR, De Cristofaro MT, Pupi A, Meldolesi U. High-performance computing and networking as tools for accurate emission computed tomography reconstruction. Eur J Nucl Med 1997; 24: 390-397.

92. Comittee on Advanced Cardiac Imaging and Technology, Council on Clinical Cardiology, American Heart Association; Cardiovascular Imaging Comittee, American College of Cardiology; and Board of Directors, Cardiovascular Council, Society of Nuclear Medicine. Standarization of Cardiac Tomographic Imaging. Circulation 1992; 86: 338-399.

93. Cooke CD, Garcia EV, Cullom SJ, Faber TL, Pettigrew RI. Determining the accuracy of calculating systolic wall thickening using a fast Fourier transform approximation: a simulation study based on canine and patient data. J Nucl Med 1994; 35: 1185-1192.

94. Fukuchi K, Uehara T, Morozumi T et al. Quantification of systolic count increase in technetium-99m-MIBI gated myocardial SPECT. J Nucl Med 1997; 38: 1067-1073.

95. Germano G, Kiat H, Kavanagh PB et al. Automatic quantification of ejection fraction from gated myocardial perfusion SPECT. J Nucl Med 1995; 36: 2138-2147.

96. Germano G, Erel J, Kiat H, Kavanagh PB, Berman DS. Quantitative LVEF and qualitative regional function from gated thallium-201 perfusion SPECT. J Nucl Med 1997; 38: 749-754.

97. Nichols K, DePuey EG, Rozanski A. Automation of gated tomographic left ventricular ejection fraction. J Nucl Cardiol 1996; 3: 475-482.

98. DePuey EG, Nichols K, Dobrinsky C. Left ventricular ejection fraction assessed from gated technetium-99m-sestamibi SPECT. J Nucl Med 1993; 34: 1871-1876.

99. Maunoury C, Chen CC, Chua KB, Thompson CJ. Quantification of left ventricular function with thallium-201 and technetium-99m-sestamibi myocardial gated SPECT. J Nucl Med 1997; 38: 958-961.

2. CRITERIA FOR SPET INTERPRETATION

JOAN CASTELL-CONESA and JOSEFA CORTADELLAS-ANGEL

Currently, the majority of myocardial perfusion scintigraphy studies are performed using SPET since there are clear advantages over planar studies: better localisation as well as the evaluation of the extent of myocardial ischaemia [1,2]. For a correct interpretation, however, it is important to familiarise oneself with the standard studies so as to appreciate the variations of normality, to systematically evaluate the characteristics of perfusion defects and to be aware of circumstances related to technical problems (mechanical or even inherent in the patient) of image acquisition which can lead to an erroneous diagnosis.

1. Image analysis

To standardise cardiac SPET, three principal planes of image slices are recommended: the vertical long axis (VLA) parallels the inter-ventricular septum and follows the long axis of the heart; the horizontal long axis (HLA) perpendicular to the VLA; the short axis (SA) perpendicular to the HLA and the VLA. Their presentation, below, are according to the consensus [3] of the American Heart Association, the American College of Cardiology, and the American Society of Nuclear Medicine (Plate 2.1):
- The VLA slices are horseshoe shaped and are presented, generally, with the cardiac apex to the right of the observer as viewed from the wall across the septum with the anterior face placed above and the diaphragm below. Usually, the sections are numbered from the septum to the lateral face.
- The HLA slices, as well, are horseshoe shaped and are presented with the apex in the upper part of the image. With the septum placed to the left and the lateral face to the right, the sections are numbered from bottom to top.
- The SA slices are circular and are observed from the apex. With the septum placed to the left with the lateral face to the right and the anterior to the top with the inferior to the bottom, the sections are numbered from the apex to the base.

The correct interpretation of the images depends on their quality at the moment of acquisition. It is important to assess the images on the screen as well as in the cinematographic form before processing them. This facilitates the detection of artefacts that would otherwise contribute to an erroneous interpretation [4].

J. Candell-Riera et al. (eds.), Myocardium at Risk and Viable Myocardium, 27–43.
© 2001 *Kluwer Academic Publishers. Printed in the Netherlands.*

2. Normal perfusion scintigraphy

In a normal perfusion scintigraphy, tracer uptake is, generally, homogeneous but, occasionally, the number of counts can be decreased in the apex due to the myocardium in this zone being very thin. On the other hand, tracer uptake in the septum is usually lower than that of the lateral wall and, in its basal portion, is practically zero since this is a membranous zone. Usually, the wall of the right ventricle can be identified and the size evaluated and, depending on the quality of the image, the perfusion defects can be detected.

The distribution of normal ventricular activity is somewhat different in males and females due to the differences in tissue distributions leading to differences in signal attenuation. In both genders the maximum uptake is located in the lateral wall and the lowest in the anterior and inferior regions. In quantifying ventricular activity using polar maps, we observed that, in females, there were no significant differences between the uptakes in these two territories probably because the attenuation caused by the diaphragm was balanced by that caused by breast tissue. In men, conversely, there were significant differences between the anterior and the inferior regions which is attributable to the attenuation caused by the diaphragm and the absence of the attenuating effect of breast tissue on the anterior face. (Plate 2.2). These differences diminish when attenuation correction systems are employed to individually correct for activity from the left ventricle [5,6].

Before evaluating the possible presence of perfusion defects, the tomographic images need to be inspected to obtain an overall impression with respect to the size of the cardiac chambers and of the relationship of myocardial uptake relative to the neighbouring structures. Patients with concentric ventricular hypertrophy present with, in general, a small ventricular cavity that can, on occasions, almost disappear while patients with a very dilated ventricular cavity present with a diffuse thinning of the walls that appear to be more intense in the apical region [7].

It is very important to be aware that there are individual variations in the distribution of the epicardial coronary arteries [8,9]. The anterior descending artery irrigates the anterior wall, the septum and, in general, the apex. Depending on the location of the lesion, the septum could be free from ischaemia while, conversely, it is less usual that with the septum being affected that the anterior wall would be free from ischemia. The inferior distal region and the portion inferior to the septum may be irrigated by the anterior descending artery when necessary on occasions, or by the posterior descending artery proceeding from the left circumflex or from the right coronary artery. In 85% of the population the right coronary artery is dominant and gives rise to the posterior descending artery which irrigates the inferior wall of the heart. In the other 15% of the population the posterior descending artery proceeds from the left circumflex coronary artery. When the right coronary is dominant, the circumflex irrigates the basal portions of the lateral face and the inferior (and possibly the basal) septum, while the lateral wall is irrigated by the side branches of this artery. In general, then, the anterior wall and the septum are zones irrigated by the anterior descending artery and the lateral wall by the left circumflex artery, but the inferior face of the heart can be irrigated by the right coronary or by the left circumflex artery (Plate 2.3). The defects of the apex can correspond to either of these arteries.

3. Evaluation of perfusion defects

In clinical practice, perfusion defects are considered significant when they are observed in several consecutive sections. These can be observed in the short axis and in one of the long axes such as, for example, septal and lateral defects in the HLA and anterior and inferior defects in the VLA. Asymmetry of uptake visible in only one axis should be evaluated with caution because of the possibility that the planes of the sections do not exactly follow the axes of the left ventricle. Apical defects are identified in the long axes because short axis slices do not facilitate correct visual evaluation from the apex. The only basal alterations are the equivocal evaluations, especially in the short axis, because of the variability in length of the ventricular walls and the loss of resolution of the image in the deeper zones of the thorax.

Normalisation of scale type (grey or colour) being used on the screen should be taken into account in the evaluation of the images. The four types most commonly used are:

- Normalisation to a single maximum irrespective of whether the study images are of stress or rest. This presentation is a useful complement in studies performed with ^{201}Tl because it facilitates easy approximation of the phenomenon of "washout" for each ventricular region.
- Normalisation to two maxima (one for each of the two acquisitions) with the maximum activity common to the three sets of sections. It is a system recommendable for technetium tracers as well as for thallium. This presentation ensures that the maximum intensities of uptake in stress and at rest are equal independent of the quantity of the dose administered (long protocol, short protocol, re-injection etc.). Also, the zones with the same grade of hyper-uptake in the opposite walls are visible in the long axis sections.
- Normalisation individualised for image or for set. This system has a drawback in that each of the images (or set of sections) has its own maximum and may not reflect the extents of the decreases in the perfusions that affect the distinct territories represented in each of the tomographic sections. The typical maximum specific to each of the six sets of sections is that which is most frequently employed in the processing programs made available by the gammacamera manufacturers.

Perfusion defects are evaluated in a subjective manner taking into account the following characteristics: extent, severity, reversibility and involvement of one or more territories. In general a large gradation in intensity exists from hypo-uptake (slight defect), an intensity of uptake which is clearly above that of background (moderate defect) and the severe defects in which the uptake is almost undifferentiated from that of background activity. Reversibility is recorded as total, partial or null and different examples are shown in Plate 2.4. Following the scheme of interpretation of planar studies, totally reversible defects can be considered as ischaemic patterns. Those that increase resting activity correspond to zones without ischaemia and, hence, the defect can be attributed to the presence of infarct (most frequent cause) or other alterations of the myocardial tissue of the permanent type (fibrosis, degeneration, space-occupying lesions) as discussed in the Chapter 4. The partial reversible defects are interpreted as areas in which myocardial ischaemia and scar tissue (generally zones of infarct) co-exist although this could be due, as well, to the existence of very severe ischaemia that results in the delayed redistribution phenomenon of >3-4 hours when ^{201}Tl is used [10-13]. When technetium tracers are employed the regions with critical reduction of coronary flow, as well, can occasion a null or partial resting reversibility [14-16].

Reverse redistribution ise defined as those post-perfusion defects that are accentuated at rest. The significance is very variable because the causal factors are, themselves, numerous [17]. Firstly, mere technical factors need to be discarded such as the attenuation effect caused by the diaphragm in the inferior-basal region or in the anterior and inferior basal zones. More important, perhaps, are those visible in the VLA and which are seen in individuals with an ample thorax and those in whom the zones that are most distant from the detector show a poorer image representation. All these perfusion defects_can be more accentuated at rest due to the lower myocardial extraction of the perfusion tracers in basal conditions of myocardial oxygen consumption. Moreover, in the case of ^{201}Tl this can, under normal conditions, present a loss of myocardial concentration <50% at rest, after 3-4 hours of the injection, due to the normal washout process [18-20].

Reverse redistribution has been described in a variety of diseases of the myocardium but are of greatest interest in coronary artery disease [18-21]. Reverse redistribuion is observed between stress and at rest and between images of redistribution and those of re-injection or between the initial image after an injection at rest of ^{201}Tl and the delayed image [22-24]. It can be said, as a general concept, that in all cases this pattern indicates that the myocardium is viable [22,25,26]. This reverse phenomenon is less studied using technetium agents. We reviewed 1124 consecutive SPECT ^{99m}Tc-tetrofosmin studies with a prevalence of reverse pattern of 3.6% (42 patients, 21 with and 21 without previous myocardial infarction). In 3 out of 8 patients without myocardial infarction in whom the coronary angiography was performed, the coronary arteries were angiographically normal and 5 had stenosis between 50% to 70% in the vessels related with the reverse segments (Plate 2.5 A). In patients with previous myocardial infarction the reverse patters was located in the region of infarct and in nine of 11 patients in whom a coronary angiography was performed out, patency of the related artery was verified [27] (Plate 2.5 B).

The two most frequent causes for a rapid clearance of ^{201}Tl being produced in some regions with a lower uptake at rest are:

-   Presence of zones in which there had been non-transmural necrosis and which are perfused by a patent vessel or by a good collateral circulation which is capable of a greater uptake when the radio-tracer is injected during physical or pharmacological stimulation [23]. Even when no documented antecedents exist of previous myocardial necrosis, we have detected a greater prevalence of these patterns in territories irrigated by moderately-stenosed vessels [26].
-   Reverse patterns have been described in early phases following episodes of ischaemia-necrosis and permeable vessels, following thrombolysis or coronary re-vascularisation [24,27]. Possibly the metabolic derangement associated with the perturbation predisposes to an incapacity to retain the radio-tracers at the intracellular level since this requires a consumption of energy which is transitorily lacking in post-ischaemic tissue [28,29]. Whatever the explanation, the reverse pattern is reversible within a few weeks and, as such, has a high predictive value since it implies a recuperation or re-perfusion of the myocardium.

4. Indirect signs of severe coronary disease

Although the sensitivity of tomographic assessment is high for the detection of disease in the three principal coronary vessels and, also, the sensitivity of detection of coronary artery disease is greater when the disease is more extensive [30,31], the investigation can, very occasionally, generate a false negative in the presence of globally diminished coronary flow. In these cases, and taking into account the clinical status as well as the electrocardiography results of the stress test (including the functional capacity), it is useful to note certain indirect data detected in the perfusion study. As discussed in Chapter 6, data such as abnormal pulmonary uptake, slow myocardial clearance of ^{201}Tl and transitory left ventricular dilatation, are signs of severity of the coronary artery disease and of poor prognosis.

4.1. INCREASED LUNG ^{201}Tl UPTAKE

When ^{201}Tl is used as a perfusion tracer, the increased pulmonary uptake during stress is an index of depression of left ventricular function, severe coronary disease and bad prognosis caused by the increment of end-diastolic volume of the left ventricle [32-34]. In general, pulmonary uptake is already assessed in the ciné mode presentation before proceeding to the tomographic reconstruction. Nevertheless, it is advisable to quantify the relationship between the pulmonary and cardiac activity in a static image before initiating the SPET or, at least, in an anterior image from the SPECT acquisition prior to the tomography acquisition. When the ratio of maximum pulmonary activity to maximum myocardial activity is >0.55, it is considered abnormal.

Perfusion tracers labelled with ^{99m}Tc are less sensitive in the detection of pulmonary activity. Nevertheless, a ratio of pulmonary to cardiac activity >0.40 at 30-40 minutes of the stress test has been described as being associated with the severe coronary disease and decrease in ventricular function [35,36]

4.2. TRANSIENT LEFT VENTRICULAR DILATATION

In patients with severe coronary disease a transient ischaemic dilatation of the ventricular cavity can be observed in relation to a decrease in ventricular function during the stress test and secondary to the increase in left ventricular volume. Ventricular dilatation persists during post-stress SPET detection; always occurring early as with ^{201}Tl [37-39]. When tracers labelled with ^{99m}Tc are use, the dilatation of the left ventricular cavity is only detected in the situation of very severe ischaemia since image acquisition is not performed until some 30 minutes after the conclusion of the stress.

4.3. SLOW WASHOUT OF ^{201}Tl

Some investigators suggest slow diffuse or regional clearance of ^{201}Tl as an indicator of myocardial ischaemia [40-41]. The pharmaco-kinetics of the radionuclide are such that, in very severe ischaemia, incorporation of the isotope into the myocardium during exercise following intravenous injection is greatly reduced. However, the continuance of the ^{201}Tl in the blood enables that, over time, the ischaemic regions begin to slowly incorporate it and the uptake, although delayed, is above baseline. The slow-down, absence or inversion of the phenomenon of clearance can be objectively assessed using perfusion studies to visually (qualitatively) analyse ventricular uptake (normalisation to a single maximum) or quantitatively assessed using washout polar maps [42-44].

Nevertheless, various factors exist that interfere in myocardial washout of the tracer (regional metabolism, prandial status, pharmacological agents...) [45-49], the most important of which is the level of tachycardia attained [50,51]. If it does not reach high enough levels (above 80%) the subsequent washout of the radionuclide cannot be analysed. In practice, then, these data cannot be used in isolation as an indication of myocardial ischaemia when localised perfusion defects are not evident. The value is complementary to the other signs of ischaemic ventricular dysfunction and can help in the diagnosis of diffuse vascular disease when accompanied by scintigraphy and electrocardiographic signs of severe ischaemia [17,52,53].

5. Perfusion defects in patients without coronary disease

Certain situations exist in which alterations in the distribution of the tracer may be detected without this corresponding to coronary disease. With left bundle branch block, the uptake of the tracer in the septum can be reduced in the presence of normal coronary arteries [54,55]. The mechanism is not well understood, but it is thought that it is due to the asynchronicity of contraction and relaxation of the septum relative to the rest of the ventricle. As a result, the coronary flow takes place, essentially, during diastole and, at the septal level, this interval is cut-short in patients with left branch block; septal perfusion being especially decreased during the exercise and the diastole being more shortened. In general, this type of septal defect is of moderate intensity, fixed or discretely reversible [56] (Plate 2.6). With planar methodology and ^{201}Tl we have observed a high number of patients (46%) with left bundle branch block and normal coronary arteries. Corresponding to forms of congestive cardiomyopathy, dilatation of the ventricular cavity and heterogeneous uptake by the ventricular walls is observed together with persistent septal hypo-activity both in stress as well as rest [57].

To preclude false positives of ischaemia in the anterior-septal territory, the suggestion has been to conduct, in these patients, a test with a pharmacological agent such as dipyridamole instead of the exercise [58-62]. With it, the duration of diastole is, practically, non-shortened and the incidence of false positive reversible defects will be minimised. Nevertheless, the most common cause of perfusion defects in patients with left bundle branch block continues to be coronary disease [63] especially when not isolated in effect from the inter-ventricular septum [64]. As discussed in Chapter 4, we continue to use exercise as a provocation in these patients since, in our experience, the negative predictive value of the test is very high.

Detectable localised increases in the uptake of the tracer have been described in patients with left ventricular hypertrophy [65,66] (Plate 2.7). However, as discussed in Chapter 4, in verifying true alterations of myocardial perfusion in these patients [67,68] it is frequently observed that the regions that appear hypo-perfused correspond to the normal myocardium which is hypo-active relative to the hyper-trophic zones. This increase in regional activity is, in general, more obvious during the provocation test whether with exercise or a pharmacological agent. Normalising the images relative to the higher uptake zone can appear as decreased fixed or reversible perfusions in other zones of the myocardium. This can give rise to false positives in the diagnosis of coronary artery disease. However, correct detection of the origin of the differences in uptake between the ventricular walls becomes, in general, easier with greater experience in evaluating these patterns.

Equally, as happens in patients with hypertrophic cardiomyopathy, the dilated cardiomyopathy can present perfusion defects, as well [69]. Although some studies have suggested that the presence of extensive perfusion defects indicate that the origin of the cardiomyopathy will be ischaemic, it is not easy to distinguish those cases which are secondary to coronary artery disease from those of idiopathic origin when the defects are not reversible [70-71]. It is probable, nevertheless, that the ischaemic patterns of SPET, including the idiopathic cardiomyopathy with normal epicardiac coronary arteries, represent ischaemia, as has been demonstrated in some studies that encountered anomalies in the coronary reserve of these patients [71].

6. Interpretation of Gated-SPET studies

Evaluation by tomography synchronised with the ECG of the patient can be very simple methodologically but very valuable information can accrue from it [72]. The cinematograpic presentation of the cardiac cycle images in the three ventricle axes provides information on the contractility and the thickening of the left ventricular walls. This is the principal objective of the "gated" SPECT technique and, as such, achievable in any conventional scintigraphic facility for which a minimum "software" for reconstruction of the sections synchronised with the ECG is available [73].

This type of acquisition is performed, generally, when a high dose of the technetium-labelled tracer has been administered. However, applicability of the technique has been described in studies with ^{201}Tl and with low doses of ^{99m}Tc-MIBI or tetrofosmin (10 mCi; the ideal quality in a reasonable acquisition time is obtained with doses of 20-25 mCi) [74]. Depending on the chosen protocol, gated-SPET studies can be applied at rest, in stress or both.

It needs to be borne in mind that the dynamic images obtained always represent the ventricular movement at rest even when the myocardial distribution of the tracer corresponds to its injection in stress. In this sense, and with a preferentially-focalised indication in the assessment of myocardium viability, the most useful exploration would be the gated-SPET in the resting phase of the study since the uptake in the walls will be at maximum. When there is an intense ischaemia and the post-stress defects are extensive and severe, the evaluation of the contractility above that of the post-stress study can be very difficult or equivocal and results from the absence of a visible ventricular wall.

Another application of the synchronised studies is the differentiation of fixed defects localised in regions that are frequently subject to physiological attenuation [75,76], as in the improved evaluation of septal defects due to left bundle branch block [77]. The thinning of the basal zone, especially, is a frequent finding in males, as is the anterior-lateral hypo-activity in females. On occasions, a complication is to decide if the fixed defect is due to attenuation or, if there really is an area of scar tissue, whether it is slight, extensive or non-transmural. This is especially so if one takes into account that the majority of non-Q wave infarcts are located in the inferior-lateral region on ECG. The motility response and conserved systolic enlargement help to confirm the absence of a myocardial lesion.

Software is available for quantification methods [78,79] for the majority of gamma cameras. By integrating the area contained within the endocardial border of the short axis slices the end-diastolic, end-systolic volumes and the ejection fraction values can be obtained (Plate 2.8). Although this method represents a methodological basis distinct from that of the first-pass or equilibrium ventriculography for the evaluation of ventricular function, the correlations that have been obtained are satisfactory. In this quantitative evaluation, other image parameters such as polar maps representative of motility, ejection fraction and regional systolic thickening are also included. Limitations in the quantification of ventricular volumes and of ejection fractions reside in the definition of the ventricular borders when there is no uptake by the wall or as a result of extensive scar areas. Nevertheless, recently published mathematical algorithms for the determination of ventricle outline achieve excellent results when compared to other traditional methods for the calculation of ventricular function [80].

7. Artefacts secondary to technical problems

In evaluating images one needs to constantly bear in mind a series of technical artefacts that can alter the interpretation of the results [81,82]:

7.1. LACK OF UNIFORMITY OF THE DETECTOR OR BEYOND-RANGE CENTRE OF ROTATION

As discussed in Chapter 1, it is not possible to perform tomographic studies if the minimum technical requirements guarantying reliability of the images are not fulfilled. In this sense, apart from the periodic checks of uniformity of the detector and of the centre of rotation, it is recommendable to obtain images of irregular sources of known characteristics such as the cardiac models that represent figures similar to those of the walls of the left ventricle.

7.2. DEFECTS RESULTING FROM SLICE RECONSTRUCTION, INAPPROPRIATE FILTER SELECTION AND VENTRICLE ORIENTATION

Operator inexperience constitutes a clear limitation in the technique. There is a learning curve in which every procedure needs to be supervised in the initial training if interpretable images are to be guaranteed in subsequent practice [83].

7.3. ECG IRREGULARITY

The studies synchronised with the ECG of the patient (gated SPET) require consistency of the electrical tracing that, in general, is obtained in all patients in sinus rhythm. Although marked respiratory arrhythmia can exist in younger patients, the wide tolerance in the R-R variation employed in this type of investigation (40-99%) allows problem-free acquisition [82].

The presence of cardiac arrhythmias such as atrial fibrillation, ventricular bigeminy, atrial-ventricular blocks etc. impede gated-SPET studies. Also, one needs to guard against the deterioration of the ECG during the acquisition. For example, although the initial signals may be correct, movements in the attached electrodes during the detector rotation can alter the electrical signal transmission to the computer. Should this occur without warning, the non-synchronised SPET can be lost as well since the majority of hardware equipment cannot store the scintigraphic data when the ECG is not correctly detected.

7.4. ANOMALOUS EFFECT OF ATTENUATION CORRECTION

Despite correcting for attenuation using polar maps of simultaneous transmission, and which present some notable advantages over conventional acquisition [5,6], there are still some drawbacks that need to be taken into account [84]. On occasions the attenuation due to the diaphragm exercises an advantageous effect by contributing to the diminution in the intensity of the extra-cardiac sub-diaphragmatic uptakes especially by the intestines when technetium-labelled tracers are used. As a consequence of the action of correcting the emission image by that of transmission, the difficulty in obtaining vertical sections with an activity scale that contains only that of the cardiac uptake is increased and, further, the effect of disperse radiation on the cardiac walls is increased. Probably, a combined correction for attenuation and for disperse radiation will be a better method for approximating the real cardiac uptake in the near future [84].

7.5. PATIENT MOVEMENT DURING ACQUISITION

This type of alteration in the series of images acquired can be difficult to avoid despite explaining to the patient the need for immobility even though the position adopted may be uncomfortable. Measures can be adopted that would reduce repetitions of the exploration and, as a consequence, minimum discomfort for the patient. For example, placing a bolster under the knees can reduce the patient's dorso-lumbar discomfort. In seeking "improved" image quality, a slow and deliberate image acquisition may, paradoxically, worsen the final result because of the patient's inability to remain immobile over a protracted period. Similarly, when it is traumatic to raise the left arm, it may be preferable to accept images that have the upper extremity interposed.

The artefact due to movement during the SPET procedure is clearly seen at two instances: the rotating ciné display of all the images acquired and in the sinogram image summation. Movement or discontinuity in the helical image of the sinogram may necessitate a repeat acquisition.

Ventricular displacement immediately post-stress (upward creep) is specific to the studies with ^{201}Tl that are performed too soon after exercise [85]. Initially, the heart has a more distal position with a more intense movement during the cardiac cycle. While the detection is being performed, the patient normalises the movement of the diaphragm and, progressively, the heart adopts a slightly more elevated position. These positional modifications can produce an effect similar to that of upward movement of the thorax by the patient.

If, in the reconstruction phase, movement has not been detected, the tomographic tomograms reflect an imbalance in activity distribution that tends to show as acceleration of a part of the left ventricle. There appears, in the long axes, a disconnection of the ventricle walls at the apex (Plate 2.9) and, in the coronal slices, a circular rupture with the upper part overhanging the lower like a "fringe". Polar maps, as well, highlight this peculiar artefact. The imbalance is seen as an image that has been termed the "hurricane sign" because of its similarity to the symbol for hurricane used on meteorological maps [86].

Although the majority of commercial software programs incorporate corrections for movement, in a high proportion of cases the problem is not resolved. In this respect, the advantage of the technetium-labelled tracers resides in the option of repeating the acquisition without the myocardial distribution of the tracer having been modified.

7.6. DIFFERENCES IN HOMOGENEITY OF MYOCARDIAL UPTAKE OF RADIO-TRACERS

When ^{201}Tl is used, a high initial myocardial concentration is observed especially when adequate physical exercise has been performed and the cardiac effort is elevated. At 3-4 hours, the activity in the myocardium has been considerably washed-out (>50% under normal conditions) and the redistribution image may be of low quality. Although, in principle, this should not be a diagnostic problem since increased myocardial washout is associated with perfusion normality, paradoxical patterns can be produced in the zones of low, post-stress uptake that appear as still lower uptake in the delayed image because of the lower count effect [87].

Nowadays, a short protocol with the technetium-labelled tracers is used with increasing frequency [88,89]. The study can be completed in a single work session and speeds-up the data entry. But in this method the second image contains a greater activity than the first and which results from a higher dose together with the summed effect of the two injections. When the first dose (about 8-10 mCi) is administered during stress, the higher photon flow of the second image corresponds to that at rest (about 20-25 mCi) and can produce an effect of improving the myocardial uptake in the irregular zones visible in the stress study that, in reality, is due to a lower quality of the image [90-92].

The solutions to this problem are various. One can opt for inverting the protocol and begin with SPECT test at rest. This has the inconvenience that all the patients need to be subjected to the double injection-detection even though the stress images are normal. Alternatively, the long protocol applied over two days with high doses can be used and which would be recommendable in obese patients or those with an elevated mammary attenuation. Whenever the short protocol is employed it is necessary to compensate, at the time of acquisition, for the difference in the doses administered and to adjust the reconstruction filters to the characteristics of the acquired image. Generally, with low doses the study time is doubled and the filters employed are smoother so as to obtain comparable images.

8. Artefacts inherent in the patient

8.1. SOFT-TISSUE ATTENUATION

A knowledge of the physical characteristics of the patient [81,82] is fundamental in the interpretation of SPET since secondary attenuation by soft tissue can, in many cases, cause diagnostic errors.

Large breasts can simulate an anterior-lateral perfusion defect. To ensure that the defect detected remains fixed, the breasts need to be aligned exactly the same in the stress test as in that at rest. Hence, before diagnosing an anterior-lateral fixed perfusion defect in a woman with large breasts, the possibility of the detection being an artefact must always be considered. Reversible defects are more difficult to interpret since this can result merely from changes in the position of the left breast relative to angle of elevation of the left arm.

Obesity, as well, can be a source of errors since adipose tissue of the thoracic wall can give rise to an attenuated image, especially of the lateral face.

The left hemi-diaphragm is one of the most frequent causes of erroneous interpretation of perfusion studies in males. It is not clear why this type of artefact is more frequent in men than in women but it could be attributable to the diaphragm in the male being more muscular and that of the female fatter. Or, perhaps that the men use the abdominal musculature more for breathing than do women and, as such, produce a marked elevation during respiration. Usually, perfusion attenuation takes place in the inferior face and more markedly in the basal portions. Nevertheless, perfusion attenuation can be observed, on occasions, in the inferior-basal, inferior-septal and inferior-apical zones. In general, the diminution of perfusion observed, in stress as at rest, when gastric distension by aerophagia during exercise is produced and the diaphragm remains in a more elevated position than in the at-rest scintigraphy. This would be seen as a reversible defect and can give rise to a false diagnosis of ischaemia. This can happen with a greater frequency when the exploration is performed with ^{201}Tl and the stress scintigraphy detection is performed too early.

8.2. CONCENTRATION OF THE TRACER IN THE ABDOMINAL VISCERA

Activity of the tracer in the abdominal viscera close to the heart can give rise to errors of interpretation. If the extra-cardiac activity is included in the normalisation of the images, the overall concentration of the tracer in the heart will appear to be decreased. When ^{201}Tl is used, the activity in the abdominal viscera is limited, generally, to the liver while if the ^{99m}Tc-labelled tracers were used and which are excreted by the hepato-biliary system, the activity is concentrated in the biliary vesiculae, intestine and, occasionally, in the stomach when gastro-duodenal reflux is present. (Plate 2.10). To minimise hepatic uptake it is desirable that the level of exercise performed should be the maximum possible since, under these conditions, there is a diminution of the hepatic flow relative to the myocardium and the peripheral muscles. Hence, at the conclusion of the pharmacolological test with dipyridamole also, it is advisable that the patient performs a grade of exercise up to his limit.

When tracers labelled with ^{99m}Tc are used, the patient is advised to ingest milk or some fatty meal once the stress test is completed and before the acquisition of the images so as to minimise the hepato-biliary and intestinal activity. However, in some cases this give rise to an increase in the concentration of the radio-labelled pharmacological agent in the intestinal ansae and excessive activity is observed. Hence, before initiating the image acquisition it is advisable to have the patient ingest one or two glasses of water to accelerate the transit through the intestine while, at the same time, to delay the exploration for about 30 minutes.

9. Reproducibility in myocardial perfusion studies

Data on intra- and inter-observer agreement in interpreting thallium-201 studies have been reported. Okada et al. [93] and Atwood et al. [94] reported good observer agreement when studies were interpreted in a simple dichotomous fashion (normal or abnormal) with kappa values ranging from 0.56 to 0.74. Watson et al. [95] reported on quantitative computer assisted analysis of planar ^{99m}Tc sestamibi studies acquired in a different institution. They found high (90%) agreement between interpreters and between computer operators. In the MSSMI study (Multicenter Study on Silent Myocardial Ischemia), 556 planar ^{201}Tl images were interpreted in 24 clinical centers and in a Radionuclide Core Laboratory.

Studies assessing reproducibility of myocardial SPET have generally been limited to an unblinded analysis of intra- and inte-robserver comparisons of the same scan [96,97], or to a series including patients with previous myocardial infarction [98,99]. Hendel et al. [98] found an overall concordance of 86% (kappa value = 0.669) with ^{99m}Tc furifosmin perfusion imaging studies in a series of 150 patients including 53% with previous myocardial infarction, and Golub et al. [99] described a moderate to excellent interpretative reproducibility (87-94%) with stress ^{99m}Tc sestamibi SPECT imaging among nuclear cardiologists with a wide range of training and experience.

In our experience in 150 SPET myocardial perfusion studies from 5 hospitals in patients without previous myocardial infarction and a prevalence of 60% of coronary artery disease, we obtained an agreement in 87% of patients (kappa value 0.626). The agreement in left anterior descending artery territory was 81%, 79% for the right coronary artery territory and 91% in the left circumflex artery territory. Agreement was similar in patients with one- two- and three-vessel coronary artery disease (91%, 88% and 86% respectively). The overall sensitivity and specificity were 82% and 87% respectively [100,101].

References

1. Fintel DJ, Links JM, Brinker JA et al. Improved diagnostic performance of exercise thallium-201 single photon emission computed tomography over planar imaging in the diagnosis of coronary artery disease: A receiver operating characteristic analysis. J Am Coll Cardiol 1989; 13: 600-612.

2. Maddahi J, Kiat H, Berman DS. Myocardial perfusion imaging with technetium-99m-labeled agents. Am J Cardiol 1991; 67: 27D-34D.

3. Committee on Advanced Cardiac Imaging and Technology, Council on Clinical Cardiology, American Heart Association; Cardiovascular Imaging Committee, American College of Cardiology; and Board of Directors, Cardiovascular Council, Society of Nuclear Medicine. Standardization of Cardiac Tomographic Imaging. Circulation 1992; 86: 338-339.

4. DePuey EG, García EV. Optimal specificity of thallium-201 SPECT through recognition of imaging artifacts. J Nucl Med 1989; 30: 441-449.

5. Ficaro EP, Fessler JA, Shreve PD, Kritzman JN, Rose PA, Corbett JR. Simultaneous transmission/emission myocardial perfusion tomography. Diagnostic accuracy of attenuation-corrected ^{99m}Tc-sestamibi single-photon emission computed tomography. Circulation 1996; 93: 463-473.

6. Kluge R, Sattler B, Seese A, Knapp WH. Attenuation correction by simultaneous emission-transmission myocardial single-photon emission computed tomography: impact on diagnostic accuracy. Eur J Nucl Med 1997; 24: 1107-1114.

7. Iskandrian AS, Verani MS (1996) Exercise perfusion imaging in coronary artery disease: physiology and diagnosis, in Iskandrian AS and Verani MS (eds.), Nuclear Cardiac Imaging: Principles and Applications. F.A. Davis Company, Philadelphia; pp. 73-143.

8. Slomka, PJ, Hurwitz GA, St. Clement G, Stephenson J. Three-dimensional demarcation of perfusion zones corresponding to specific coronary arteries: application for automated interpretation of myocardial SPECT. J Nucl Med 1995; 36: 2120-2126.

9. Segal GM, Atwood JE, Botvinick EH. Variability of normal coronary anatomy: implications for the interpretation of thallium-SPECT myocardial perfusion images in single-vessel disease. J Nucl Med 1995; 36: 944-951.

10. Brunken R, Schwaiger M, Grover-McKay M, Phelps ME, Tillisch J, Schelbert HR. Positron emission tomography detects tissue metabolic activity in myocardial segments with persistent thallium perfusion defects. J Am Coll Cardiol 1987; 10: 557-567.

11. Kiat H, Berman DS, Maddahi J et al. Late reversibility of tomographic myocardial thallium-201 defects: An accurate marker of myocardial viability. J Am Coll Cardiol 1988; 12: 1456-1463.

12. Gutman J, Berman DS, Freeman M et al. Time to complete redistribution of thallium-201 in exercise thallium-201 scintigraphy: relationship to the degree of coronary artery stenosis. Am Heart J 1983; 108: 989-995.

13. Yang LD, Berman DS, Kiat H et al. The frequency of late reversibility in SPECT thallium-201 stress-redistribution studies. J Am Coll Cardiol 1990; 15: 334-340.

14. Cuocolo A, Pace L, Ricciardelli B, Chiariello M, Trimarco B, Salvatore M. Identification of viable myocardium in patients with chronic coronary artery disease: comparison of thallium-201 scintigraphy with reinjection and technetium-99m-methoxyisobutylisonitrile. J Nucl Med 1992; 33: 505-511.

15. Altehoefer C, Kaiser HJ, Doerr R et al. Fluorine-18 deoxyglucose PET for assessment of viable myocardium in perfusion defects in ^{99m}Tc-MIBI SPET: a comparative study in patients with coronary artery disease. Eur J Nucl Med 1992; 19: 334-342.

16. Berman DS, Kiat H, VanTrain KF, Friedman J, Garcia EV, Maddahi J. Comparison of SPECT using technetium-99m agents and thallium-201 and PET for the assessment of myocardial perfusion and viability. Am J Cardiol 1990; 66: 72E-79E.

17. Leppo J. Thallium washout analysis: fact or fiction?. J Nucl Med 1987; 28: 1058-1060.

18. Silberstein EB, DeVries DF. Reverse redistribution phenomenon in thallium-201 stress test: angiographic correlation and clinical significance. J Nucl Med 1985; 26: 707-710.

19. Brown KA, Benoit L, Clements JP, Wackers FJT. Fast washout of thallium-201 from area of myocardial infarction: possible artifact of background subtraction. J Nucl Med 1987; 28: 945-949.

20. Lear JL, Raff U, Jain R. Reverse and pseudo redistribution of thallium-201 in healed myocardial infarction and normal and negative thallium-201 washout in ischemia due to background oversubtraction. Am J Cardiol 1988; 62: 543-550.
21. Candell-Riera J, Ortega-Alcalde D. Reverse redistribution pattern of thallium-201 stress test in subjects with normal coronary angiograms. J Nucl Med 1986; 27: 1377.
22. Pace L, Cuocolo A, Maurea S et al. Reverse redistribution in resting thallium-201 myocardial scintigraphy in patients with coronary artery disease: relation to coronary anatomy and ventricular function. J Nucl Med 1993; 34: 1688-1692.
23. Marin-Neto JA, Dilsizian V, Arrighi JA et al. Thallium reinjection demonstrates viable myocardium in regions with reverse redistribution. Circulation 1993; 88: 1736-1745.
24. Pace L, Cuocolo A, Marzullo P et al. Reverse redistribution in resting thallium-201 myocardial scintigraphy in chronic coronary artery disease: an index of myocardial viability. J Nucl Med 1995; 36: 1968-1973.
25. Dilsizian V, Freedman NMT, Bacharach SL, Perrone-Filardi P, Bonow RO. Regional thallium uptake in irreversible defects. Magnitude of change in thallium activity after reinjection distinguishes viable from nonviable myocardium. Circulation 1992; 85: 627-634.
26. Romero-Farina B, Candell-Riera J, Aguadé S et al. Significado de los defectos paradójicos segmentarios en la tomogammagrafía miocárdica con ^{99m}Tc-tetrofosmina. Rev Esp Med Nuclear 1999; 18: 348-355.
27. Weiss AT, Maddahi J, Lew AS et al. Reverse redistribution phenomenon in thallium-201: a sign of nontransmural myocardial infarction with patency of the infarct-related coronary artery. J Am Coll Cardiol 1986; 7: 61-67.
28. Bonow RO, Dilsizian V. Tallium-201 for assessment of myocardial viability. Sem Nucl Med 1991; 21: 230-241.
29. Piwnica-Worms D, Krounage JF, Chiu ML. Uptake and retention of hexakis (2-methoxyisobutyl isonitrile) technetium (I) in cultured chick myocardial cells. Mitochondrial and plasma membrane potential dependance. Circulation 1990; 82: 1626-1836.
30. Berman DS, Kiat H, VanTrain KF et al. Technetium-99m-sestamibi in the assessment of chronic coronary artery disease. Sem Nucl Med 1991; 21: 190-212.
31. Castell J, Santana C, Candell J et al. La tomogammagrafía miocárdica de esfuerzo en el diagnóstico de la enfermedad coronaria multivaso. Rev Esp Cardiol 1997; 50: 635-642.
32. Boucher CA, Zir LM, Beller GA et al. Increased lung uptake of thallium-201 during exercise myocardial imaging: clinical, hemodynamic and angiographic implications in patients with coronary artery disease. Am J Cardiol 1980;46:189-196.
33. Levy R, Rozanski A, Berman DS et al. Analysis of the degree of pulmonary thallium washout after exercise in patients with coronary artery disease. J Am Coll Cardiol 1983; 2: 719-728.
34. Villanueva FS, Kaul S, Smith WH et al. Prevalence and correlates of increased lung/heart ratio of thallium-201 during dipyridamole stress imaging for suspected coronary artery disease. Am J Cardiol 1990; 66: 1324-1335.
35. Giubbini R, Campini R, Milan E et al. Evaluation of technetium-99m-sestamibi lung uptake: correlation with left ventricular function. J Nucl Med 1995; 36: 58-63.
36. Saha M, Farrand TF, Brown KA. Lung uptake of technetium 99m-sestamibi. Relation to clinical exercise, hemodynamic, and left ventricular function variables. J Nucl Cardiol 1994; 1: 52-56.
37. Weiss AT, Berman DS, Lew AS et al. Transient ischemic dilation of the left ventricle on stress thallium-201 scintigraphy: A marker of severe and extensive coronary artery disease. J Am Coll Cardiol 1987; 9: 752-759.
38. Stolzenberg J. Dilation of the left ventricular cavity on stress thallium scan as an indicator of ischemic disease. Clin Nucl Med 1980; 5: 289-292.
39. Chouraqui P, Rodrigues E, Berman D, Maddahi J. Significance of dipyridamole induced transient dilation of the left ventricle during thallium-201 scintigraphy in suspected coronary artery disease. Am J Cardiol 1990; 66: 689-698.
40. Sklar J, Kirch D, Johnson T et al. Slow late myocardial clearance of thallium: A characteristic phenomenon in coronary artery disease. Circulation 1982; 65: 1504-1510.
41. Bateman TM, Maddahi J, Gray RJ et al. Diffuse slow washout of myocardial thallium-201: a new scintigraphic indicator of extensive coronary artery disease. J Am Coll Cardiol 1984; 4: 55-64.

42. Maddahi J, Abdulla A, García EV, Swan HJC, Berman D. Noninvasive identification of left main and triple vessel coronary artery disease: Improved accuracy using quantitative analysis of regional myocardial stress distribution and washout of thallium-201. J Am Coll Cardiol 1986; 7: 53-60.

43. VanTrain KF, Berman DS, Garcia EV et al. Quantitative analysis of stress thallium-201 myocardial scintigrams: a multicenter trial. J Nucl Med 1986; 27: 17-25.

44. Kasabali B, Woodard ML, Beckerman C et al. Enhanced sensitivity and specificity of thallium-201 imaging for the detection of regional ischemic coronary disease by combining SPECT with Bull's Eye' analysis. Clin Nucl Med 1989; 14: 484-491.

45. Van Train KF, Garcia EV, Cooke CD, Areeda J (1995) Quantitative analysis of SPECT myocardial perfusion, in De Puey E.G., Berman D.S. and Garcia E.V.(eds.), Cardiac SPECT Imaging, New York, Raven Press Ltd, pp. 49-74.

46. Brown KA, Benoit L, Clements JP, Wackers FJT. Fast washout of thallium-201 from area of myocardial infarction: possible artefact of background subtraction. J Nucl Med 1987; 28: 945-949.

47. O'Byrne GT, Rodrigues EA, Maddahi J et al. Comparison of myocardial washout rate of thallium-201 between rest, dipyridamole with and without aminophyline, and exercise states in normal subjects. Am J Cardiol 1989; 64: 1022-1028.

48. Wilson RA, Okada RD, Strauss HW et al. Effect of glucose-insulin-potassium infusion on thallium myocardial clearance. Circulation 1983; 68: 203-209.

49. Schachner ER, Oster ZH, Sacker DF, Som P, Atkins HL. The effect of procainamide, lidocaine and diphenylhydantoin on thallium-201 chloride uptake. Nucl Med Biol 1987; 14: 497-498.

50. Kaul S, Chesler DA, Pohost GM, Strauss HW, Okada RD, Boucher CA. Influence of peak exercise heart rate on normal thallium-201 myocardial clearance. J Nucl Med 1986; 27: 26-30.

51. Massie BM, Wisneski J, Kramer B, Hollenberg M, Gertz E, Stern D. Comparison of myocardial thallium-201 clearance after maximal and submaximal exercise: implications for diagnosis of coronary disease: concise comunication. J Nucl Med 1982; 23: 381-385.

52. Wackers FJT, Fatterman RC, Mattera JA, Clements JP. Quantitative planar thallium-201 stress scintigraphy: a critical evaluation of the method. Semin Nucl Med 1985; 15: 46-66.

53. McCarthy DM, Makler PT. Potential limitations of quantitative thallium scanning. Am J Cardiol 1985; 55: 215-217.

54. Hirzel HO, Senn M, Nuesch K et al. Thallium-201 scintigraphy in complete bundle branch block. Am J Cardiol 1984; 53: 764-769.

55. DePuey EG, Guertler-Krawcynska EG, Robbins WL. Thallium-201 SPECT in coronary artery disease patients with left bundle branch block. J Nucl Med 1988; 29: 1479-1485.

56. Tawahara K, Kurata Ch, Taguchi T, Kobayashi A, Yamazaki N. Exercise testing and thallium-201 emission computed tomography in patients with intraventricular conduction disturbances. Am J Cardiol 1992; 69: 97-102.

57. González JM, Castell J, Arana R et al. Utilidad de la gammagrafía planar con 201-Talio en pacientes con bloqueo de rama izquierda. Rev Esp Med Nucl 1993; 12: 41.

58. Burns RJ, Galligan L, Wright LM et al. Improved specificity of myocardial thallium-201 single photon emission computed tomography in patients with left bundle branch block by dipyridamole. Am J Cardiol 1991; 68: 504-508.

59. Rockett JF, Chadwick W, Moinnddin M et al. Intravenous dipyridamole thallium-201 SPECT imaging in patients with left bundle branch bolock. Clin Nucl Med 1990; 15: 401-407.

60. Larcos G, Brown ML, Gibbons RJ. Role of dipyridamole thallium-201 imaging in left bundle branch block. Am J Cardiol 1991; 68: 1097-1100.

61. Jukema JW, Van der Wall EE, Van der Vis-Melsen MJ et al. Dipyridamole thallium-201 scintigraphy for improved detection of left anterior descending coronary artery stenosis in patients with left bundle branch block. Eur Heart J 1993; 14: 53-56.

62. Jazmati B, Sadaniantz A, Emaus SP, Heller GV. Exercise thallium-201 imaging in complete bundle branch block and the prevalence of septal perfusion defect. Am J Cardiol 1991; 67: 46-49.

63. Matzer L, Kiat H, Friedman JD et al. A new approach to the assesment of tomographic thallium-201 scintigraphy in patients with left bundle branch block. J Am Coll Cardiol 1991; 17: 1309-1317.

64. DePuey EG, Guertler-Krawczynska E, Perkins JV, Robbins WL, Whelchel JD, Clements SD. Alterations in myocardial thallium-201 distribution in patients with chronic systemic hypertension undergoing single-photon emission computed tomography. Am J Cardiol 1988; 62: 234-238.

65. O´Gara PT, Bonow RO, Maron BJ et al. Myocardial perfusion abnormalities in patients with hypertrophic cardiomyopathy: assesment with thallium-201 emission computed tomography. Circulation 1987; 76: 1214-1223.

66. Romero-Farina G, Candell-Riera J, Pereztol-Valdés O et al. Clasificación morfológica de la miocardiopatía hipertrófica mediante tomogammagrafía miocárdica. Comparación con la clasificación ecocardiográfica. Rev Esp Cardiol 2000; 53: 511-516.

67. Cannon RO, Dilzisian V, O'Gara PT et al. Myocardial metabolic, hemodynamic, and electrocardiographic significance of reversible thallium-201 abnormalities in hypertrophic cardiomyopathy. Circulation 1991; 83: 1660-1667.

68. Dunn RF, Uven RF, Sadick N et al. Comparison of thallium-201 scanning in idiopathic dilated cardiomyopathy and severe coronary artery disease. Circulation 1982; 66: 804-810.

69. Yamaguchi S, Tsuik K, Hayasaka M, Yasui S. Segmental wall motion abnormalities in dilated cardiomyopathy: Hemodynamic characteristics and comparison with thallium-201 myocardial scintigraphy. Am Heart J 1987; 113: 1123-1128.

70. Pasternac A, Noble J, Strenlens Y et al. Pathophysiology of chest pain in patients with cardiomyopathy and normal coronary arteries. Circulation 1982; 65: 778-789.

71. Nitenberg A, Koult JM, Blanchet F, Zouioueche S. Multifactorial determinants of reduced coronary flow reserve after dipyridamole in dilated cardiomyopahy. Am J Cardiol 1985; 55: 748-754.

72. Chua T, Kiat H, Germano G et al. Gated technetium-99m sestamibi for simultaneous assessment of stress myocardial perfusion, post-exercise regional ventricular function and myocardial viability: correlation with echo-cardiography and rest thallium-201 scintigraphy. J Am Coll Cardiol 1994; 23: 1107-1114.

73. Berman DS, Germano G. Evaluation of ventricular ejection fraction, wall motion, wall thickening, and other parameters with gated myocardial perfusion single-photon emission computed tomography. J Nucl Cardiol 1997; 4: S169-S171.

74. Germano G, Erel J, Kiat H, Kavanagh PB, Berman DS. Quantitative LVEF and qualitative regional function from gated thallium-201 perfusion SPECT. J Nucl Med 1997; 38: 749-754.

75. DePuey EG, Rozanski A. Gated Tc-99m sestamibi SPECT to characterize fixed defects as infarct artefact. J Nucl Med 1995; 36: 952-955.

76. Mannting F, Morgan-Mannting M. Gated SPECT with technetium-99m sestamibi for assessment of myocardial perfusion abnormalities. J Nucl Med 1993; 34: 601-608.

77. Sugihara H, Tamaki N, Nozawa M et al. Septal perfusion and wall thickening in patients with left bundle branch block assessed by technetium-99m-sestamibi gated tomography. J Nucl Med 1997; 38: 545-547.

78. Germano G, Kiat H, Kavanagh PB et al. Automatic quantification of ejection fraction from gated myocardial perfusion SPECT. J Nucl Med 1995; 36: 2138-2147.

79. Miron SD, Finkelhor R, Penuel JH, Bahler R, Bellon EM. A geometric method of measuring the left ventricular ejection fraction on gated Tc-99m sestamibi myocardial imaging. Clin Nucl Med 1996; 21: 439-444.

80. Nichols K, De Puey EG, Rozansky A, Salensky H, Friedman MI. Image enhancement of severely hypoperfused myocardia for computation of tomographic ejection fraction. J Nucl Med 1997; 38: 1411-1417.

81. Nichols KJ, Galt JR (1995) Quality control for SPECT imaging, in E.G. De Puey, D.S. Berman and E.V. Garcia (eds.) Cardiac SPECT Imaging. New York, Raven Press Ltd, pp. 21-48.

82. García EV, Cooke CD, Van Train KF. Technical aspects of myocardial SPECT imaging with technetium-99m sestamibi. Am J Cardiol 1990; 66: 23E-31E.

83. Lancaster JL, Starling MR, Kopp DT, Lasher JC, Blumhardt R. Effect of errors in reangulation on planar and tomographic thallium-201 washout profile curves. J Nucl Med 1985; 26: 1445-1455.

84. Hutton BF. Cardiac single-photon emission tomography: is the attenuation correction enough? Eur J Nucl Med 1997; 24: 713-715.

85. Friedman J, VanTrain K, Maddahi J et al. "Upward creep" of the heart: a frequent source of false-positive reversible defects during thallium-201 stress-redistribution SPECT. J Nucl Med 1989; 30: 1718-1722.

86. Sorrell V, Figueroa B, Hansen CJ. The "hurricane sign": evidence of patient motion artefact on cardiac single-photon emission computed tomographic imaging. J Nucl Cardiol 1996; 3: 86-88.

87. Liu P, Burns RJ. Easy come, easy go: time to pause and put thallium reverse redistribution in perspective. J Nucl Med 1993; 34: 1692-1694.

88. Taillefer R. Technetium-99m sestamibi myocardial imaging: same-day rest-stress studies and dipyridamole. Am J Cardiol 1990; 66: 80E-90E.

89. Jain D, Wackers FJT, Mattera J, McMahon M, Sinusas AJ, Zaret BL. Biokinetics of Technetium-99m-Tetrofosmin: myocardial perfusion imaging agent: Implications for a one-day imaging protocol. J Nucl Med 1993: 43: 1254-1259.

90. Buell U, Dupont F, Uebis R et al. 99mTc-methoxy-isobutyl-isonitrile SPECT to evaluate a perfusion index from regional myocardial uptake after exercise and at rest: Results of a four hour protocol in patients with coronary heart disease and in controls. Nucl Med Commun 1990; 11: 77-94.

91. Taillefer R, Gagnon A, Laflame L et al. Same day injections of Tc-99m methoxy isobutyl isonitrile (hexamibi) for myocardial tomographic imaging: Comparison between rest-stress and stress-rest injection sequences. Eur J Nul Med 1989; 15: 113-117.

92. Sridhara B, Sochor H, Rigo P et al. Myocardial single-photon emission computed tomographic imaging with technetium 99m tetrofosmin: Stess-rest imaging with same-day and separate-day rest imaging. J Nucl Cardiol 1994; 1: 138-143.

93. Okada RD, Boucher CA, Kirshenbaum HK et al. Improved diagnostic accuracy of thallium-201 stress test using multiple observers and criteria derived from interobserver analysis of variance. Am J Cardiol 1980; 46: 619-624.

94. Atwood JE, Jensen D, Froelicher V et al. Agreement in human interpretation of analog thallium myocardial perfusion images. Circulation 1981; 64: 601-609.

95. Watson DD, Smith WH, Beller GA, Vinson EL, Taillefer R. Blinded evaluation of planar technetium-99m-sestamibi myocardial perfusion studies. J Nucl Med 1992; 33: 668-675.

96. Mahmarian JJ, Boyce TM, Goldberg RK, Cocanougher MK, Roberts R, Verani MS. Quantitative exercise thallium-201 single-photon emission computed tomography for the enhanced diagnosis of ischemic heart disease. J Am Coll Cardiol 1990; 15:318-29.

97. Mahmarian JJ, Pratt CM, Nishimura S, Abreu A, Verani MS. Quantitative adenosine Tl-201 single-photon emission tomography for the early assessment of patients surviving acute myocardial infarction. Circulation 1993; 87: 1197-210.

98. Hendel RC, Verani MS, Miller D et al. Diagnostic utility of tomographic myocardial perfusion imaging with technetium 99m furifosmin (Q12) compared with thallium 201: Results of a phase III multicenter trial. J Nucl Cardiol 1996; 3: 291-300.

99. Golub RJ, Ahlberg AW, McClellan JR et al. Interpretative reproducibility of stress Tc-99m sestamibi tomographic myocardial perfusion imaging. J Nucl Cardiol 1999; 6: 257-269.

100. Candell-Riera J, Santana-Boado C, Bermejo B et al. Impacto de los datos clínicos y concordancia interhospitalaria en la interpretación de la tomogammagrafía miocárdica de perfusión Rev Esp Cardiol 1999; 52: 892-897.

101. Candell-Riera J, Santana-Boado C, Bermejo B et al. Interhospital observer agreement in interpretation of 99mTc-tetrofosmin myocardial exercise SPECT studies. J Nucl Cardiol (in press).

3. METHODS OF QUANTIFICATION

SANTIAGO AGUADÉ-BRUIX and JOAN CASTELL-CONESA

1. Concept and extent of quantification

Quantification, by definition, is the measurement or evaluation of a given magnitude in real and reliable terms. Logically, in relation to studies of myocardium perfusion, we refer to the evaluation, in an objective manner, of the quantity of tracer present in the myocardium. It is possible, also, to evaluate tracer variations as a function of clinical situations (exercise, pharmacological stress, rest, pacemaker...) or, in Gated-SPET studies, to evaluate other parameters such as ventricular function, ventricular volumes, myocardial mass, ventricular wall thickening and movement of the wall [1].

The radiotracer used influences the type of quantification to be performed. For example, in using Thallium-201 the parameters to be quantified are post-stress myocardial activity, myocardial activity in the redistribution phase and variation in stress/redistribution activity (washout or clearance) that is representative of the coronary reserve flow [2].

If technetium tracers are used, MIBI or tetrofosmin, it is only possible to quantify the activities of stress and at rest, and since the parameter of clearance cannot be obtained, the quantification of coronary reserve is more complicated and is assessed in an indirect manner [3].

Once the parameter to be quantified is defined and the methodology to be employed is selected for the optimum interpretation and evaluation of the results, it is a requirement to determine the levels or limits of normality for this parameter i.e. to generate some tables of data of normality that identifies a value as normal or pathological within a grade of acceptable certainty.

The end interest of quantification, apart from obtaining numerical values, lies in the better standardisation of the procedures and in the better comparison with other techniques and which is clearly superior to the semi-quantitative methods of evaluation of myocardial perfusion [1].

2. Absolute quantification: PET

The only non-invasive technique that allows for quantification of myocardial perfusion, in absolute terms, is positron emission tomography (PET). The emission of pairs of photons of 511 keV with opposite direction that is produced by the annihilation reaction of the positrons (e^+), antimatter of the electron in its combination with electrons and which suffers minimum tissue attenuation.

J. Candell-Riera et al. (eds.), Myocardium at Risk and Viable Myocardium, 45–67.
© *2001 Kluwer Academic Publishers. Printed in the Netherlands.*

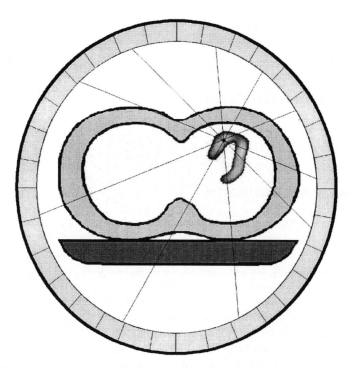

Figure 1: Scheme of the PET detector ring. The detection is performed in several adjacent rings formed into detection blocks where each block is composed of 8 scintillation crystals mounted below two photo-multiplier tubes.

Disperse radiation is minimised because the system of detection with which the equipment is provided for the formation of images, takes into account only the emissions detected simultaneously at 180° (coincidence detection). These units are formed by groups of detector rings to which the information is directed so as to determine the point in space at which emission of the positron has been produced (Figure 1) [4,5].

These are the qualities that facilitate determining the absolute quantity of tracer present in the tissue as a function of the quantity of radiation detected and, with a correct analysis of the kinetics, of the positron concentrations in the tissues.

Currently there are available several radionuclides which are emitters of positrons and which are useful in the study of the myocardium (Table 1) and which are used in marking physiological substrates for assessing tissue metabolism. These are, essentially, ^{18}F-deoxyglucose, ^{11}C-acetate and ^{11}C-palmitate, and are used either directly as indicators of myocardial perfusion or in the evaluation of regional blood flow. Taken as "gold standard" of perfusion is the measurement of flow using microspheres of albumin injected into the coronary tree by catheterisation. The values established are 90 ± 30 ml/min/100mg in healthy coronary arteries and vary between 0 and 60 ml/min/100mg in ischaemic and necrosed regions [6-8]. The values obtained with PET are practically the same, using perfusion tracers such as ammonium labelled with nitrogen-13 (^{13}NH$_3$), rubidium-82 (^{82}Rb) or water labelled with oxygen-15 (H$_2$^{15}O).

TABLE 1: Radionuclide positron emitters used in the evaluation of the myocardium with PET.

Radionuclide	$T^{1}/_{2}$ (minutes)	Energy (MeV)	Radio-pharmaceutical
^{11}C	20.38	0.690	Acetate, Palmitate
^{13}N	9.96	1.198	Ammonium (NH_3)
^{15}O	2.03	1.732	Water (H_2O), CO_2
^{62}Cu	9.73	2.917	PTSM
^{82}Rb	1.27	3.150	ClRb

The first tracer used for the measurement of blood flow with PET was $^{13}NH_3$ [9,10], which has a high myocardial first-pass extraction (90%). The relationship of flow measured with microspheres and that by $^{13}NH_3$ is linear over a wide range of flows of between 44-200 ml/min/100mg [11]. The lack of linearity over greater ranges could be due to the progressive decrease of incorporation of the diffusible tracers at high flows and/or the metabolic entrapment of ammonia by the myocardium [12,13]. This dependency on cellular integrity for myocardial fixation of the tracer is, potentially, an inconvenience for its use as a pure indicator of perfusion but, nevertheless, carries with it considerable additional information regarding tissue viability.

Rubidium-82 (^{82}Rb) is a potassium analogue, as is thallium, whose uptake by the myocardium depends on the blood flow [14]. The advantage is that it is not a direct product of the cyclotron but is obtained from a strontium/rubidium generator. Its short half-life of 76 seconds permits repeat studies within 10-minute intervals [15]. The values of regional blood flow obtained with ^{82}Rb are similar to those measured by $^{13}NH_3$ but as well, shows saturation at high flows [16]. Conversely, the high energy of the positron emitted by ^{82}Rb has an effect on a lower spatial resolution of the images obtained [17].

Due to its metabolic independence and to its 100% extraction by the myocardium, water labelled with oxygen-15 ($H_2^{15}O$) is an excellent tracer of flow [18-21]. However, there are detection inconveniences originating from the intensity of activity of the vascular and pulmonary bases that reduce the contrast of the myocardial image obtained and enormously complicates the quantification [22].

Fluoro-18-deoxyglucose (^{18}FDG) competes with glucose transport and intracellular phosphorylation but does not participate in glycolysis or glycogen synthesis and, due to its low membrane permeability, remains trapped in the cytosol [23,24]. In ischaemic territories, the consumption of energy is preferentially form anaerobic glycolysis and, hence, the uptake of ^{18}FDG is increased relative to normo-perfused tissues and, as such, quantification of tissue consumption of glucose can identify the ischaemic tissues [25-27]. Necrotic areas do not incorporate the tracer.

The pattern of ischaemia in PET is defined as a defect of incorporation of a flow tracer (^{13}N, ^{82}Rb, ^{15}O) in conditions with or without stress which show an increase of uptake or a normal uptake in the exploration with ^{18}FDG. The presence of ^{18}FDG activity signifies, further, the existence of viable myocardium [28].

3. Relative quantification: SPET

The studies of myocardial perfusion that conventionally can be performed in units of nuclear cardiology employ low energy gamma emitters: [201]Tl (70-80 KeV, 135 KeV, 167 KeV) and [99m]Tc (140 KeV). Detection by sodium iodide crystal is affected by attenuation caused by interpolation of anatomical structures between the myocardium and the surface of the scintillation counter (i.e. impedes the arrival of the gamma photons at the detector) and which precludes absolute quantification of the activity of the tracer located in the myocardium. This attenuation can be partially corrected-for by using various methods. The best, albeit more complex, is the attenuation correction by transmission tomography SPET [29,30].

Quantification of the absolute activity in the myocardium requires very complex methodology with appropriate technical skills of the teams and without which the clinical benefit obtained will be seen to differ from that obtained using the system of relative quantification. In practice, the studies of myocardial perfusion with relative quantification provide excellent results in terms of diagnosis of the extent of coronary artery disease [31,32] and, in the evaluation of the viable myocardium, are comparable to the PET studies [33,34].

Two forms exist for the relative quantification of myocardial perfusion. The first is based on the activity detected in the heart compared to that in other organs (lung, liver…) detected simultaneously. The technique follows that of myocardial perfusion studies with [201]Tl [35], in which, if the correct grade of exercise is reached during the test, the radioactivity concentration at the level of the lung is low (<50% of the heart) while its increase under these conditions is indicative of left ventricular dysfunction in stress, with increased intra-pulmonary pressure and consequent elevation of the availability of thallium to the lung [36,37].

The second form of quantification is obtained comparing the activity of a given region of the myocardium relative to the region with the maximum uptake in the same organ (normalisation to the maximum activity in the heart) during the study. Logically, the value of the myocardial activity at the maximum will not be the same in the post-stress/exercise images as those at rest/redistribution, but the images are presented normalised to their own maximum value while only taking into account the relative increases or decreases in the activity. A particular form of normalisation is performed with the Thallium-201 studies in that the images of redistribution are normalised to the maximum of the stress images with the corresponding correction for the decay in activity, due to the dose having been injected only during stress[38].

The use of this second form of quantification has certain advantages, applying equally for the Thallium as for the technetium tracers, in that the technique is performed automatically and clearly for the operator. It facilitates the evaluation of sections independent of their thickness as well as comparisons of studies performed with different doses and of variable technical quality.

4. Factors that influence quantitative studies

In quantitative studies the images undergo a series of computational manipulations which need to be profoundly understood. It is necessary to bear in mind all the factors that affect the specific kinetics of the tracer and of the methods employed to assess them. If these conditions are not fulfilled, the quantitative techniques can result in erroneous results and would negatively affect the patient's diagnosis. Table 2 contains the principal aspects that influence the quantitative analyses of myocardial perfusion studies with single photon emitters [2].

TABLE 2: Factors that influence myocardial perfusion study quantification.

Factors inherent in the patient
Insufficient stress level
Concomitant medication
Individual variation (age, weight, cardiac rhythm)
Movement
Attenuation (breast, diaphragm)
Superimposition of extra-cardiac activities
External factors
Defects of the equipment (colimator, uniformity of detector)
De-alignment of the centre of rotation
Variations in rotation distance
Inadequate dose administration
Processing factors
Artefacts of reconstruction
Inadequate filters
De-alignment of reorientation axes.
Tomographic section selection

Initially, the quality control requirements for the equipment need to be fulfilled so as to ensure correct quality for the study [39-41]. Also, the correct procedures for acquiring, processing and reconstructing the tomographic images need to be standardised so as to ensure good reproducibility of the final quantification. A high degree of automation is advisable so that human operator variability is minimised [42].

The usefulness of a quantitative study is based, in a large part, on the analysis of myocardial clearance/washout of Thallium-201 or of the identification of defects that increase its relative uptake at rest (fill-in). As such, the level of exercise performed by the patient determines the maximum uptake at stress and facilitates a correct evaluation of the grade of clearance/fill-in [43-44].

Concomitant medications need to be taken into account in evaluating the response to a pharmacological agent. Dipyridamole, for example, can be inhibited by the xantines in the form of the agent teophylline, and stimulated by other beverages. Hence, it is necessary to bear the prandial status in mind and to avoid food ingestion between detection at stress and redistribution in Thallium-201 studies, while recommending food intake between the dose administration at rest and the subsequent detection in technetium tracers studies [45].

Extravasation during administration must be avoided so as to preclude the delayed arrival of the tracer to the myocardium. This point is critical in the short protocols with technetium and the classical protocols with Thallium.

Another aspect to consider is the existence of considerable individual variations with respect to age [46], weight (greater attenuation, greater radius of detection, insufficient dose…) as well as variations in cardiac rhythm (pacemakers, left bundle branch block) and myocardial asymmetries (hypertrophic myocardiopathy).

In the course of acquiring the tomographic images it is a basic necessity to maintain patient immobility. Artefacts produced by movement of the patient are the most frequent causes of errors in perfusion studies [47].

Attenuation correction solves the problems of alterations produced by the individual's own body structures that decrease the photon flow of the tracer arriving at the detector [46]. However, it is not possible to modify the superimposition of the extra-cardiac tissue activities (liver, intestine…) that can accrue despite the attenuation correction [48]. Although methods for masking these activities exist and which help in tomographic reconstruction, when capable of being superimposed on a myocardial region, these activities produce alterations in the quantitative values in the region.

5. Quantification methodology

The method used for the quantification of the tomographic images has received the name of "bull's eye" polar map (due to the images being circular and concentric) and represents a plane of activity of the different myocardial sections. The method was initially described by Caldwell et al. [49] in an experimental study in 1984 and was developed for use in patients by the group at Cedars-Sinai Medical Centre [50] in 1985 and followed by certain modifications by the group of Emory University [51]. More recently, image quantification has been standardised in a three dimension "CEqual" method (Cedars and Emory quantitative analysis) [1,52] with a representation of the myocardial perfusion on its surface [53,54]. The visualisation is much more informative than the two-dimensional polar map [55].

All the methods of quantification globally estimate, in practice, all the aspects of the process of the investigation of myocardial perfusion, from the type of stress used, the minimum level of stress necessary for its evaluation, parameters of detection (time, collimator…), reconstruction filters, processing and finally quantification [1]. This overall control necessary for the myocardial perfusion study compels the operator to use certain protocols and procedures (similar to those which have already been described in previous chapters) which come supplied with the purchase of the hardware such as the various types of gamma cameras (Cedars, CEqual) [42] many of which have the warranty of approval by the FDA.

5.1. POLAR MAP

5.1.1 *Cedars-Sinai method* [1,50,56,57]:
Generation of the polar map begins with the tomographic slices in stress and in redistribution studies with Thallium-201 since this is a method that evolved from the quantification systems of planar studies with Thallium-201 [58].

Although there are small individual variations in each processing system the operator, in effect, selects the number and the boundaries of subendocardiac, apical and basal sections of the short axis that are to be quantified over a slice of the vertical long axis in which the ventricular cavity has its greatest area. The subendocardiac apex needs to be selected to exclude the apical zone and the basal boundary. Approximately the last three slices of the short axis are excluded because of the large variation that exists in the zone more basal to the septal and inferior levels.

For the apical zone assessment, a more apical slice of the vertical long axis is selected and automatically scanned ± 30° starting from the apical mark.

The greater diameter short axis slice, normally in the middle zone of the cavity, defines the centre and the exterior boundary of the ventricle. For a better evaluation, subsequent to the assignment of defects with respect to arterial territories, it is advisable to reorientate the rotation of the bulls eye so that the start of the septum from the inferior wall (approximately 102° from the middle zone of the lateral wall) is set to coincide always with the position previously fixed by convention (90°).

The profile of maximum activity is automatically calculated for each section of the short axis. Starting with a sample of 60 sectors per slice (6° per sector) and beginning in the middle zone of the lateral wall the scan follows clockwise from the most apical section to the most basal. The information so obtained is collated in bidimensional form in successive layers, from the most apical zone (interior) to the most basal zone (exterior). The calculation of the apical zone is performed using the averaged profiles of maximum counts ± 30° beginning from the apical line, in the sections of the vertical long axis and the horizontal long axis, and remains placed in the centre of the polar image and, hence, the polar image is shown as an apical plot (Figure 2).

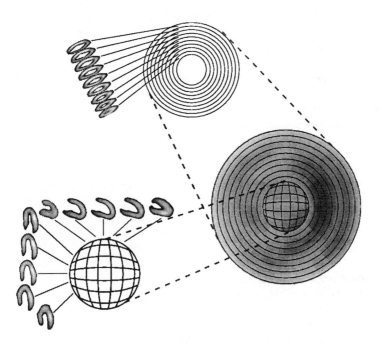

Figure 2: CEDARS method: Scheme for generation of polar maps split by the short axis slices and using a radial sample together with averaged vertical and horizontal long axes slices to generate the apical region.

The normalisation of the final polar image is with the point of maximum myocardial activity being assigned the value of 100. Irrespective of the heart size, an identical polar image is obtained. However, the greater the size of the heart the greater the number of slimmer concentric circles.

5.1.2. *Emory method* [1,51,59]:

The generation of the polar map starts from tomographic slices performed in stress and in redistribution studies with Thallium-201.

The slices selected for the generation of the polar map are those from the short axis and built-up covering the apical region with variable thicknesses as a function of heart size (about 12 slices for a heart of normal size). The profile of maximum activity is calculated automatically for each of the short axis slices and generated beginning with a sample of 40 sectors per slice (9° per sector), starting in the middle zone between the anterior and lateral face (at 45° from the vertical) and continuing anticlockwise from the third apical section to the more basal. The two most apical sections are expressed as a single value representing the maximum value of counts in this section. The information so obtained is placed in bidimensional format generated by interpolation of 15 curves independently of the number of short axis slices existing and are shown as successive concentric layers from the more apical zone (centre) to the more basal zone (exterior) (Figure 3).

The final polar image, composed always of 15 concentric circles, retains the maximum values of the slice counts and is only normalised when the values are needed to be compared against groups of normality.

The polar images in 2D dimensions generated by both methods keep the thickness or representations of the sections fixed so a linearity is maintained with respect to the situation of the defects but produces an overestimation in the basal zones and underestimation in the apical zones; an angular sector effect [55]. It is possible to perform a correction for the polar image such that each radial segment is representative of the same expanse of the myocardium (correcting the angular sector effect) and is achieved by varying the thickness of the sections in proportion to the radius [55].

Clearly different from the methods described so far, is the polar map generating method

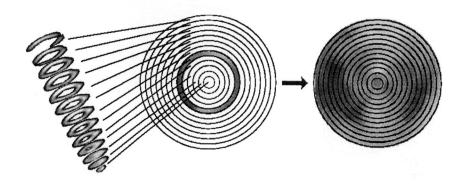

Figure 3: EMORY method: Scheme for generating polar maps starting only from the short axis slices. The more apical zone is represented by the two central circles and expresses the mean activity of the more apical short axis slices. The rest of the short axis slices are expressed as radial samples.

using radial sectors which is based on radial sections generated using the long axis as the axis of rotation [60] and with the assumption of an elliptical outline for the myocardium [61].

5.2.   3D PARAMETRICAL IMAGES

5.2.1. *CEqual method* [1,52,62-64]:
The generation of the polar map starts from the tomographic slices obtained in stress and at rest studies with technetium tracers. Specifically, the studies at rest/stress are designed to be conducted with ^{99m}Tc-MIBI in only one day.

The methodology for the processing is considerably automated with very little intervention from the operator (only for validation of certain values and limits). The processor defines the epicardial limits of the left ventricle, automatically re-orientates the long axis of the heart, extracts the short axis slices out of those on which the quantification is based [42].

In the quantification, all the short axis slices are placed superimposed, isolating the apex from the rest of the myocardium for a differentiated sample. Circumferential profiles of maximum counts are performed in the apical zone based on spherical co-ordinates (on the assumption that the apical region is a hemisphere), while the rest of the myocardium profiles are with cylindrical co-ordinates generating 40 sectors per slice (9°) [1] (Figure 4).

These sampling differences facilitate correcting the aberrations and distortions that are generated when creating a 2D polar image starting from 3D information [55]; a clear tendency to underestimate the more apical defects and to overestimate those more basal.

The polar image in 3D retains the maximum value of the counts of each slice and, as with the Emory method, is only normalised when there is a need for comparison with normal group data [1].

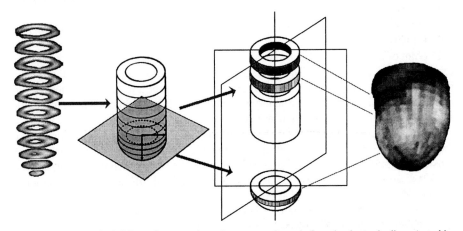

Figure 4: CEQUAL method: Scheme for generating polar maps starting only from the short axis slices. A stacking of short axis slices is performed divided into two groups: the apical zone on which the sampling performed follows hemispherical co-ordinates and the rest of the myocardium where the sampling is based on cylindrical co-ordinates. The resulting presentation is three-dimensional.

For comparison with the 2D methods, a simplified representation exists in which the cylindrical sectors are grouped in 16 segments and the apical sectors in 2 segments. The presentation generated is similar to the 2D polar map [55].

6. Polar map analysis

In addition to obtaining polar maps of stress and redistribution in the case of Thallium-201, one can obtain a polar image representing wash-out and fill-in that, with increasing effectiveness, can help in the interpretation of the study.

In a technetium tracers studies, polar maps of stress and rest are generated and normalised (each to its own maximum) and each map correspond to a different tracer injection. The polar maps normalised for reversibility are generated from these and which graphically show the regions that gain activity at rest with respect to exercise [65-67] and of paradoxical distribution [68]; that of activity loss relative to that at rest.

These polar maps have been validated in selected groups of subjects with low probability of coronary disease (<5% according to the criteria of Diamond and Forrester [69,70] so as to define the limits of normality for the quantitative values. The Cedars method employed 35 subjects (20 male and 15 female) [56], the Emory method 36 subjects (20 male and 16 females) [51] and the CEqual method employed 60 subjects (35 male and 25 female) [63]. The results from these groups are shown as the values grouped in zones with means and standard deviation values and segregated with respect to gender.

These results form the database of normality are included in the nuclear medicine software packages distributed by the manufacturer.

For optimum comparison, the patterns of normality need to be specific to the population with respect to gender, age, race etc and, if possible, generated in the same investigation centre with the same detection equipment and processor. The majority of patterns of normality that are available with the current equipment are of Anglo-Saxon origin and are not totally applicable to the Mediterranean population [71].

The principal advantage of comparison with patterns of normality is that not only are the localisation, extent and severity being quantified but also that the grade of uptake of each point of the polar image is evaluated relative to that of the reference and the result is expressed in number of standard deviations from the mean [63,72,73]. In this way, a territory does not need to have a level of uptake of 100% for it to defined as normal [74] and that the zones with great variability of activity (such as the inferior face, in middle-aged males) results in a higher standard deviation.

The expression of normality in terms of standard deviations allows for the expression of the gravity of the defects in terms of statistical probability. This, together with localisation and extent, is the basis of the Expert Systems analysis in the interpretation of myocardial perfusion studies [53,75-77]. Recent studies [76] validated the automatic quantitative segmental myocardial perfusion and automated perfusion scores (summed stress score and summed rest score) using three-dimensional quantitative algorithm, as a basis of computer aided diagnosis.

Another form of evaluation of polar maps is based on the analysis of the levels of uptake [77-80], always conducted on normalised maps, where for each polar map (stress, rest or reversibility) a range of levels of uptake is defined. In our hospital we designed a methodology for the analysis of the levels of uptake with a definition of range appropriate for each polar image and, within this range of intervals, a polar map mask for each interval level. The area of the map is quantified beyond the value of the section of the interval [45,77] or area of the defect; whichever is convenient (Plate 3.1). This type of analysis is used to quantify myocardial viability on the resting polar map and for the evaluation of the myocardium at risk of ischaemia on the reversibility map [77].

6.1. ASSIGNMENT OF TERRITORIES TO CORONARY ARTERIES

Several studies have been performed using the different methodologies and with patients with single vessel coronary artery disease so as to determine, on the polar map, the extent of territory perfused by each coronary artery.

The Cedars method was based on the study of 44 patients with single vessel disease [56] and defined (Figure 5A) certain areas of interest that fall within the zones of the polar map in which there could be a probability >80% that the perfusion depended on one or other specific coronary arteries [1,56]. This left areas of up to 30% of the polar map without assignment.

The same process was repeated with the Emory method on 45 patients with single vessel coronary artery disease [51]. Again, certain areas of interest where the probability of dependence on a particular artery is very high (Figure 5B) but, as well, considerable

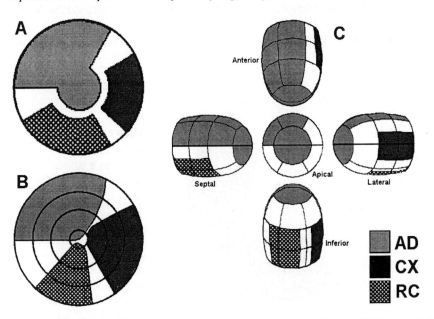

Figure 5:   Assignment of territories to coronary vessel: A) Assignment according to the Cedars method with zones of the polar map of probability >80% of being the territory irrigated by a specific coronary artery. B) Assignment according to the method of Emory without expression of the shaded zones (variable assignment). C) Assignment according to the CEqual method, very similar to the Cedars but expressed in three-dimensions. AD: Anterior descending, CX: Circumflex, RC: Right coronary.

zones of superimposed territories are present [1,51] due to the individual variability in dominance of the different coronary arteries.

For the CEqual method, 53 patients with single vessel coronary artery disease [63] was used in attempting to define the areas of interest of high probability of assignment of specific coronary territories on a tri-dimensional image (Figure 5C) and which sufficiently resembles distribution of regions of the polar map of Cedars. Other authors [81] have defined very similar zones based on patients with single vessel disease.

Logically it is easier to directly assign territories (anterior, septal, inferior, lateral and apical) purely on anatomical grounds with the orientation on the cardiac axes (short axis) and to have all of them in direct correspondence with respect to sites on the polar maps (Figure 6). Further, this type of areas-of-interest would cover whole of the polar map without leaving any zones unassigned [45,77].

6.2. EVALUATION OF EXTENT

The evaluation of extent of defects using methods with reference to values of normality, are based on determining the area of the defect [80] described as the polar map zone below a certain limit.

For the Cedars method, two cut-off points at 10% and 20% below normality were used to define 4 levels of uptake: normal uptake, diminished up to 10%, from 10% to 20%, and >20% and are expressed in the form of the polar map with each level a different colour. On such a map (Plate 3.2), all defects > –10% of the normal level for this region are recorded as defects [56].

The Emory method defined the defects using the criterion of –2.5 standard deviations from the normal value for this region [51].

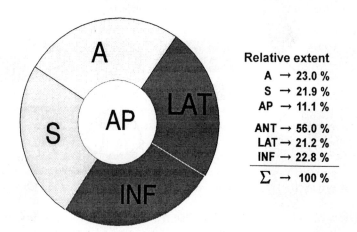

Relative extent

A   → 23.0 %
S   → 21.9 %
AP → 11.1 %

ANT → 56.0 %
LAT → 21.2 %
INF → 22.8 %

Σ   → 100 %

Figure 6:   Scheme for the assignment of territories according to the method that we follow in the Hospital General Universitari Vall d'Hebron. The whole polar map is divided into 5 regions (A: anterior, AP: apical, S: septal, LAT: lateral and INF: inferior). To facilitate identifying the associated vascular territories, a weighted sum calculation of the area of the anterior, septal and inferior regions is performed so as to obtain the territory of the anterior descending artery (ANT) while assigning the lateral region to the circumflex artery and the inferior region to the right coronary artery.

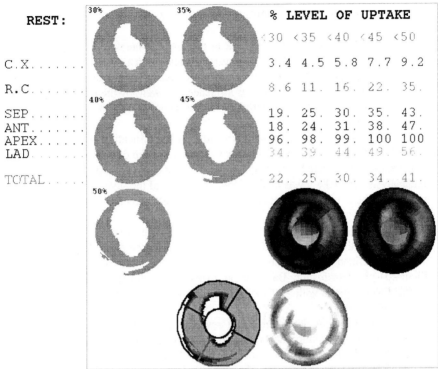

REST:

	% LEVEL OF UPTAKE				
	<30	<35	<40	<45	<50
C.X.......	3.4	4.5	5.8	7.7	9.2
R.C.......	8.6	11.	16.	22.	35.
SEP.......	19.	25.	30.	35.	43.
ANT.......	18.	24.	31.	38.	47.
APEX......	96.	98.	99.	100	100
LAD.......	34.	39.	44.	49.	56.
TOTAL.....	22.	25.	30.	34.	41.

Figure7:   Analysis of the level of uptake method on the resting polar map: masks of the selected levels of uptake are presented between 30% and 50% levels (at intervals of 5%). For each level a certain percentage of the region of interest is calculated (areas of interest defined in Figure 6) that do not reach the selected level. The total weighting is the summed weighting of the areas of each territory (LAD: left anterior descending, CX: circumflex, RC: right coronary).

The CEqual method is more complex in defining values in terms of standard deviations and as a function of the site of the defect; 1.75 x SD for the inferior wall, 3.0 x SD for the anterior face and up to 3.75 x SD in the lateral wall (values applicable to males) [63].

Once the defect is defined and its extent (area) is quantified by planimetry, the results are presented numerically as a function of the affected coronary artery territories.

For analysis of reversibility maps, evaluation of extent is done on the defect zone in the stress map which recovers its normal activity in the rest map [59] and the extent of the reversible zone is determined in rest polar image. Superimpositioning of this area on the stress polar image clearly distinguishes reversible territory from the non-reversible. With the method of Emory [67], a minimum area of 15% of recuperation defines significant reversibility.

In the analysis of uptake levels method, the assessments of extent and severity are performed in the same data set in which the extent is quantified in some masked levels of the polar image generated by certain required levels of uptake and which vary according to the polar image selected [82]. The resulting information is expressed as a percentage of the territory affected and as a percentage of the total myocardium for each masked level analysed (Figure 7).

6.3. EVALUATION OF SEVERITY

Severity is directly related to the decrease in the level of uptake of the hypoperfused region. So, to evaluate the severity of a reversible defect (ischaemia) or to evaluate the severity of a non-reversible defect (necrosis), the quantification of viability is from extrapolating these data. However, this is influenced, as well, by the extent of the defect in that, for the same level of hypoperfusion, the severity will be greater when the extent of the defect is greater.

The methods with database comparisons facilitate a quantification of the severity as a function of the number of standard deviations that separate the defect from the zone with normal uptake and, as such, is able to quantify the extent of each standard deviation level.

In the analysis of uptake levels method, the assessment of the severity is marked by the progression of the extend values obtained in the different levels of uptake evaluated [77] (Figure 8).

The level of uptake needs to be clearly defined if acceptable and reproducible results are to be obtained. With our method and polar image at rest for the evaluation of myocardial viability, we defined as optimum, the levels of 40% for MIBI [82] and 45% for Thallium-201 plus tetrofosmin. Based on our experience with MIBI [83], we consider as non-viable those regions with >50% of territory having an uptake <40% relative to the maximum [84].

Another useful point in determining the severity is the polar map of reversibility, particularly for the technetium tracers, since this represents a quantification of the level of ischaemia shown by the test [59,67] and, given its objectivity, allows for comparison of levels of ischaemia measured in the same patient using different stress tests (exercise/dipyridamole [45], dobutamine,...).

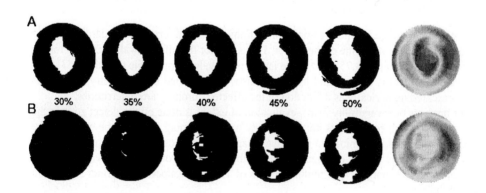

Figure 8:   Evaluation of the severity in the analysis of levels of uptake method:
A)   Severe anterior-apical defect that is maintained whatever level of section is selected (fixed defect, without progression/level change).
B)   Severe anterior-apical defect at 45% and 50% levels that progressively disappear to values below the levels of the section (defect with rapid progression with level change) indicative of maintenance of tissue viability.

3.7. Quantification of Gated-SPET

Image acquisition from myocardial perfusion SPET synchronised with the electrocardiographic signal allows slices to be obtained in the three cardiac axes and to indicate the position and uptake along the representative cardiac cycle; as discussed in Chapter 1. Information on the movement of the ventricular walls and increment of systolic activity can be assessed in a qualitative manner. Visual inspection of the movie pictures of the tomographic slices provides sufficient information for the analysis of ventricular contractility [85,86] but results that are evident in certain images of the representative cardiac cycle can provide quantitative information regarding ventricular volumes and units for the calculation of ejection fraction (EF); a parameter which is fundamental as a prognostic indicator of coronary artery disease.

The first quantitative approximation in the estimation of the overall systolic function is performed using the manual definition of the ventricular outline during the representative cardiac cycle [87]. In 1994 Goris et al. [88] obtained, for the first time, quantitative data using a semiautomated system that assumes that the position of the ventricular wall can be located using a statistical analysis of the density distribution of the counts. The method requires the manual adjustment of the myocardial wall to an ellipsoidal mask of the ventricle outline. In this way the operator excludes the activity arriving from the right ventricle and from the neighbouring structures. The average count is calculated in a small region of interest drawn in the base of the left ventricle in the end-diastole image. The manual mask is applied and the baseline activity is subtracted leaving the image only with the activity corresponding to the left ventricular myocardial wall. The distance from the wall to the centre of the cavity is calculated using the separation at the point of maximum slope calculated from the distribution of count rate along the long radius and the centre of the cavity and from which an ellipsoidal figure of calculable volume can be generated. Evaert et al. [89] applied this method to SPET with tetrofosmin in 50 patients and obtained excellent intra- and inter-observer reproducibility. In 30 patients a correlation of r=0.92 was observed with the values obtained in an equilibrium isotopic ventriculograph. There was no significant tendency toward systematic under- or over-estimation. The standard deviation of the differences between both explorations was 3.1%.

Other methods have appeared [90,91] to evaluate, more or less automatically, ventricular function since Germano et al. [92] published in 1995, a program that calculates ventricular volumes totally automatically. In essence, the algorithm starts with segmentation of the left ventricle in the non-gated images and the determination of the maximum counts in each group of voxels. Starting from the central mass of the ventricle, a series of sample radii build a profile of activity. The first lengthways maximum of the profile indicates the mid-point of the myocardium and, following this, an ellipsoid adjustment is made to the series of maxima obtained. The process of determining the endocardiac and epicardiac borders starts with the projection from the centre of the ventricular mass in the long axis of the ellipsoid and, starting from this, a further system of sample co-ordinates is generated. The limits of the walls are defined using the asymmetric Gaussian adjustment to the profile of counts of each radial co-ordinate. Once all the points have been determined, two new ellipsoids are adjusted around the endo- and epi-cardium whose volumes are calculated geometrically. This method showed and excellent correlation with the volumes of a model and with the EF calculated from the ventriculographs of first-pass MIBI at rest in a population of 65 patients (45 male and 20 female). Subsequently, several publications have demonstrated the values of these methods based on Gated-SPET studies whether with MIBI [93,94] tetrofosmin [95,96] or even with Thallium-201 [97,98] although the lower photon flow and lower tracer dose administered appears less than ideal for the acquisition of these characteristics.

The precision of the method proposed by the University of Stanford [88] has been compared with that by Cedars Sinai Medical Centre [92]. In 40 patients with coronary artery disease and studied with tetrofosmin, no differences were observed between the two methods and their correlations with the ventriculagraph were r=0.93 and r=0.94, respectively. Neither were there differences with the method of reference with respect to high and low values of the range nor, more importantly, in the patients with more severe or extensive perfusion defects. There only appeared to be differences in the absolute values of ventricular volumes with the Stanford method having higher values due, possibly, to taking the zone of maximum activity of the wall as the ventricular border and which only corresponds to the middle zone of the myocardium. The Cedars Sinai method, conversely, uses the endocardial border as the limit of the cavity [99].

A possible methodological limitation of the functional evaluations obtained using Gated-SPET perfusion studies is the limited number of images per cycle (normally 8) that are obtained in each projection. This is a compromise between the quality of each of the images and the total time of the exploration. Distress to the patient and the logistics preclude prolonging the tomographic studies beyond 25-30 minutes. The quality of the images of the cardiac cycle depends, principally, on the time of detection and the doses administered. In general, exploratory strategies envisage synchronised acquisition with administration of high doses of technetium tracers (20-25 mCi) and, since current gamma cameras require a minimum of 22-25 seconds per image, the quality of a study with 8 images/cycle will be adequate. Inevitably, dual-headed cameras reduce exploration time by half or allows for an increase to 16 images /cycle. Also, the importance of acquiring images ever 3 or 6 degrees has been questioned. In a methodology evaluation exercise, Germano et al. [100] did not encounter significant differences in global function parameters (volumes and EF) and segmental assessment of contractility between acquisition of 30 and 60 images (every 6 or 3 degrees). However, the studies with a total of 15 images showed a notable loss of quality that made it difficult to evaluate regional contractility. Nevertheless, these same authors claim that rapid studies (5-7 minutes) can be done with a correct estimation of the EF and of regional contractility [101,102]. It is known that the accuracy of the EF value is related to the number of images that form the ventricular volume curve [103]. Equilibrium radionuclide ventriculography employs 24 to 32 images/cycle to proportion a spatial resolution of some 25 milliseconds; ideal for determining, with precision, the times of peak filling rate (diastole) and peak emptying rate (systole) and value of peak filling rate and peak emptying rate. These characteristics are, currently, unattainable, for the Gated-SPET with perfusion tracers. However, comparative studies show excellent concordance with equilibrium radionuclide ventriculography [94,101,104] and with other imaging techniques [93,96,105,106] when volumes and EF need to be calculated. As yet there is little experience with respect to other parameters that may be derived from the ventricular volume curve.

Calculations of volumes based on systems adjusted to figures of known volume have limitations when the ventricular cavity is remodelled as a consequence of ischaemic disease and drifts away from volumes of regular geometric figures [107]. In studies with other perfusion tracers, other circumstances provide more difficulties for ventricular definition. Perfusion defects that extend to all of the ventricular wall or those that affect a large apical area with divergent morphology of the walls with preserved uptake (normally the basal zones) the algorithms locating the ventricular borders can err and, consequently, proportionally incorrect levels of the functional parameters are derived. It is imperative, then, to visually inspect the adjustment of the contours of the myocardial wall to obtain good results of EF and ventricular volumes [108]. Some methods have been proposed to correct for normalisation, the maximum on the grey scale, the point with highest activity of count profile of each of the radial segments that divide the ventricular wall. In this way an image of wall is created that is practically independent of perfusion variations and facilitates improving the

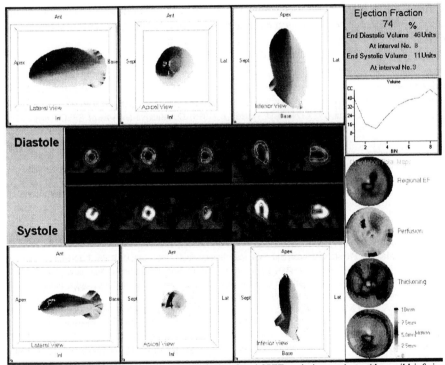

Figure 9:   Presentation of the results of a quantitative Gated-SPET study in a patient with a mild inferior myocardial infarct. Images at end-diastole (upper) and end-systole (lower) in three slices of the short axis (apical, mid ventricle and basal) and mid-ventricle sections vertical and horizontal long axes, and 3D views. To the right, the polar maps regional ejection fraction (upper), of perfusion uptake at rest, systolic thickening and motility (lower), and upper then, the parameters of ventricular volumes and ejection fraction together with the ventricular volume curve.

ventricular definition in regions of very low uptake [109]. More recently, the group at the University of Virginia [110,111] have developed a method based on the variation of counts in the ventricular wall such that the EF is calculated on the basis of count increment, or thickening regional systole without the need for ellipsoid adjustment or other types of geometric figures.

Quantification of regional contractility is performed, generally, by determining the movement of the ventricular wall and the systolic thickening at the base to the displacement of the ventricular edges lengthways in the cardiac cycle and of the increment in counts by radio-tracer pixels detected in the centre of the ventricular cavity [110,112,113]. The form of presentation is usually that of polar maps which represent the regional EF, the wall motion and the wall thickening (Figure 9).

With special software, as well as Emory Cardiac Toolbox®, is possible assess the unification of the Gated-SPET information with the coronary tree obtained by digital coronary angiography, in the same patient [114](Plate 3.3).

In conclusion, the acquisition of values of overall and regional systolic function constitutes an important additional value to the analysis of tomographic slices at stress and at rest. This study has an excellent cost-benefit profile since the most relevant variables for a patient with coronary artery disease can be evaluated in a single day: severity and location of the ischaemia, EF, ventricular volumes and evaluation of the regional myocardial viability as measured by the analysis of contractility and systolic thickening [108].

References

1.   Van Train KF, Garcia EV, Cooke CD, Areeda J. (1995) Quantitative analysis of SPECT myocardial perfusion, in De Puey EG, Berman DS, Garcia EV (eds.), Cardiac SPECT imaging. Raven Press Ltd., New York, pp. 49-74.

2.   Castell-Conesa J. (1994) Methods for quantifying myocardial perfusion, in Candell-Riera J and Ortega-Alcalde D (eds.), Nuclear Cardiology in everyday practice, Kluwer Academic Publishers, Dordrecht, pp. 88-108.

3.   Kiat H, Maddahi J, Roy LT et al. Comparison of technetium 99m methoxy isobutyl isonitrile and thallium-201 for evaluation of coronary artery disease by planar and tomographic methods. Am Heart J 1989; 117:1-11.

4.   Koeppe RA, Hutchins GD. Instrumentation for positron emission tomography: tomographs and data processing and display systems. Semin Nucl Med 1992; 22:162-181.

5.   Galofré-Mora P. Physicochemical and technical fundamentals. En: Candell-Riera J, Ortega-Alcalde D, editores. Nuclear Cardiology in everyday practice. Dordrecht: Kluwer Academic Publishers, 1994; 1-28.

6.   Wisenberg G, Schelbert HR, Hoffman EJ, et al. In vivo quantification regional myocardial blood flow by positron-emission computed tomography. Circulation 1981; 63: 1248-58.

7.   Wilson RA, Shea MJ, De Landsheere CM et al. Validation of quantitation of regional myocardial blood flow in vivo with 11C-labeled human albumin microspheres and positron emission tomography. Circulation 1984; 70: 717-23.

8.   Wolters-Geldof MJA, Manger Cats V, Bruschke AVG. Clinical methods to determine coronary flow and myocardial perfusion. Int J Cardiac Imag 1997; 13:79-94.

9.   Schelbert HR, Phelps ME, Hoffman EJ, Huang SC, Selin CE, Kuhl DE. Regional myocardial perfusion assessed with N-13-labeled ammonia and positron emission computerized axial tomography. Am J Cardiol 1979;43: 209-218.

10. Schelbert HR, Phelps ME, Huang SC et al. Nitrogen-13 ammonia as an indicator of myocardial blood flow. Circulation 1981; 63:1259-1272.

11. Hutchins GD, Schwaiger M, Rosenspire KC, Krivokapich J, Schelbert H, Kuhl DE. Noninvasive quantification of regional blood flow in the human heart using N-13 ammonia and dynamic positron emission tomographic imaging. J Am Coll Cardiol 1990; 15:1032-1042.

12. Krivokapich J, Smith GT, Huang SC et al. Nitrogen-13-ammonia myocardial imaging at rest and with exercise in normal volunteers. Circulation 1989; 80:1328-1337.

13. Beanlands RSB, Melon PG, Muzik O et al. N-13 ammonia PET identifies reduced perfusion reserve in angiographically normal regions of patients with CAD. Circulation 1992; 86: I-184 (Abstr).

14. Mullani NA, Goldstein RA, Gould KL et al. Perfusion imaging with rubidium-82: I. Measurement of extraction and flow with external detectors. J Nucl Med 1983;24:898-906.

15. Goldstein RA, Mullani NA, Marani SK, Fisher DJ, Gould KL, O'Brien HA Jr. Myocardial perfusion with rubidium-82. II. Effects of metabolic and pharmacologic interventions. J Nucl Med 1983; 24:907-915.

16. Herrero P, Markham J, Shelton ME, Weinheimer CJ, Bergmann SR, Noninvasive quantitation of regional myocardial blood flow with rubidium-82 and positron emission tomography: exploration of a mathematical model. Circulation 1990; 82: 1377-1386.

17. Schwaiger M. Myocardial perfusion imaging with PET. J Nucl Med 1994; 35:693-698.

18. Bergmann SR, Fox KAA, Rand AL et al. Quantification of regional myocardial blood flow in vivo with H215O. Circulation 1984; 70:724-733.

19. Iida H, Kanno I, Takahashi A et al. Measurement of absolute myocardial blood flow with H215O and dynamic positron-emission tomography. Strategy for quantification in relation to the partial-volume effect. Circulation 1988; 78:104-115.

20. Schelbert HR, Czernin J, Huang SC. Quantitation of regional myocardial blood flow: oxygen-15-water versus nitrogen-13-ammonia. J Nucl Med 1990; 31: 1431-3.

21. Bergmann SR, Herrero P. Markham J. Weinheimer CJ, Walsh MN. Noninvasive quantitation of myocardial blood flow in human subjects with oxygen-15-labeled water and positron emission tomography. J Am Coll Cardiol 1989; 14:639-652.

22. Huamg SC, Schwaiger M, Carson RE et al. Quantitative measurement of myocardial blood flow with oxygen-15 water and positron computed tomography: an assessment of potential and problems. J Nucl Med 1985; 26:616-625.

23. Phelps ME, Hoffman EJ, Selin CE et al. Investigation of [18F]2-fluoro-2-deoxyglucose for the measure of myocardial glucose metabolism. J Nucl Med 1978; 19: 1311-1319.

24. Ratib O, Phelps ME, Huang SC, Henzse E, Selin CE, Schelbert HR. Positron tomography with deoxyglucose for estimating local myocardial glucose metabolism. J Nucl Med 1982; 23: 577-586.

25. Marshall RC, Tillisch JH, Phelps ME et al. Identification and differentiation of resting myocardial ischemia and infarction in man with positron computed tomography 18F-labeled fluorodeoxyglucose and N-13 ammonia. Circulation 1983; 67: 766-778.

26. Camici P, Araujo Ll, Spinks T et al. Increased uptake of 18F-fluorodeoxyglucose in postischemic myocardium of panents with exercise-induced angina. Circulation 1986; 74: 81-88.

27. Tamaki N, Ohtani H, Yamashita K et al. Metabolic activity in the areas of new fill-in after thallium-201 reinjection: comparison with positron emission tomography using fluorine-18-deoxyglucose. J Nucl Med 1991; 32: 673-678.

28. Maddahi J, Schelbert H, Brunken R, Di Carli M. Role of Thallium-201 and PET imaging in evaluation of myocardial viability and management of patients with coronary artery disease and left ventricular dysfunction. J Nucl Med 1994; 35: 707-715.

29. Ficaro EP, Fessler JA, Ackermann RJ et al. Simultaneous transmission-emission thallium-201 cardiac SPECT: effect of attenuation correction on myocardial tracer distribution. J Nucl Med 1995; 36: 921-931.

30. Ficaro EP, Fessler JA, Shreve PD, Kritzman JN, Rose PA, Corbett JR. Simultaneous transmission/emission myocardial perfusion tomography. Diagnostic accuracy of attenuation-corrected 99mTc-sestamibi single-photon emission computed tomography. Circulation 1996; 93: 463-473.

31. Go RT, Marwick TH, McIntyre WJ et al. A prospective comparison of rubidium-82 PET and thallium-201 SPECT myocardial perfusion imaging utilizing a single dipyridamole stress in the diagnosis of coronary artery disease. J Nucl Med 1990; 31: 1899-1905.

32. Stewart R, Schwaiger M, Molina E et al. Comparison of rubidium-82 positron emission tomography and thallium-201 SPECT imaging for detection of coronary artery disease. Am J Cardiol 1991; 67:1303-1310.

33. Tamaki N, Ohtani H, Yamashita K et al. Metabolic activity in the areas of new fill-in after thallium-201 reinjection: comparison with positron emission tomography using fluorine-18-deoxyglucose. J Nucl Med 1991; 32: 673-678.

34. Ludgnani G, Paolini G, Landoni C et al. Presurgical identification of hibernating myocardium by combined use of technetum-99m hexakis 2-methoxyisobutylisonitrile single photon emission tomography and 18F-fluoro-2-deoxy-D-glucose positron emission tomography in patients with coronary artery disease. Eur J Nucl Med 1992; 19: 874-881.

35. Boucher CA, Zir LM, Beller GA et al. Increased lung uptake of thallium-201 during exercise myocardial imaging: clinical, hemodynamic and angiographic implications in patiens with coronary artery disease. Am J Cardiol 1980; 46: 189-196.

36. Kushner FG, Okada RD, Kirschenbaum HD. Botcher CA. Strauss HW. Pohost GM. Lung thallium-201 uptake after stress testing in patients with coronary artery disease. Circulation 1981; 63: 341-347.

37. Levy RD, Rozanski A, Garcia EV et al. Combined quantitation of pulmonary thallium washout and myocardia thallium activity analysis enhances the detection of coronary artery disease. Clin Nucl Med 1981; 17: 467-472

38. Alexander C, Oberhausen E. Myocardial scintgraphy. Sem Nucl Med 1995; 25: 195-201.

39. Graham LS. Quality control for SPECT systems. Radiographics 1995; 15: 1471-1481.

40. Baron JM, Chouraqui P. Myocardial single-photon emission computed tomographic quality assurance. J Nucl Cardiol 1996; 3: 157-166.

41. Kijewski MF, Muller SP, Moore SC. Nonuniform collimator sensitivity: improved precision for quantitative SPECT. J Nucl Med 1997; 38:151-156.

42. Germano G, Kavanagh PB, Chen J et al. Operator-less processing of myocardial perfusión STECT studies. J Nucl Med 1995; 36: 2137-2132.

43. Wakers FJTh. Exercise myocardial perfusion imaging. J Nucl Med 1994; 35: 726-729.

44. Santana-Boado C, Candell-Riera J, Castell-Conesa J et al. Importancia de los parámetros ergométricos en los resultados de la tomogammagrafía de perfusión miocárdica. Med Clín (Barc.) 1997; 109: 406-409.

45. Candell-Riera J, Santana-Boado C, Castell-Conesa J et al. Simultaneous dipyridamole/maximal subjective exercise with 99mTc-MIBI SPECT: Improved diagnostic yield in coronary artery disease. J Am Coll Cardiol 1997; 29: 531-536.

46. Cohen M, Touzery C, Cottin Y et al. Quantitative myocardial thallium single-photon emission computed tomography in normal women: demonstration of age-related differences. Eur J Nucl Med 1996; 23: 25-30.

47. De Puey EG. How to detect and avoid myocardial perfusion STECT artifacts. J Nucl Med 1994; 35: 699-702.

48. Prvulovich EM, Lonn AH, Bomanji JB, Jarritt PH, Ell PJ. Effect of attenuation correction on myocardial thallium-201 distribution in patients with a low likelihood of coronary artery disease. Eur J Nucl Med 1997; 24: 266-275.

49. Caldwell J, Williams D, Harp G et al. Quantitation of size of relative myocardial perfusion defect by single-photon emission computed tomography. Circulation 1984; 70: 1048-1056.

50. Garcia EV, Van Train K, Maddahi J et al. Quantification of rotational thallium-201 myocardial tomography. J Nucl Med 1985; 26: 17-26.

51. DePasquale E, Nody A, DePuey G et al. Quantitative rotational thallium-201 tomography for identifying and localizing coronary artery disease. Circulation 1988; 77: 316-327.

52. Garcia EV, Cooke CD, Van Train KF et al. Technical aspects of myocardial SPECT imaging with technetium-99m sestamibi. Am J Cardiol 1990; 66: 23E-31E.

53. Cooke CD, Faber TL, Garcia EV. (1995) Advanced computer methods in cardiac SPECT, in De Puey EG, Berman DS, Garcia EV (eds.), Cardiac SPECT imaging, Raven Press Ltd, New York, pp. 75-89.

54. Faber TL, Cooke CD, Peifer JW et al. Tree-dimensional displays of left ventricular epicardial surface from standard cardiac SPECT perfusion quantification techniques. J Nucl Med 1995; 36: 697-703.

55. Cooke CD, Vansant JP, Krawczynska EG, Faber TL, Garcia EV. Clinical validation of three-dimensional color-modulated displays of myocardial perfusion. J Nucl Cardiol 1997; 4: 108-116

56. Maddahi I, Van Train KF, Prigent F et al. Quantitative single photon emission computerized thallium-201 tomography for the evaluation of coronary artery disease: optimization and prospective validation of a new technique. J Am Coll Cardiol 1989; 14: 1689-1699.

57. Van Train KF, Maddahi J, Berman DS et al. Quantitative analysis of tomographic stress thallium-201 myocardial scintigrams: a multicenter trial. J Nucl Med 1990; 31: 1168-1179.

58. Maddahi J, Garcia EV, Berman DS, Waxman A. Improved noninvasive assessment of CAD by quantitative analysis of regional stress myocardial distribution and washout of thallium-201. Circulation 1981; 64: 924-935.

59. Dilsizian V, Rooco TP, Freedman NM et al. Enhanced detection of ischemic but viable myocardium by the reinjection of thallium after stress-redistribution imaging. N Engl J Med. 1990; 333: 141-146.

60. Nuyts J, Mortelmans L, Suetens P, Oosterlinck A, de Rou M. Model-based quantification of myocardial perfusion images from SPECT. J Nucl Med 1989; 30: 1992-2001.

61. Benoit T, Vivegnis D, Foulon J, Rigo P. Quantitative evaluation of myocardial single-photon emission tomographic imaging: application to the measurement of perfusion defect size and severity. Eur J Nucl Med 1996; 23: 1603-1612.

62. Berman DS, Kiat H, Van Train KF et al. Technetium 99m sestamibi in the assessment of chronic coronary artery disease. Semin Nucl Med 1991: 21: 190-212.

63. Van Train KF, Areeda J, Garcia EV et al. Quantitative same day rest-stress technetium-99m-Sestamibi SPECT: Definition and validation of stress normal limits and criteria for abnormality. J Nucl Med 1993; 34: 1494-1502.

64. Van Train KF, Garcia EV, Maddahi J et al. Multicenter trial validation for quantitative analysis of same-day rest-stress technetium-99m-sestamibi myocardial tomogramas. J Nucl Med 1994; 35: 609-618.

65. Luna E, Klein L, Garcia EV et al. Reversibility bullseye polar map: accuracy in detecting myocardial ischemia. J Nucl Med 1987; 29(5): 951 (Abstr).

66. Garcia EV, DePuey EG, Sonnemaker RE et al. Quantification of the reversibility of stress induced SPECT thallium-201 myocardial perfusion defects: A multicenter trial using Bull's-eye polar maps and standard normal limits. J Nucl Med 1990; 31:1761-1765.

67. Klein JL, Garcia EV, DePuey EG et al. Reversibility bullseye: A new polar Bull's-eye map to quantify reversibility of stress induced SPECT-Tl-201 myocardial perfusion defects. J Nucl Med 1990; 31: 1240-1246.

68. Lera JL, Raff U, Jain R. Reverse and pseudo redistibution of thallium-201 in healed myocardial infarction and normal and negative thallium-201 washout in ischemia due to background over substraction. Am J Cardiol 1988; 62: 543-550.

69. Diamond GA, Forrester JS. Analysis of probability as an aid in the clinical diagnosis of coronary artery disease. N Engl J Med 1979; 300: 1350-1358.

70. Rozanski A, Diamond GA, Forrester JS et al. Alternative referent standards for cardiac normality. Implications for diagnostic testing. Ann Intern Med 1984; 101: 164-171.

71. Toft J, Hesse B, Rabol A. The occurrence of false-positive technetium-99m sestamibi bull's eye defects in different reference databases. A study of an age- and gender-stratified healthy population. Eur J Nucl Med 1997; 24: 179-183.

72. Eisner RL, Tamas Stl, Cloninger K et al. Normal SPECT thallium-201 Bull's-eye display: gender differences. J Nucl Med 1988; 29: 1901-1909.

73. Lette J, Caron M, Cerino M et al. Normal qualitative and quantitative Tc-99m sestamibi myocardial SPECT: spectrum of intramyocardial distribution during exercise and at rest. Clin Nucl Med 1994; 19: 336-343.

74. Van Train K, Berman DS, Garcia EV et al. Quantitative analisis of stress Tl-201 myocardial scintigrams: a multicenter trial validation utilizing standard normal limits. J Nucl Med 1986; 27: 17-25.

75. Garcia EV, Herbst MD, Cooke CD et al. An expert system for automatically interpreting three-dimensional myocardial perfusion imaging. 2nd international symposium on computer applications in Nuclear Medicine and cardiac Magnetic Resonance imaging. Rotterdam, 1991: 64 (Abstr).

76. Germano G, Kavanagh PB, Waechter P et al. A new algorithm for the quantitation of myocardial perfusion SPECT. I: Technical principes and reproducibility. J Nucl Med 2000; 41: 712-719.

77. Aguadé S. (1994) Automatización, cuantificación y sistemas expertos en Cardiología Nuclear, in SPECT en Cardiología Nuclear, Sociedad Gallega de Medicina Nuclear (eds.). Artes gráficas Portella, SL, Vigo, pp. 87-112.

78. Verani MS, Jeoroundi MO, Mahamarian JJ et al. Quantification of myocardial infartion during coronary occlusion and myocardial salvage after reperfusion using cardiac imaging wiht technetium-99m hexaquis-2-methoxyisobutil isonitrile. J Am Coll Cardiol 1988; 12: 1573-1581.

79. O'Conor MK, Hammel T, Gibbsons RJ. In vitro validation of a simple tomographic technique for estimation of porcentage myocardium at risk using methoxyisobutil isonitrile technetium 99m (sestamibi). Eur J Nucl Med 1990; 16: 69-76.

80. Ceriani L, Verna E, Giovanella L et al. Assessment of myocardial area at risk by technetium-99 sestamibi during coronary artery occlusion: comparison between three tomographic methods of quantification. Eur J Nucl Med 1996; 23: 31-39.

81. Slomka PJ, Hurwitz GA, Clement GS, Stephenson J. Three-dimensional demarcation of perfusion zones corresponding to specific coronary arteries: Aplication for automated interpretation of myocardial STECT. J Nucl Med 1995; 36: 2120-2126.

82. Tamosiunas G, Castell J, Candell-Riera J, Fraile M, Aguadé S, García-Burillo A. Contractilidad y viabilidad miocárdicas. Estudio mediante tomogammagrafía con isonitrilos marcados con tecnecio-99m. Rev Esp Cardiol 1995; 48: 473-479.

83. Candell-Riera J, González JM, Castell J et al. Cuantificación de la extensión de miocardio viable mediante 99mTc-MIBI SPET de reposo. Rev Esp Cardiol 1997; 50 (Suppl..6): 56 (Abstr.).

84. Santana C, Candell-Riera J, Aguadé S et al. Extensión del territorio no viable en el infarto anterior, inferior y no Q. Estudio con ^{99m}Tc-MIBI SPET de reposo. Rev Esp Cardiol 1997; 50 (Suppl.6): 79 (Abstr.).

85. Berman DS, Germano G, Kiat H, Friedman J. Simultaneous perfusion/function imaging. J Nucl Med 1995; 2: 271-273.

86. Chua T, Kiat H, Germano G et al. Gated technetium-99m sestamibi for simultaneousassessment of stress myocardial perfusion, postexercise regional ventricular function and myocardial viability: correlation with echocardiography and rest thallium-201 scintigraphy. J Am Coll Cardiol 1994; 23: 1107-1114.

87. De Puey EG, Nichols K, Dobrinsky C. Left ventricular ejection fraction assessed fron gated technetium-99m-sestamibi SPECT. J Nucl Med 1993; 34: 1871-1876.

88. Goris ML, Thompson C, Maolone L, Franken PR. Modeling the integration of myocardial regional perfusion and function. Nucl Med Commun 1994; 15: 9-20.

89. Everaert H, Franken PR, Flamen P, Goris M, Momen A, Bossuyt A. Left ventricular ejection fraction from gated SPET myocardial perfusion studies: a method based on the radial distribution of count rate density across the myocardial wall. Eur J Nucl Med 1996; 23: 1628-1633.

90. Yang KTA, Chen HD. A semi-automated for edge detectionin the evaluation of left ventricular function usingECG-gated single-photon emission tomography. Eur J Nucl Med 1994; 21: 1206-1211.

91. Boonyaprapa S, Ekmahachai M, Thanachaikum N, Jaipresert W, Sukthomya V, Poramatikul N. Measurement of left ventricular ejection fraction from gated technetium-99m sestamibi myocardial images. Eur J Nucl Med 1995; 22: 528-531.

92. Germano G, Kiat H, Kavanagh PB et al. Automatic quantification of ejection fraction from gated myocardial perfusion SPECT. J Nucl Med 1995; 36: 2138-2147.

93. Williams KA, Lang RM, Reba RC, Taillon LA. Comparison of technetium-99m sestamibi-gated tomographic perfusion imaging with echocardiography and electrocardiography for determination of left ventricular mass. Am J Cardiol 1996; 77: 750-755.

94. Nichols K, De Puey EG, Rozanski A. Automation of gated tomographic left ventricular ejection fraction. J Nucl Cardiol 1996; 3: 475-482.

95. Mochizuki T, Murase K, Tanaka H, Kondoh T, Hamamoto K, Tauxe WN. Assessment of left ventricular volume using ECG-gated SPECT with technetium-99m-MIBI and technetium-99m tetrofosmin. J Nucl Med 1997; 38: 53-57.

96. Gunning MG, Anagnostopoulos C, Davies G, Forbat SM, Ell PJ, Underwood SR. Gated technetium-99m-tetrofosmin SPECT and cine MRI to assess left ventricular contraction. J Nucl Med 1997; 38: 438-42.

97. Germano G, Erel J, Kiat H, Kavanagh PB, Berman DS. Quantitative LVEF and qualitative regional function from gated thallium-201 perfusion SPECT. J Nucl Med 1997; 38: 749-754.

98. Lee DS, Ahn JY, Kim SK et al. Limited performance of quantitative assessment of myocardial function by thallium-201 gated myocardial single-photon emission tomography. Eur J Nucl Med 2000; 27: 185-191.

99. Everaert H, Bossuyt A, Franken PR. Left ventricular ejection fraction and volumes from gated single photon emission tomographic myocardial perfusion images: Comparison between two algorithms working in thee-dimensional space. J Nucl Cardiol 1997; 4: 472-476.

100. Germano G, Kavanagh PB, Berman DS. Effect of the number of projections collected on quantitative perfusion and left ventricular ejection fraction measurements from gated myocardial perfusion single-photon emission computed tomographic images. J Nucl Cardiol 1996; 3: 395-402.

101. Mazzanti M, Germano G, Kiat H, Friedman J, Berman DS. Fast technetium 99m-labeled sestamibi gated single-photon emission computed tomography for evaluation of myocardial function. J Nucl Cardiol 1996; 3: 143-149.

102. Everaert H, Vanhove C, Franken PR. Gated-SPET myocardial perfusion acquisition within 5 minutes usinf focussing collimators and tree-head gamma camera. Eur J Nucl Med 1998; 25: 587-593.

103. Parker DA, Thrall JH, Froelich JW. (1987) Radionuclide ventriculography: Methods, in Gerson MC (ed.). Cardiac Nuclear Medicine. McGraw-Hill Book Company, New York, pp. 67-84.
104. Miron SD, Finkelhor R, Penuel JH, Bahler R, Bellon EM. A geometric method of measuring the left ventricular ejection fraction on gated Tc-99m sestamibi myocardial imaging. Clin Nucl Med 1996; 21: 439-444.
105. Cwajg E, Cwajg J, He ZX et al. Gated myocardial perfusion tomography for the assessment of left ventricular function and volumes: Comparison with echocardiography. J Nucl Med 1999; 40: 1857-1865.
106. Vallejo E, Dione DP, Bruni WL et al. Reproducibility ans accuracy of Gated SPECT for determination of left ventricular volumes and ejection fraction: Experimental validation using MRI. J Nucl Med 2000; 41: 874-882.
107. Nichols K, De Puey EG, Rozanski A, Salensky H, Friedman MI. Image enhancement of severely hypoperfused myocardia from computation of thomographic ejection fraction. J Nucl Med 1997; 38: 1411-1417.
108. Udelson JE, Fares MA. How accurate is quantitative Gated SPECT? J Nucl Med 2000; 41: 883-886.
109. Smith WH, Kastner RJ, Calnon DA, Segalla D, Beller GA, Watson DD. Quantitative gated single photon emission computed tomography imaging: A counts-based method for display and measurement of regional and global ventricular systolic function. J Nucl Cardiol 1997; 4: 451-463.
110. Calnon DA, Kastner RJ, Smith WH, Segalla D, Beller GA, Watson DD. Validation of a new counts-based gated single photon emission computed tomography method for quantifying left ventricular systolic function: Comparison with equilibrium radionuclide angiography. J Nucl Cardiol 1997; 4: 464-471.
111. Fukuchi K, Uehara T, Morozumi T et al. Quantification of systolic count increase in technetium-99m-MIBI gated myocardial SPECT. J Nucl Med 1997; 38: 1067-1073.
112. Germano G, Erel J, Lewin H, Kavanagh PB, Berman DS. Automatic quantitation of regional myocardial wall motion and thickening from gated technetium-99m sestamibi myocardial perfusio single-photon emission computed tomography. J Am Coll Cardiol 1997; 30: 1360-1367.
113. Berman DS, Germano G. Evaluation of ventricular ejection fraction, wall motion, wall thickening, and other parameters with gated myocardial perfusion single-photon emission computed tomography. J Nucl Cardiol 1997; 4: S169-S171.
114. Aguadé S, Candell-Riera J, Angel J et al. Superposición en tres dimensiones de las imágenes de perfusión miocárdica y de la coronariografía. Rev Esp Med Nuclear 1999; 18: 137 (Abstr.).

4. DIAGNOSTIC ACCURACY OF SPET

CESAR SANTANA-BOADO and JAUME CANDELL-RIERA

1. Diagnosis of coronary disease with conventional exercise test and planar scintigraphy

The accuracy precision of the stress electrocardiogram has been assessed using a meta-analysis of 147 studies that included a total of 24,074 patients [1,2]. The mean values for the sensitivity and specificity in the 58 studies that included only patients without antecedents of myocardial infarction were 67% and 72%, respectively. As can be seen in Table 1, the results improve when patients who have ST segment depression in the basal ECG, those who are being treated with digoxin and those who have criteria of left ventricular hypertrophy are excluded. These values highlight that the conventional exercise test is an investigation that is more specific than sensitive. Fortunately its sensitivity is lower only with respect to patients with less serious coronary artery disease such as those with single vessel disease.

Table 1. Meta-analysis of conventional exercise stress test [1,2].

	Number of series	Number of patients	SEN (%)	SPE (%)	GV (%)
ET Conventional	147	24047	68	77	73
Without previous infarct	58	11691	67	72	69
With basal ↓ ST	22	9135	69	70	69
Without basal ↓ ST	3	840	67	84	75
With digoxin	15	6338	68	74	71
Without digoxin	9	3548	72	69	70
With LV hypertophy	15	8016	68	69	68
Without LV hypertrophy	10	1977	72	77	74

GV = global value; SEN = sensitivity; SPE = specificity; ET = exercise test; LV = left ventricular

Studies of perfusion in conjunction with the stress test began in Spain around 1980 [3-10]. The sensitivity results have been shown consistently to be superior to that of conventional exercise test. Gibson et al. [11] published results on 22 studies with ^{201}Tl planar scintigraphy in which the mean sensitivity was 83% and the specificity was 90%; significantly better than the conventional stress test (58% and 83%, respectively). Port et

J. Candell-Riera et al. (eds.), Myocardium at Risk and Viable Myocardium, 69–93.
© 2001 *Kluwer Academic Publishers. Printed in the Netherlands.*

al. [12] confirmed these results by assessing 47 patients with single vessel disease (stenosis >70%) and without previous myocardial infarction; 52% and 91% being positive on exercise test and ^{201}Tl, respectively.

We have published a series of studies in which the exercise test was combined with ^{201}Tl planar scintigraphy [4-6] and with ^{99m}Tc-MIBI SPET [7,9,10]. In all of them the results of the scintigraphy studies were better than the conventional stress test (Figure 1).

The low values of sensitivity and specificity for the conventional stress test are explained, among other reasons, by the characteristics of the patients that are admitted into the Nuclear Medicine Department to have a perfusion scintigraphy performed. In the majority of these patients, a stress test had been previously performed and the results of which were inconclusive or were discrepant with regards to the patient's clinical condition (electrocardiographically positive in asymptomatic patients and negative in patients with typical angina) [1,4-10,13]. Thus, some degree of selection bias exists for the conduct of perfusion scintigraphy.

The better results from perfusion studies have been confirmed by extensive studies such as that of Gerson et al. [14] analysing the results obtained in 2,473 patients corresponding to 30 series and conducted with non-quantitative ^{201}Tl planar scintigraphy. The mean sensitivity and specificity was found to be 84%.

Although at the expense of a degree of reduction in specificity, Maddahi et al. [15] obtained an improvement in the values of sensitivity by using a consistent quantitative method in the evaluation of the ^{201}Tl clearance from the myocardium. This tendency continues when each of the coronary arteries are considered separately; the sensitivities being superior for the quantitative analyses and specificities for the visual analyses. Another cause of variability in the results of sensitivity and specificity in these tests is the grade of coronary stenosis considered as significant. The sensitivity of ^{201}Tl is greater for

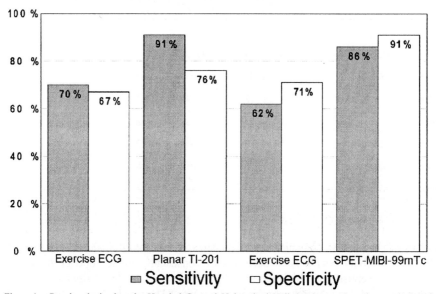

Figure 1. Results obtained at the Hospital General Universitari Vall d'Hebron using planar scintigraphy with [201]Tl [4-6] and SPET with ^{99m}Tc-MIBI [7, 9, 10].

stenosis >70% (84% for quantitative and 61% for visual analysis) than for stenosis >50% (79% for quantitative and 52% for visual analysis).

2. Diagnosis of coronary artery disease with SPET

The diagnostic accuracy of SPET [16-22], particularly if technetium compounds are employed (isonitriles [23-26] and tetrofosmin [27-35], is superior to the planar studies. This is due to the fact that the problems of superimposition of regions that can occur with planar studies are resolved. In Table 2 are the results of a meta-analysis published by Kolter et al. [36] of 3,258 planar studies and of 361 SPET studies with ^{201}Tl together with the results of 5 series published by Penell et al. [37] in which planar ^{201}Tl and SPET were compared.

Table 2. Diagnostic accuracy of planar scintigraphy and SPET with ^{201}Tl.

	Sensitivity		Specificity	
	Planar	**SPET**	**Planar**	**SPET**
Kolter et al.[36]	87%	96%	87%	83%
Pennell et al. [37]	77%	93%	82%	88%

The initial studies performed with ^{99m}Tc-MIBI [38-58] had values for sensitivity and specificity very similar to those with Thallium-201 with a high level of concordance between both types of investigations [38-47] but with lower specificity for Thallium-201 as can be seen in Table 3. A mean sensitivity and specificity of 92% and 68% respectively was obtained in a compilation of results obtained with 201Tl in 1,447 patients [59-64] and which confirmed a lower specificity for Thallium-201.

Table 3. Diagnostic accuracy of SPET with ^{201}Tl and with ^{99m}Tc-MIBI.

	Sensitivity		Specificity	
	^{201}Tl	**^{99m}Tc-MIBI**	**^{201}Tl**	**^{99m}Tc-MIBI**
Kiat et al. [44]	80%	93%	75%	75%
Iskandrian et al. [45]	82%	82%	82%	100%
Kahn et al. [46]	84%	95%	---	---

In the studies published by the investigators of the Emory University and Sinai Cedars Hospital using ^{99m}Tc-MIBI, the values of normal uptake for the different regions of the myocardium were determined using a quantitative method applied to polar maps [48]. These values were then applied in a multicenter study to 161 patients corresponding to 7 hospital centers in the USA [49]. The sensitivity of this method was 87% but the specificity (36%) was very low compared to studies in which visual interpretation was conducted by experts (Table 4) [44,45,49-51].

                         C. Santana-Boado and J. Candell-Riera.

Table 4. Diagnostic accuracy of SPET with ^{99m}Tc-MIBI.

	Sensitivity	Specificity
Kiat et al. [44]	93%	75%
Iskandrian et al. [45]	82%	100%
Van Train et al. [49]	95%	56%
Maddahi et al. [50]	89%	91%
Maddahi et al. [51]	90%	93%

The results for sensitivity of SPET with ^{99m}Tc-MIBI [7,9,10] and ^{99m}Tc-tetrofosmin [30, 31] of the different series of studies conducted in our centre are very similar and are shown in Figure 2. With ^{99m}Tc-tetrofosmin [30,31] we adopted a short protocol in which the complete study (stress and resting) was performed within approximately 2 hours while for the ^{99m}Tc-MIBI we adopted a long protocol (stress and resting on different days) which represented a considerable logistic limitation [7,9,10].

The energy characteristic of ^{99m}Tc, that of greater penetration of tissue, explains why a lower diaphragmatic attenuation in men and breast in women was achieved and with consequent improvement of the images [53-58, 65-72].

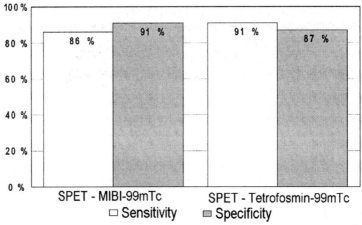

Figure 2. Results obtained at the Hospital General Universitari Vall d'Hebron using SPET with ^{99m}Tc-MIBI [7, 9, 10] and with ^{99m}Tc-tetrofosmine [30, 31].

3.   Diagnostic accuracy of SPET with respect to the number of vessels and the affected coronary arteries

Perfusion studies are superior to the rest of the non-invasive studies in the diagnosis of single vessel disease. In a review of 33 series performed with ^{201}Tl and planar methodolgy [37], sensitivities of 78% were obtained for single vessel, 89% for double vessel and 92% for triple vessel disease. The results reported in the literature for SPET are similar [49,62] as are those from a series of 147 patients investigated at the Hospital General Universitari Vall d'Hebron [9] (Table 5).

Table 5. Sensitivity of SPET in the diagnosis of coronary disease of one, two and three vessels.

	1 vessel	2 vessels	3 vessels
Mahmarian et al. [62]	74%	85%	100%
Van Train et al. [49]	84%	91%	96%
Castell et al. [9]	81%	84%	93%

In our series we observed that undiagnosed single vessel lesions corresponded, in the majority of cases, to non-severe stenosis of the left anterior descending coronary artery; in all cases being <90%. In another series conducted in this hospital with ^{99m}Tc-MIBI [7], we observed that, although the levels of sensitivity were slightly superior when levels of stenosis were >70% compared to 50%, the differences were not statistically different. These results coincide with reports in other series [49].

It needs to be noted here, and will be discussed in Chapter 5, that the accuracy of perfusion scintigraphy for the diagnosis of coronary disease in patients with 2 or 3 vessels is high while the accuracy of this investigation for multivessel disease has more limitations.

In the diagnosis of stenosis corresponding to each coronary artery, the perfusion defects of the anterior-septal region are attributable to the left anterior descending, those of the lateral to the left circumflex and those of the inferior region to the right coronary artery. These criteria have limitations due, particularly, to the attributes and distribution of the coronary arteries in individual patients.

In Table 6 are the results obtained with ^{99m}Tc-MIBI in different published series [26,48, 49,70] and those obtained by us in 2 series using two-day protocol [7,9]. As can be seen in the overall diagnosis by vessel, adequate results for the right coronary artery and the left anterior descending are obtained but the diagnosis of the left circumflex presented more limitations [7,9,49,70,73-75]. These were due, probably, to the posterior-lateral region being situated further from the detector and/or to the superimposition of the more anterior territories [38]. As such, the territory irrigated by the left circumflex is less extensive when this artery is not dominant and which is the situation that occurs in 85-90% of patients.

In our experience, difficulties are present when the stenosis of the left circumflex is accompanied by greater severity in the other arteries in that no false negatives are observed when only the left circumflex is lesioned. It needs to be taken into account that perfusion scintigraphy is not a study that permits an exact quantitative determination of the ischaemia but only an evaluation of segments with less perfusion relative to those better perfused, which are not always normally perfused. The left circumflex artery, on the other hand, is the one with the best specificity.

C. Santana-Boado and J. Candell-Riera.

Table 6. Diagnostic accuracy of ^{99m}Tc-MIBI-SPET for each of the coronary arteries.

	Sensitivity			Specificity		
	LAD	CX	RC	LAD	CX	RC
Wackers et al. [70]	70%	25%	73%	--	--	--
Van Train et al. [26]	74%	70%	71%	82%	88%	86%
Van Train et al. [63]	69%	50%	77%	76%	74%	85%
Van Train et al. [49]	78%	70%	77%	67%	82%	80%
Santana et al. [7]	68%	33%	65%	91%	96%	90%
Castell et al. [9]	74%	45%	79%	85%	96%	85%

CX = left circumflex; LAD = left anterior descending; RC = right coronary

4. Application of Bayes' theorem to SPET results

Until quite recently, it had been accepted that the sensitivity and the specificity of a test are constant in a methodology that does not vary and are independent of the population in which the methodology is applied. It is now accepted that the sensitivity and the specificity of the stress test vary as a function of other factors. These include maximum heart rate achieved, the number of vessels affected, the type of pain, the age and gender of the patients selected for the evaluation of a particular test and on the result of a previously-conducted diagnostic test. As such, the post-test probability for a patient after a particular test has been performed can be converted into a pre-test probability for the subsequent test [5,7,76-79].

The predictive value of a diagnostic test cannot be evaluated precisely without knowledge of the prevalence of the disease in the patient population [80-82]. Following the various publications in which the prevalences of coronary disease were investigated in asymptomatic populations (n = 23,996) using necropsy studies [83] and in symptomatic patients (n = 3,317) using angiography [68, 84-86], the theoretical prevalence, or pre-test probability, for a particular patient based on age, gender and symptomatology is known.

According to the Reverend Bayes, an English mathematician and Presbyterian priest of the 18th Century, the predictive value of a test depends on the pre-test probability, or prevalence, of the disease in the study population and, as such, the predictive value of a test varies with the prevalence of the disease in the population in which it is applied [80-83].

The probability of having the disease with a positive test (positive predictive value; PPV) is given by:

$$PPV = \frac{prevalence \times sen\,sitivity}{(prevalence \times sen\,sitivity) + (1 - prevalence) \times (1 - specificty)}$$

The probability of having the disease with a negative test (negative predictive value; NPV) is given by:

$$NPV = \frac{(1-\text{sen } sitivity) \times prevalence}{(1-\text{sen } sitivity) \times prevalence + specificty \times (1 - prevalence)}$$

Hence, a positive results in an individual from a population with low prevalence of coronary disease (asymptomatic, without risk factors) has a greater possibility of being a false positive than if the same result was obtained in a patient from a population with a high probability of coronary disease (typical pain, risk factors). Similarly, a negative result in a patient with the latter characteristics would have a much higher probability of being considered a false negative than if the same result was obtained in a patient with a low probability of coronary disease.

Applying the formula of this theorem [85-87] graphs can be constructed in which the pre-test probability or prevalence is expressed on the abscissa and the post-test probability on the ordinate axis. Hence, knowing the sensitivity, the specificity and the prevalence or the pre-test probability it is possible to calculate the post-test probability of coronary disease in any particular patient, based on the result of the test being positive or negative. The shape of the curve depends on the sensitivity and of the specificity of the test. In Figure 3, the upper curve represents the positive results and the lower the negative results. There are other graphs (Figure 4) which represent the difference between both curves and are termed "difference of post-test probability". The levels of these curves indicate the discriminatory capacity of the test between positive and negative results as well as the levels of prevalence in which the discriminatory power is maximal [7].

To evaluate the levels of prevalence of coronary disease at which the best diagnostic benefit of a perfusion SPET study can be obtained, we applied the Bayesian analysis to

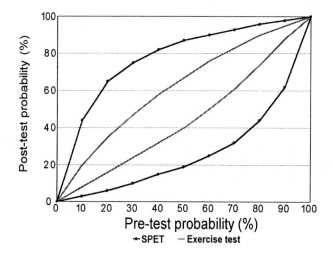

Figure 3. Application of Bayes' theorem to the results of the conventional stress test and to the SPET with ^{99m}Tc-MIBI at the Hospital General Universitari Vall d'Hebron [7].

the results from the stress test and the SPET test in a series of 159 patients who had performed a maximum subjective stress test. From the curves obtained (shown in Figures 3 and 4) we deduced that the best diagnostic profitability of ^{99m}Tc-MIBI SPET would be encountered in a population that had a prevalence of coronary disease between 30% and 70%. This prevalence range corresponds, based on the studies of Diamond and Forrester [80], to patients with one or other of the risk factors, atypical thoracic pain, and with a diagnostically non-successful conventional stress test. These results coincide with those of other authors [88] and are similar to those that we obtained [6, 89] when applying the Bayesian theorem to the results of isotopic ventriculography and of myocardial perfusion with [201]Tl.

Paterson et al. [88] applied sequential Bayesian analysis to a stress test with sensitivity of 82% and specificity of 62% and to a ^{201}Tl perfusion scintigraphy test with a sensitivity of 88% and a specificity of 74%. The higher diagnostic benefit was obtained in the range of coronary disease prevalence similar to ours (30%-70%). Several studies [90, 91] have highlighted that, in a considerable percentage of the diagnostic indications for perfusion scintigraphy, the Bayesian criteria described above had not been taken into account and had been performed in patients beyond the coronary disease prevalence range of between 30% and 70%. Diamond et al. [91], in a review of diagnostic indications in more than 7000 patients, observed that, from the Bayesian perspective, the indication for perfusion scintigraphy was inadequate in more than a third of the cases. This type of retrospective analysis has many limitations: considering tha the indication of perfusion scintigraphy for prognostic purposes is increasingly common [92-94], it is not unreasonable that the population with a high pre-test probability of coronary disease is seen to increase.

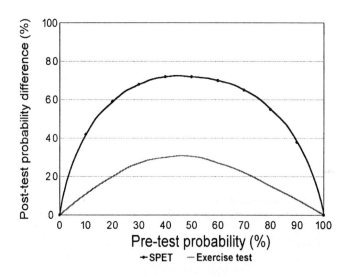

Figure 4. Difference of probability subsequent to the conventional stress test and of the SPET with ^{99m}Tc-MIBI applied to the results from the Hospital General Universitari Vall d'Hebron [7].

5. SPET results in women and men

The diagnosis of coronary artery disease in women presents certain limitations which are related, above all, to the underestimation of pre-test probabilities in the Bayesian analysis of coronary disease as well as with the low specificity of the conventional stress test [95-97].

Hence, several authors have, in reference to the different management of coronary disease in males and females, proposed that the latter would benefit less from complex non-invasive investigations, from coronary angiographic studies and from re-vascularisation procedures or from coronary angioplasty [98-103]. The bias introduced by not conducting coronary angiography in all of the patients prior to the use of non-invasive explorations could influence the results [5,82,104,105].

On the other hand, in planar ^{201}Tl perfusion scintigraphic studies there are difficulties in interpretation of the images due, essentially, to the interposition of mammary tissue [14,106]. With quantitative ^{201}Tl SPET, as well, a lower uptake in the anterior region in women [107,108] has been observed. It is not unreasonable to suppose that these limitations could be resolved, in part, by using perfusion tracers of greater energy characteristic such as ^{99m}Tc, which could generate SPET images of greater quality [109-112].

Different studies have demonstrated that conventional exercise test is less exact in the study of coronary disease in women relative to men. False positive results are more frequent in women because the specificity of the conventional stress test is much lower [112,113]. Iskandrian et al. [108] observed, as well, that the positive predictive value of ST segment depression is much lower in women (47% vs 77%; p< 0.05).

Using the methodology and criteria of interpretation that is standard in our clinical practice, we evaluated the diagnostic accuracy of ^{99m}Tc-MIBI myocardial SPET in women and men. Taking into account the bias introduced by the selection of more men than women for the cardiac catheterization, we assessed not only those patients in whom a coronary angiography had been performed (selected minority) but also all those patients who had been investigated with myocardial SPET over the same period of time but had not had a coronary angiography performed (silent majority) [10].

We studied 702 consecutive patients (44% women) without previous myocardial infarction in whom a ^{99m}Tc-MIBI perfusion SPET was performed. Of these patients, 539 had not had coronary angiography (silent majority) and 163 had had a coronary angiography (select minority) within an interval of less than 3 months of the SPET. Of the group of 163 patients, 63 were women.

We calculated the sensitivity, specificity, global value, positive predictive value and negative predictive value of the SPET for the total group as well as segregated by gender. We applied the corrections proposed by Diamond [104] for sensitivity and specificity taking into account the probability of positive results in the silent majority as follows:

$$SEN = PPR \times PPV/(PPR \times PPV) + (CoNPV \times [1 - PPR]$$

$$1 - SPE = PPR \times CoPPV/(PPR \times CoPPV) + (NPV \times [1 - PPR]$$

$$\text{Positive predictive value (PPV)} = TP/TP + FP$$

Complenentary PPV (CoPPV) = FP/FP + TP

Negative predictive value (NPV) = TN/TN + FN

Complementary NPV (CoNPV) = FN/FN + TN

Probability of positive results (PPR) = Positive results/Total population

SEN = Sensitivity; SPE = Specificity; TP = True positives; TN = True negatives; FP = False positives; FN = False negatives.

In the analysis of the diagnostic accuracy of the conventional stress test in all the patients with coronary angiography (select minority) and in both genders, we observed that the values for sensitivity (69% vs 60%; p = 0.02), specificity (79% vs 67%; p = 0.03), positive predictive value (93% vs 43%; p = 0.003) were significantly better in men than in women. Only the negative predictive value was significantly higher in the women than in the men (38% vs 78%; p = 0.009).

Results for sensitivity (93% vs 85%; p = 0.01) and of positive predictive value (97% vs 81%; p = 0.005) for SPET were significantly better in the men only when the select minority were considered. As seen in Table 7, women showed a higher negative predictive value (93% vs 74%; p = 0.003).

Table 7. Diagnostic accurracy of myocardial SPET in the select minority [10].

	SEN	SPE	PPV	NPV	GV
Women	85%	91%	81%	93%	89%
Men	93% *	89%	97% **	74%***	92%

* p = 0.01, ** p = 0.005; *** p = 0.003 vs women
GV = global value; SEN = sensitivity; SPE = specificity; PPV = positive predictive value; NPV = negative predictive value

In our series with ^{99m}Tc-MIBI SPET, there were no significant differences in specificity between genders in those patients that had been catheterised. With the methodology used by us, there were not greater numbers of false positives with respect to the anterior region in women and which, probably, was due to the higher energy and penetration of ^{99m}Tc relative to [201]Tl.

Nevertheless, as has already been stated, the sensitivity of SPET in women (85%) in our series was significantly lower than that in men (93%). This can be explained by the lower prevalence and severity of coronary disease in women and, as well, by the lower level of METs achieved during the stress test and which would explain a high number of false negatives [111-114]. Other factors that can contribute to this lower sensitivity of SPET in the women could be that they represent a lower proportion in whom coronary angiography had been conducted as well as the higher prevalence of positive SPET results in the men.

The number of women in our series who had undergone catheterization was clearly lower than that of the men; in the overall group (9% vs 14%) as well as in the select minority group (39% vs 61%). On the other hand, the presence of positive scintigraphy studies in the men was greater than that in the women; in the silent majority (65% vs 34%) as well as in the select minority (77% vs 33%)

The lower percentage of positive results in women, due to the lower prevalence of the disease as well as to the lower number of women who had undergone catheterization, is a factor common to the various studies of this type [113,114]. Shaw et al. [115], in a series of 840 patients (47% women) with suspected coronary disease in whom the initial studies conducted were less complex (exercise test and planar ^{201}Tl scintigraphy) but performed in equal numbers of women and men (22% vs 19%), the coronary angiograph indicated a higher frequency in men compared to the women (62% vs 38%; $p < 0.01$). Lauer et al. [116], in a series of 2351 men and 1318 women studied using ^{201}Tl perfusion SPET, found the women had less coronary angiography performed than the men (6% vs 14%) and that the severity of the coronary disease and the prevalence of positive studies was greater in the men (29% vs 8%).

We applied the silent majority correction, as proposed by Diamond [104], to our results of ^{99m}Tc-MIBI-SPET to assess whether these differences could have been influenced by the higher prevalence of coronary disease in men relative to women and/or to the different percentages of positive tests in patients (of either gender) who had not been catheterised.

As can be seen in Figure 5, no significant differences between men and women are observed once the correction is applied. It is usually accepted that both values are fixed and that the variations observed in the positive and negative predictive values are due to the application of the test to populations with different prevalences of the disease. Hence, we used the Bayesian approach to obtain corrected values of positive and negative predictive values as a function of the prevalence. It is well known that the variability in sensitivity and specificity depend not only on technical characteristics or on the

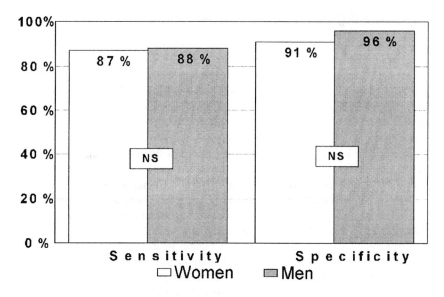

Figure 5. Results of SPET with ^{99m}Tc-MIBI in the silent majority of men and women studied at the Hospital General Universitari Vall d'Hebron [10].

utilisation of diverse criteria of evaluation of a diagnostic test but also on the probability of positive results of the test within a determinate population sample [5]. The Diamond [104] modification of the Bayesian analysis in the calculation of sensitivity and specificity attempts to approximately apply the "gold standard" derived from a test conducted in a "select minority" to a "silent majority" in which the actual prevalence of the disease is unknown. In a wide group of patients such as this, it would be invaluable to have an evaluation of the probability of positive results that is very close to the prevalence. From a comparison of the probability of positive results between the select minority and the silent majority, a first approximation of the capacity of the test to identify patients to be submitted to the "gold standard" can be obtained.

Using the formulation proposed by Diamond [104], and despite its limitations [115], the calculation of sensitivity and specificity adjusted for the probability of positive results of the overall population in which the test has been applied, allows for an estimation of probability superior to its actual diagnostic accuracy. In the case of SPET, this type of analysis shows clearly that its efficiency is the same not only for those patients who had undergone catheterization but also when the overall patient population is evaluated. The higher probability of positive results, linked to the higher prevalence of coronary disease in men, introduces a post-selection test bias that is conducive to a greater proportion of men than women being referred for a coronary angiographic study than the proportions having a SPET test performed. All things considered, it would appear that speculations on the technical limitations of SPET in women have little or no repercussion on its diagnostic accuracy, at least in our patient population, and are merely statistical aspects related patient selection that cause moderate differences in values of sensitivity and specificity.

6.   Non-atherosclerotic causes of perfusion defects

Coronary atherosclerosis is, without doubt, the most frequent cause of myocardial ischaemia. However, other non-atherosclerotic causes exist that can produce reversible defects in perfusion scintigraphy and which can result in chest pain and changes in ST segment indicative of cardiac origin. Table 8 summarises the different causes of perfusion defects of false ischaemic origin [118-134] and/or other possible causes of ischaemia of non-atherosclerotic origin [135-148].

False perfusion defects of non-atherosclerotic causes have a high tendency in clinical practice. Those that are caused by technical problems or by attenuation of tissues have been amply commented upon in previous chapters. Of greater interest are those caused by substitution of myocardial tissue by tumours or by infiltration and, above all, those related to disruptions of flow through, principally, left bundle branch block.

Perfusion defects at the septal level in patients with left bundle branch block have been described [149-155]. These could be related to dynamic alterations in the interventricular septum [156] which may be observed in left bundle branch block and which induce metabolic compensations with a consequent reduction in coronary flow. Some authors have proposed the use of dipyridamole [157,158], adenosine [159] and dobutamine [160] as provocation manoeuvres because of their greater specificity compared to the stress test. Other authors have observed that, using detailed analyses of the perfusion defects, a better differential diagnosis can be made between purely septal defects attributable to left bundle branch block and the anterior-apical septal defects corresponding to stenosis of the left anterior descending coronary artery [161].

Table 8. Non-atherosclerotic causes of reversible perfusion defects.

FALSE ISCHAEMIA
Breast attenuation [118]
Diaphragmatic attenuation [119]
Movement artefacts [120-123]
Inadequate SPET filter [124]
Mitral ring calcification [125]
Cardiac fibroma [126]
Left bundle branch block [127]
Right bundle branch block [128]
Chronic obstructive respiratory disease [129]
Congestive cardiomyopathy [130]
Cardiac amyloidosis [131]
Cardiac sarcoidosis [132, 133]
Chagas disease [134]
OTHER CAUSES OF ISCHAEMIA
Syndrome X [135]
Left ventricular hypertrophy [136]
Hypertrophic cardiomyopathy [137]
Coronary bridge [138]
Coronary spasm [139]
Coronary ectasia/aneurysm [140]
Coronary of anomalous origin [141, 142]
Spontaneous coronary dissection [143]
Coronary fistula [144, 145]
Coronary embolism [146]
Systemic sclerosis [147]
Cocaine [148]

With respect to left bundle branch block, we prefer the exercise test (+ dipyridamole when exercise is suboptimal) as the provocation manoeuvre [162]. This is so that we do not lose important prognostic information derived from exercise test. This recommendation is based on the results of our own series of 509 patients (456 without LBBB and 53 with LBBB) without previous infarction who had a coronary angiography performed within < 3 months of the scintigraphic study [163]. The same stress procedures were followed in all patients: 1/ Only exercise when it was sufficient, and 2/ exercise + simultaneous administration of dypiridamole if exercise was insufficient. Twenty-five percent of patients had a negative study and less than 20% had reversible defects in septal region (Plate 4.1). Although lower values of global sensitivity (81%) and specificity (73%) were obtained in patients with LBBB, there were no significant differences with respect to the patients without LBBB (89% and 86%, respectively). Specificity values for the diagnosis of stenosis of left anterior descending (78%), left circumflex (96%) and right coronary artery (74%) in patients with LBBB were lower, but without significant statistical differences with respect patients without LBBB (90%, 96%, and 82%, respectively). Bayes' curves obtained from these results also showed only slightly better results for patients without LBBB

(Figure 6). This highlights that, should the scintigraphy results be negative, the presence of coronary disease can be ruled out with a high degree of probability and that the percentage of patients with difficulties of differential diagnosis is not high. If to this is added the clinical prognostic value (since the electrocardiograph is not assessable in the presence of left branch blockage) from the conduct of a stress test, we believe that this should be the first-line provocation test in combination with SPET.

Within the ischaemic perfusion defects of non-atherosclerotic causes are those that may be observed in patients with left ventricular hypertrophy secondary to hypertension since a high percentage of patients with coronary disease are hypertensives. Some studies have highlighted that although the sensitivity of perfusion scintigraphy is high and facilitates detection in the majority of patients with significant coronary artery disease, the specificity is less and, as such, "false positives" may be obtained especially in populations with low prevalence of coronary artery disease [164].

DePuey et al. [165] observed that a frequent finding in the hypertensive patients was the decrease in the septal and lateral uptake ratio not only in the stress images but also in those of redistribution. This can create the false visual impression of a lateral defect without redistribution i.e. an image that appears exactly like that of possible lateral necrosis. These findings have contributed to the repeatedly-cited view that hypertension can cause fixed defects in the lateral region which can look like necrosis.

Prisant et al. [166] studied 92 hypertensive patients with chest pain or an abnormal electrocardiogram using ^{201}Tl planar stress or stress + dipyridamole (if the product of cardiac frequency x systolic pressure was <20,000). All had had coronary angiography. The sensitivity of the perfusion scintigraphy in the diagnosis of coronary stenosis >50% was 94%, the specificity was 63.5%, the positive predictive value was 38.6%, the negative predictive value was 97.9% and the global value was 69.9%. The authors affirm that these values of sensitivity and negative predictive value are so high that a negative scintigraphy with thallium excludes the presence of significant epicardiac coronary disease in hypertensive patients. However, these results also highlight the low specificity and positive predictive value of this study and which suggests that a positive result does confirm that one is dealing with a patient with significant coronary disease. The fact that these observations are obtained by planar techniques can contribute to the increase in the number of false positives.

On the other hand Cecil et al. [167] demonstrated, in a group of 16 hypertensive patients with left ventricular hypertrophy and without chronic renal disease, that the septal to lateral activity ratio was not significantly different from that of a group of 46 normotensive individuals and that none of the hypertensive patients had fixed defects in the visual interpretation of the SPET.

In our experience in the application of perfusion SPET, the specificity of the technique has significantly improved and, despite the changes on stress ECG suggestive of ischaemia, false positive results are rare (Plate 4.2)[168].

With regard to the presence of an apparent increased number of false positives in perfusion scintigraphy in hypertensive patients with left ventricular hypertrophy, the questions that arise are: do these "false positive" results correspond to myocardial ischaemia despite the absence of significant coronary stenosis? Or is one dealing with microvascular angina?.

Tubau et al. [169] prospectively studied 40 asymptomatic hypertensive patients with left ventricular hypertrophy using conventional exercise test, ^{201}Tl and radionuclide ventriculography. It was observed that both the perfusion defects and abnormal ST segment response were predictive of the appearance of angina over a mean follow-up of 38 months.

Some studies attempt to clarify these possibilities. The percentage of reversible defects with myocardial perfusion scintigraphy and of anomalous responses from stress radionuclide ventriculography is clearly greater in those patients with chest pain and angiographically-healthy coronary arteries (albeit non-hypertensive) than in an asymptomatic population with low prevalence of coronary disease [170-172]. The

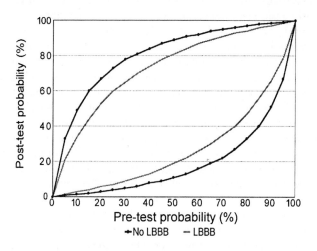

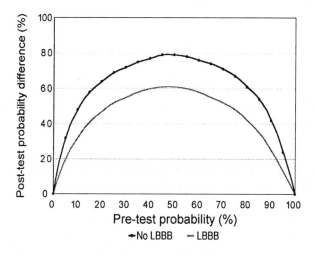

Figure 6. The pre- and post-test probability of coronary artery disease (top) and post-test probability difference curves (bottom) for patients with and without LBBB studied with exercise (+dipyridamole) myocardial perfusion SPET with technetium compounds.

patients with chest pain and angiographically-normal coronary arteries who show reversible perfusion defects with ^{201}Tl and/or contractility alterations during stress in the radionuclide ventriculography have an abnormal coronary reserve compared to those patients without abnormal radionuclide studies. Further, this decrease in coronary reserve is more manifest in the regions where the perfusion defects appear. Various factors can cause a decrease in coronary reserve in the presence of angiographically-normal coronary arteries: severe anaemia, polycythemia, hypoxia, syndrome X, prior infarct and left ventricular hypertrophy [173].

Almost all the causes of left ventricular hypertrophy are associated with decreases in the coronary reserve and which can be sufficient to produce angina. Hypertension is the most frequent cause of left ventricular hypertrophy and one of the symptoms that patients with hypertension present while still in the absence of coronary disease, is angina.

Houghton et al. [174] demonstrated that perfusion defects with planar ^{201}Tl-dipyridamole are associated with decreases in the coronary reserve in hypertensive patients with angiographically-normal coronary arteries. This coronary reserve decrease occurs, preferentially, in the patients with left ventricular hypertrophy and with increased basal coronary flow velocity. These authors evaluated the vasodilatatory response (using intravenous dipyridamole up to 0.85 mg/Kg over 6 minutes) in 48 patients with suspected coronary disease and with angiographically-normal arteries or with minimal lesions and, of whom, 40 were hypertensives or diabetics. They encountered an abnormal coronary reserve (<3:1) in half of the cases and very abnormal (<2:1) in 27% of the cases. The coronary reserve was significantly less and the left ventricular mass index significantly greater in those patients with positive perfusion scintigraphy following dipyridamole + stress.

Iriarte et al. [175] observed that stress angina in hypertensive patients with left ventricular hypertrophy could be associated with microvascular disease in 62% of cases. The same authors observed [176] that, subsequent to 18 months of treatment with enalapril (10-20 mg/d), 10 of the 11 hypertensive patients with angiographically-healthy coronary arteries were normalised in the ^{201}Tl perfusion scintigraphy.

These publications support the hypothesis that, in the absence of possible artifacts or of asymmetric ventricular hypertrophy, the perfusion scintigraphy reversible defects in hypertensive patients with left ventricular hypertrophy are, probably, due to microvascular ischaemia. As such, only the "false negative" results of the scintigraphic technique need to be taken into account rather than the "false positives" of the technique in the diagnosis of coronary disease. Future quantitative isotopic studies together with the SPET technique will be necessary to confirm these findings.

Reversible perfusion defects in planar studies with ^{201}Tl in patients with syndrome X or microvascular angina varies between 9% and 45% [177-181]. Abnormalities in the uptake and clearance of thallium have also been described in these patients [182, 183]. The fact that more than 75% of patients with syndrome X are women adds to the problem [184].

In our experience, with stress SPET and combined techniques, clear and reversible segmental perfusion defects in syndrome X patients are very infrequently observed. Only in a few cases is it possible to observe a thinning of the wall or minimal reversible defects (Plate 4.3).

A correction for attenuation [185-191], or an evaluation of wall thickening and contractility of the doubtful regions using gated SPET [192-200] will, most probably reduce false positive results of SPET and, as such, contribute to a better differentiation between perfusion defects due to artefacts and those due to authentic myocardial ischaemia of non-atherosclerotic origin.

References

1. Detrano R, Gianrossi R, Froelicher V. The diagnostic accuracy of the exercise electrocardiogram: a meta-analysis of 22 years of research. Prog Cardiovasc Dis. 1989; 32: 173-206.
2. Gianrrosi R, Detrano R, Mulvihill D et al. Exercise-induced ST depression in the diagnosis of coronary artery disease. Metaanalysis. Circulation 1989; 80: 87-98.
3. Esplugas E, Molina C, Ramos M et al. Gammagrafía miocárdica y electrocardiograma al esfuerzo en pacientes con angina y coronariografía normal. Rev Esp Cardiol 1982; 35: 393-393.
4. Candell-Riera J, Ortega D, Alijarde M et al. Gammagrafía miocárdica con ^{201}Tl: sensibilidad, especificidad y valor predictivo. Med Clín (Barc) 1984; 82: 656-660.
5. Castell J, Fraile M, Candell J et al. El rendimiento diagnóstico de la gammmagrafía de esfuerzo con talio y la "mayoría silenciosa". Rev Esp Cardiol 1988; 41: 12-19.
6. Candell-Riera J, Castell J, Ortega D et al. Diagnostic accuracy of radionuclide techniques in patients with equivocal electrocardiographic exercise testing. Eur Heart J 1990; 11: 980-989.
7. Santana-Boado C, Candell-Riera J, Castell J et al. Diagnóstico de la enfermedad coronaria mediante la tomogammagrafía de esfuerzo con isonitrilos-tecnecio-99m. Med Clín (Barc.) 1995; 105: 201-204.
8. Candell-Riera J, Bardají A, Castell-Conesa J, Jurado JA, Magriña J. IV. La cardiología nuclear en la cardiopatía isquémica crónica. Rev Esp Cardiol 1997; 50: 83-91.
9. Castell J, Santana-Boado C, Candell-Riera J et al. La tomogammagrafía miocárdica y el ECG de esfuerzo en el diagnóstico de la enfermedad coronaria multivaso. Rev Esp Cardiol 1997; 50: 635-642.
10. Santana-Boado C, Candell-Riera J, Castell J et al. Diagnostic accuracy of ^{99m}Tc-isonitrile SPET in women and in men. J Nucl Med 1998; 39: 751-755.
11. Gibson RS, Watson DD (1983) Clinical applications of myocardial perfusion scintigraphy with thallium-201, in Yu PN and Goodwin JF (eds.), Progress in cardiology, Lea & Febiger, Philadelphia, pp. 67-112.
12. Port SC, Oshima M, Ray G et al. Assessment of single vessel coronary artery disease: Results of exercise electrocardiography, thallium-201 myocardial perfusion imaging and radionuclide angiography. J Am Coll Cardiol 1985; 6: 75-83.
13. Gibson RS, Beller GA. (1983) Should exercise electrocardiographic testing be replaced by radioisotopic methods?, in Rahimtoola SH (ed.), Controversies in coronary artery disease, F. A. Davis Company, Philadelphia, pp. 1-31.
14. Gerson MC. (1987) Test accuracy, test selection, and test result interpretation in chronic coronary artery disease, in Gerson MC (ed.), Cardiac nuclear medicine, McGraw-Hill Book Company, New York, pp. 309-347.
15. Maddahi J, García EV, Berman DS. (1988) Quantitative thallium-201 myocardial perfusion scintigraphy: The method and its clinical applications in coronary artery disease, in Lyons KP (ed.), Cardiovascular nuclear medicine, Appleton & Lange, Norwalk, pp. 145-160.
16. Kim W, Lipton MJ. Exercise thallium-201 single photon emission computed tomography for the diagnosis of coronary artery disease: What should we expect from SPECT ?. J Am Coll Cardiol; 15: 330-333.
17. Berman DS, Kiat H, Germano G et al. (1995) ^{99m}Tc-Sestamibi SPECT in cardiac SPECT imaging, in De Puey EG, Berman DS, Garcia EV (eds.), Cardiac SPECT imaging, Raven Press, New York, pp. 121-146.
18. Fintel DJ, Links JM, Brinker JA et al. Improved diagnostic performance of exercise thallium-201 single photon emission computed tomography over planar imaging in the diagnosis of coronary artery disease: a receiver operating characteristic analysis. J Am Coll Cardiol 1989; 13: 600-612.
19. Kiat H, Berman DS, Maddahi J. Comparison of planar and tomographic exercise thallium-201 imaging methods for the evaluation of coronary artery disease. J Am Coll Cardiol 1989; 13: 613-616.
20. Garcia EV, Van Train K, Madahi J et al. Quantification rotational thallium-201 myocardial tomography. J Nucl Med 1985; 26: 17-26.
21. Mahmarian JJ (1999) State of the art for coronary artery disease, in Zaret BL and Beller GA (eds.), Nuclear Cardiology. State of the art and future directions, Mosby, St. Louis, pp.237-272.

22. Garcia EV, DePuey EG, Sonnemaker RE et al. Quantification of the reversibility of stress induced thallium-201 myocardial perfusion defects: a multicenter trial using bull's-eye polar maps and standard normal limits. J Nucl Med 1990; 31: 1761-1765.

23. Van Train KF, Garcia EV, Cooked AJ (1995) Quantitative analysis of SPECT myocardial perfusion, in De Puey EG, Berman DS and Garcia EV (eds.), Cardiac SPECT Imaging, Raven Press, New York, pp. 49-74.

24. Kiat H, Van Train, Maddahi J et al. Development and prospective application of quantitative 2-day stress-rest Tc-99m methoxy isobultil isonotrile SPECT for the diagnosis of coronary artery disease. Am Heart J 1990; 120: 1255-1266.

25. Wackers FJT (1995) State of the art in coronary artery disease detection: technetium-99m labeled myocardial perfusion imaging agents. Detection of coronary artery disease, in Zaret BL and Beller GA (eds.), Nuclear Cardiology. State of the art and future directions. Mosby, St. Louis, pp. 273-280.

26. Van Train KF, Areeda J, Garcia EV et al. Quantitative of same day Tc-99m-Sestamibi myocardial SPECT: Multicenter trial validation. J Nucl Med 1992; 33: 876. (Abstr.).

27. Rigo P, Leclercq B, Itti R et al. Technetium-99m-Tetrofosmin myocardial imagin: a comparison with Thallium-201 and angiography. J Nucl Med 1994; 35: 587-593.

28. Takahashi N, Tamaki N, Tadamura E et al. Combined assessment of regional perfusion and wall motion in patients with coronary artery disease with technetium 99m tetrofosmin. J Nucl Cardiol 1994; 1: 29-38.

29. Sridhara B, Sochor H, Rigo P et al. Myocardial single-photon emission computed tomographic imaging with technetium 99m tetrofosmin: Stess-rest imaging with same-day and separate-day rest imaging. J Nucl Cardiol 1994; 1: 138-143.

30. Santana Boado C, García Burillo A, Candell Riera J et al. SPET 99mTc-Tetrofosmin one day protocol in the diagnosis of CAD. QJ Nucl Med 1997; 41: 227. (Abstr.).

31. Santana Boado C, García Burillo A, Campreciós M et al. ^{99m}Tc-tetrofosmin SPECT one day protocol in the diagnosis of CAD. J Nucl Cardiol 1997; 4: 35. (Abstr.).

32. Tamaky N, Takahashi N, Kawamoto M et al. Myocardial tomography using technetium-99m-Tetrofosmin to evaluate coronary artery disease. J Nucl Med 1994; 35: 594-600.

33. Thorley PJ, Ball J, Sheard KL et al. Evaluation of ^{99m}Tc-tetrofosmin as a myocardial perfusion agent in routine clinical use. Nucl Med Commun, 1995; 16: 733-740.

34. Heo J, Cave V, Wasserleben V, Iskandrian A. Planar and tomographic imaging with technetium 99m-labeled tetrofosmin: Correlation with thallium 201 and coronary angiography. J Nucl Cardiol 1994; 1: 317-324.

35. Hendel R, Parker A, Wackers FJ et al. Reduced variability of interpretation and improved image quality with a technetium 99m myocardial perfusion agent: Comparison of thallium 201 and technetium 99m-labeled tetrosfosmin. J Nucl Cardiol 1994; 1: 509-514.

36. Kolter TS, Diamond GA. Exercise thallium-201 scintigraphy in the diagnosis and prognosis of coronary artery disease. Arch Int Med 1990; 113: 684-702.

37. Pennell DJ, Prvulovich E (1995) Imaging techniques, in Pennell DJ and Prvulovich E (eds.), Nuclear Cardiology, British Nuclear Medicine Society, London, pp. 17-33.

38. Udelson JE, Leppo JA (1994) Diagnosis of coronary artery disease, in Murray IPC, Ell PJ and Strauss HW (eds.) Nuclear Medicine, pp. 1129-1156.

39. Wackers FJ. Comparison of thallium-201 and technetium-99m methoxyisobutyl isonitrile. Am J Cardiol 1992; 70: 30E-34E.

40. Berman DS. Technetium-99m myocardial perfusion imaging agents and their relation to thallium-201. Am J Cardiol 1990; 66: 1E-4E.

41. Hicks R (1994) Myocardial perfusion scintigraphy techniques using single photon radiotracers, in I.P.C. Murray , P.J. Ell and H.W. Strauss (eds.), Nuclear Medicine, pp. 1083-1098.

42. Taillefer R, Lambert R, Dupra SG et al. Clinical comparison between thallium-201 and Tc-99m-methoxy isobutil - isonitrile (HEXAMIBI) myocardial perfusion imaging for detection of coronary artery disease. Eur J Nucl Med 1989; 15: 280-286.

43. Alexander C, Oberhausen E. Myocardial scintgraphy. Sem Nucl Med 1995; 25: 195-201.

44. Kiat H, Maddahi J, Roy LT et al. Comparison of tecnetium 99m methoxy isobutil isonitrile and thallium 201 for evaluation of coronary artery disease by planar and tomographic methods. Am Heart J 1989; 117: 1-11.

45. Iskandrian AS, Heo J, Kong B, Lyons E, Marsch A. Use of technetium-99m isonitrile (RP-30A) in assessing left ventricular perfusion and function at rest and during exercise in coronary artery disease, and comparison with coronary arteriography and exercise thallium-201 SPECT imaging. Am J Cardiol 1989; 64: 270-275.

46. Kahn JK, Mc Ghie I, Akers MS et al. Quantitative rotacional tomography with ^{201}Tl and ^{99m}Tc 2-methoxy-isobutil-isonitrile: a direct comparison in normal individual and patients with coronary artery disease. Circulation 1989; 79: 1282-1293.
47. Candell Riera J. Técnicas de imagen para la detección de isquemia miocárdica: ecocardiografía de estrés farmacológico o estudios isotópicos de perfusión? Perspectiva isotópica. Rev Esp Cardiol 1995; 48: 159-163.
48. Van Train KF, Areeda J, Garcia EV et al. Quantitative same day rest-stress technetium-99m-Sestamibi SPECT: Definition and validation of stress normal limits and criteria for abnormality. J Nucl Med 1993; 34: 1494-1502.
49. Van Train KF, García EV, Maddahi J et al. Multicenter trial validation for quantitative analysis of same-day rest-stress technetium-99m-sestamibi myocardial tomogramas. J Nucl Med 1994; 35: 609-618.
50. Maddahi J, Kiat H, Van Train KF et al. Myocardial perfusion imaging with technetium-99m sestamibi SPECT in evaluation of coronary artery disease. Am J Cardiol 1990; 66: 55E-62E.
51. Maddahi J, Kiat H, Friedman G et al. (1992) Tc-99m sestamibi myocardial perfusion imaging for evaluation of coronary artery disease, in Zaret BL, Beller GA (eds.), Nuclear Cardiology, CV Mosby, St. Louis, pp. 191-200.
52. Beller GA. Current status of nuclear cardiology techniques. Curr Prob Cardiol 1991; 16: 447-535.
53. Picard M, Dupras G, Taillefer R. Myocardial perfusion agents: Compared biodistribution of 201-Tallium, Tc-99m-tertiary butyl isonitrile (TBI) and Tc-99m-methoxy isobutil isonitrile (MIBI). J Nucl Med 1987; 28 (sulp): 654-655.
54. Piwnica-Worms D, Chiu ML, Kronauge JF. Divergent kinetics of ^{201}Tl and ^{99m}Tc-sestamibi in cultured chick ventricular myocites during ATP depletion. Circulation 1992; 85: 1531-1541.
55. Borges-Neto S, Coleman RE, Jones RH. Perfusion and function at rest and treadmill exercise using technetium-99m Sestamibi: Comparison of one and two day protocols in normal volunteers. J Nucl Med 1990; 31: 1128-1132.
56. Berman DS, Kiat H, Van Train K et al. Technetium 99m sestamibi in the assessment of chronic coronary artery disease. Sem Nucl Med 1991; 21: 190-212.
57. Sochor H. Tecnetium-99m sestamibi in chronic coronary artery disease: the european experience. Am J Cardiol 1990; 66: 91E-96E.
58. Berman DS, Kiat HS, Van Train KF et al. Myocardial perfusion imaging with technetium-99m-Sestamibi: Comparative analysis of available imaging protocols. J Nucl Med 1994; 35: 681-688.
59. Tamaki N, Yonekura Y, Kodama S et al. Stress thallium-201 transaxial emission computed tomography: Quantitative vs qualitative analysis for evaluation of coronary artery disease. J Am Coll Cardiol 1984; 4: 1213-1221.
60. De Pascuale EE, Nody AC, DePuey EG et al. Quantitative rotational thallium-201 tomography for identifying and localizing coronary artery disease. Circulation 1988; 77: 316-327.
61. Iskandrian AS, Heo J, Kong B, Lyons E. Effect of exercise level on the ability of thallium-201 tomography imaging in coronary artery disease: Analysis of 461 patients. J Am Coll Cardiol 1989; 14: 1477-1486.
62. Mahmarian JJ, Boyce TM, Goldberg RK et al. Quantitative exercise thallium-201 single fhoton emission computed tomography for the enhanced diagnosis of ischemic heart disease. J Am Coll Cardiol 1990; 15: 318-329.
63. Van Train KF, Maddahi J, Berman DS et al. Quantitative analysis of tomographic stress thallium-201 myocardial scintigrams: A multicenter trial. J Nucl Med 1990; 31: 1168-1179.
64. Maddahi J, Van Train K, Prigent F et al. Quantitative single fhoton emission computed thallium-201 tomography for detection and localization of coronary artery disease: Optimization and prospective validation of a new technique. J Am Coll Cardiol 1989; 14: 1689-1699.
65. Higley B, Smith FW, Smith T et al. Technetium-99m-1,2-bis[bis(2-ethoxyethyl)phosphino]ethane: Human biodistribution, dosimetry and sefety of a new myocardial perfusion imaging agent. J Nucl Med 1993; 34: 30-38.
66. Sinusas AJ, Beller GA, Watson DD. Cardiac imaging with technetium 99m-labeled isonitriles. J Thorac Imaging 1990; 5: 20-30.
67. Dahlberg ST, Leppo JA. Myocardial kinetics of radiolabeled perfusion agents: Basis for perfusion imaging. J Nucl Cardiol 1994; 189-197.
68. Beller GA, Watson DD. Physiological of myocardial perfusion imaging with technetium 99m agents. Semin Nucl Med 1991; 21: 173-181.

69. Taillefer MD, Dupras G, Sporin V et al. Myocardial perfusion imaging with a new radiotracer, technetium-99m-hexamibi (methoxy isobutil isonitrile): comparison with thallium-201 imaging. Clin Nucl Med 1989; 14: 89-96.

70. Wackers FJ, Berman DS, Maddahi J et al. Technetium-99m hexakis 2 methoxyisobutil isonitrile (hexamibi): Human biodistribution, dosimetry, safety, and preliminary comparison to thallium-201 for myocardial perfusion imaging. J Nucl Med 1989; 30: 301-311.

71. Garcia EV, Cooke D, Van Train KF et al. Technical aspect of myocardial SPECT technetium-99m sestamibi. Am J Cardiol 1990; 66: 23E-31E.

72. Udelson JE. Choosing a thallium-201 or technetium 99m sestamibi imaging protocol. J Nucl Cardiol 1994; 1: S99-S108.

73. Berger BC, Watson DD, Taylor GJ et al. Quantitative thallium-201 exercise scintigraphy for detection of coronary artery disease. J Nucl Med 1981; 22: 585-593.

74. Maddahi J, Garcia EV, Berman DS et al. Improved noninvasive assessment of coronary artery disease by quantitative analysis of regional stress myocardial distribution and washout thallium-201. Circulation 1981; 64: 924-935.

75. Gibbons L. The value of maximal versus submaximal treadmill testing. J Cardiac Rehab 1981; 1: 362-368.

76. Froelicher VF (1984) Standard exercise testing, in Froelicher VF (ed.), Exercise testing & training, Year Book Medical Publishers Inc., Chicago, pp. 1-11.

77. Weiner DA, Ryan TJ, McCabe CH et al. Exercise stress testing. Correlations among history of angina, ST-segment response and prevalence of coronary artery disease in the coronary artery surgery study (CASS). N Engl J Med 1979; 301: 230-235.

78. Patterson RE, Eng C, Horowitz SF. Practical diagnosis of coronary artery disease: A Bayes' theorem nomogram to correlate clinical data with noninvasive exercise tests. Am J Cardiol 1984; 53: 252-256.

79. Hlatky MA, Pryor DB, Harrell FE et al. Factors affecting sensitivity and specificity of exercise electrocardiography. Multivariable analysis. Am J Cardiol 1984; 77: 64-71.

80. Diamond GA, Forrester JS. Analysis of probability as an aid in the clinical diagnosis of coronary-artery disease. N Engl J Med 1979; 300: 1350-1358.

81. Rozanski A, Berman D. The efficacy of cardiovascular nuclear medicine exercise studies. Sem Nucl Med 1987; 2: 104-102.

82. Rozanski A. Referral bias and the efficacy of radionuclide stress tess: problems and solutions. J Nucl Med 1992; 33: 2074-2079.

83. Proudfit WL, Shirey EK, Sones FM. Selective cine coronary angiography: Correlation with clinical findings in 1000 patients. Circulation 1966; 33: 901-910.

84. Campeau L, Bourassa MG, Bois MA et al. Clinical significance of selective coronary cinearteriography. Canad M A J 1968; 99: 1063-1068.

85. Friesinger GC, Smith RF. Correlation of electrocardiographic studies and arteriographic findings with angina pectoris. Circulation 1972; 56: 1173-1183.

86. McConahay DR, McCallister BD, Smith RE. Post-exercise electrocardiography: Correlation with coronary arteriography and left ventricular hemodynamics. Am J Cardiol 1971; 28: 1-9.

87. Diamond G: Clinical diagnosis of coronary artery diseases using Bayes theorem. Myocardium 1989; 1: 9-11.

88. Patterson RE, Horowitz SF. Importance of epidemiology and biostatistics in deciding clinical strategies for using diagnostic tests: a simplified approach using examples from coronary artery disease. J Am Coll Cardiol 1989; 13: 1653-1665.

89. Olona-Cabases M. (1994) The probability of a correct diagnosis, in Candell-Riera J and Ortega-Alcalde D (eds.), Nuclear cardiology in everyday practice, Kluwer Academic Publishers, Dordrecht, pp. 348-358.

90. Gitler B, Fishbach M, Steingart RM. Use of electrocardiographic thallium exercise testing in clinical practice. J Am Coll Cardiol 1984; 3: 262-271.

91. Diamond GA, Denton TA, Berman DS, Cohen I. Prior restraint: A Bayesian perspective on the optimization of technology utilization for diagnosis of coronary artery diseas. Am J Cardiol 1995; 76: 82-86.

92. Candell Riera J (1994) Prognostic evaluation and follow-up of chronic coronary artery disease", in Candell-Riera J and Ortega-Alcalde D (eds.), Nuclear cardiology in everyday practice, Kluwer Academic Publishers, Dordrecht, pp. 216-240.

93. Steinberg EP, Klag MJ, Bakal CW et al. Exercise thallium scans: patterns of use and impact on management of patients with known or suspected coronary artery disease. Am J Cardiol 1987; 59: 50-55.

94. Mañé S, Moragas G, Martínez P et al. Evolución de las indicaciones de la prueba de esfuerzo con 201-talio en nuestro medio. Rev Esp Med Nucl 1990; 9 (Supl. 1): 9 (Abstr.).

95. Johnson LL. Sex specific issues relating to nuclear cardiology. J Nucl Cardiol 1995; 2: 339-348.
96. Miller DD. Evaluation of coronary artery disease in women. Current Opinion in Cardiolgy 1996; 11: 447-453.
97. Steingart RM, Packer M, Hamm P et al. Sex differences in the managenent of coronary artery disease. N Engl J Med 1991; 325: 226-230.
98. Hachamovitch R, Berman D, Kiat H et al. Gender-related differnces in clinical management after exercise nuclear testing. J Am Coll Cardiol 1995; 26: 1457-1464.
99. Khan SS, Nessim S, Gray R et al. Increased mortality of women in coronary artery bypass surgery: Evidence for referral bias. Ann Inter Med 1990; 112: 561-567.
100. Ayanian JZ, Epstein AM. Differences in the use of procedures between women and men hospitalized for coronary heart disease. N Engl J Med 1991; 325: 221-225.
101. Maynard C, Beshansky JR, Griffith JL et al. Influence of sex on the use of cardiac procedures in patients presenting to the emergency department. A prospective multicenter study. Circulation 1996; 94: 93-98.
102. Malenka DJ, O'Conor GT, Quinton H et al. Differences in outcomes between women and men associated with percutaneous transluminal coronary angioplasty. A regional prospective study of 13061 procedures. Circulation 1996; 94: 99-104.
103. Roeters van Lennep JE, Borm JJJ, Zwinderman AH, Pauwels EKJ, Bruschke AVG, van der Wall EE. No gender bias in referral for coronary angiography after myocardial perfusion scintigraphy with technetium-99m tetrofosmin. J Nucl Cardiol 1999; 7: 596-604.
104. Diamond GA. 'Reverend Bayes' Silent majority. An alternative factor affecting sensitivity and specificity of exercise electrocardiography. Am J Cardiol 1986; 57: 1175-1180.
105. Mullani NA, Caras D, Ahn C et al. Fewer women than men have positive SPECT and PET cardiac findings among patients with no history of heart disease. J Nucl Med 2000; 41: 263-268.
106. Strauss HW, Harrinson K, Langan JK et al. Thallium-201 for myocardial imaging to regional myocardial perfusion. Circulation 1975; 51: 641-645.
107. Leppo JA, Meerdink DJ. Comparative myocardial extraction of two technetium-labeled BATO derivatives (SQ30217), (SQ30014) and thallium. J Nucl Med 1990; 31: 67-74.
108. Iskandrian AS, Verani MS (1996) Exercise perfusion imaging in coronary artery disease: Exercise testing and physiology, in Iskandrian AS and Verani MS (eds.), Nuclear Cardiac Imaging: Principles and applications. F.A. Davis Company, Philadelphia , pp. 46-72.
109. Kelly JD, Foster AM, Higley B et al. Tecnetium-99m-Tetrofosmin as a new radiopharmaceutical for myocardial perfusion imaging. J Nucl Med 1993; 34: 222-227.
110. Val PG, Chaimant BR, Waters DD. Diagnostic accuracy of exercise ECG lead system in clinical subsets of woman. Circulation 1982; 65: 1465-1472.
111. Taillefer R, DePuey GE, Udelson J et al. Comparative diagnostic accuracy of thallium-201 and Tc-99m sestamibi (perfusion and gated SPECT) in detecting coronary artery disease in women. J Am Coll Cardiol 1997; 29: 69-77.
112. Iskandrian AE, Heo J, Nallamothu N. Detection of coronary artery disease with use of stress single-photon emission computed tomography myocardial perfusion imaging. J Nucl Cardiol 1997; 4: 329-335.
113. Chae SC, Heo H, Iskandrian AS et al. Identification of extensive coronary artery disease in women by exercise single photon emission computed tomographic (SPECT) thallium imaging. J Am Coll Cardiol 1993; 21: 1305-1310.
114. Friedman TD, Greene AC, Iskandrian AS et al. Exercise thallium-201 myocardial scintigraphy in women: Correlation with coronary arteriography. Am J Cardiol 1992; 49: 1632-1637.
115. Shaw LJ, Miller DD, Romeis JC et al. Gender differences in the noninvasive evaluation and management of patients wiht suspected coronary artery disease. Ann Intern Med 1994; 120: 559-566.
116. Lauer MS, Pashkow FJ, Snader CE et al. Gender and referral for coronary angiography after treadmill thallium testing. Am J Cardiol 1996; 78: 278-283.
117. Tavel ME, Enas NH, Woods JR. Sensitivity and specificity of tests: can the "silent majority" speak?. Am J Cardiol 1987; 60: 1167-1169.
118. Garver PR, Wasnich RD, Shibuya AM et al. Apearance of breast attenuation artifacts with thallium myocardial SPET imaging. Clin Nucl Med 1985; 10: 694-696.
119. Gordon DG, Pfisterer M, Williams R, Walaski S, Ashburn W. The effect of diaphragmatic attenuation on Tl-201 images. Clin Nucl Med; 1979: 150-151.
120. De Puey EG, Garcia EV. Optimal specificity of thallium-201 SPECT through recognition of imaging artifacts. J Nucl Med 1989; 30: 441-449.
121. Eisner R, Churchwell A, Noever T et al. Quantitative analysis of the tomographic thallium-201 myocardial bulleye display: critical role of correcting for patient motion. J Nucl Med 1988; 29: 91-97.

122. Friedman J, Van Train K, Maddahi J et al. "Upward creep" of the heart: A frequent source of false-positive reversible defects during thallium-201 stress-redistribution SPECT. J Nucl Med 1989; 30: 1718-1722.

123. Geckle WJ, Frank TL, Links JM et al. Correction for patients and organ movement in SPECT: aplication to exercise thallium-201 cardiac imaging. J Nucl Med 1986; 27: 889 (abstr).

124. Madsen MT, Park CH. Enhancement of SPECT images by Fourier filtering the projection image set. J Nucl Med 1985; 26: 395-402.

125. Wagoner LE, Movahed A, Reeves WC. Myocardial imaging artefacts caused by mitral valve annulus calcification. J Nucl Med 1991; 16: 94-97.

126. Helmer S, Abghari R, Stone AJ et al. Detection of benign cardiac fibroma on thallium-201 imaging in an adult. Clin Nucl Med 1987; 12: 365-367.

127. Lebtahi NE, Stauffer JC, Delaloye B. Left bundle branch blook and coronary artery disease: Accuracy of dipiridamole thallium-201 single-photon emission computed tomography in patients with exercise anteroseptal perfusion defects. J Nucl Cardiol 1997; 4: 266-273.

128. Shih Wj, Berk MR, Mills BJ et al. Reversible thallium-201 perfusion defects of the septal and inferoapical segments in a patient with imcomplete right bundle branch block and normal coronary angiogram. J Nucl Med 1992; 33: 1556-1557.

129. Mahrotra PP, Weaver YJ, Higginbotham EA. Myocardial perfusion defect on thallium-201 imaging in patients with chronic obstrutive pulmonary disease. J Am Coll Cardiol 1983; 2: 233-239.

130. Tamai J, Nagata S, Nishimura T. Hemodynamic and prognostic value of thallium-201 myocardial imaging in patients with dilated cardiomyopathy. Int J Cardiol 1989; 24: 219-224.

131. Arai H, Yamazaki J, Nakano H et al. A case of cardiac amyloidosis showing the ischemic change by exercise Tl-201 myocardial scintigraphy. Jpn J Nucl Med 1990; 27: 1157-1162.

132. Nishimura T, Uehara T, Kozuca T et al. A perfusion defect in the case of a sarcoid heart by thallium-201 myocardial perfusion imaging. Jpn J Clin Radiol 1981; 26: 509-512.

133. Candell-Riera J, Bardají A, Sagrista J et al. Aneurisma ventricular en la sarcoidosis. Su detección mediante la ventriculografía isotópica. Rev Esp Cardiol 1986; 39: 151-153.

134. Martin-Neto JA, Marzullo P, Marcassa C et al. Myocardial perfusion abnormalities in chronic Chagas disease as detected by thallium-201 scintigraphy. Am J Cardiol 1992; 69: 780-784.

135. Zeiher AM, Krause T, Schächinger V et al. Impaired endothelium-dependent vasodilation of coronary resistence vessels is associated with exercise-induced myocardial ischemia. Circulation 1995; 91: 2345-2352.

136. O'Gara PJ, Bonow RO, Maron BJ et al. myocardial perfusion abnormalities in patients with hypertrophic cardiomyopathy: assessment with thallium-201 emission computed tomography. Circulation 1987; 76: 1214-1223.

137. Camici P, Chiriatti G, Lorenzoni K. Coronary vasodilation is impaired in both hypertrophic and non-hypertrophic myocardium of patients with hypertrophic cardiomyopathy: a study with nitrogen-13 ammonia and positron emission tomography. J Am Coll Cardiol 1991; 17: 879-886.

138. Iskandrian AS, Verani MS (1996) Exercise perfusion imaging in coronary artery disease: Physiology and diagnosis, in Iskandrian AS, Verani MS (eds.), Nuclear cardiac imaging: principles and applications, FA Davis Company, Philadelphia, pp. 73-143.

139. Gallik DM, Mammaharian JJ, Verani MS. Therapeutic significance of exercise induced ST segment elevation in patients without previous myocardial infartion. Am J Cardiol 1993; 72: 1-7.

140. Iskandrian AS, Nallamothu N, Heo J. Nonatherosclerotic causes of myocardial ischemia. J Nucl Cardiol 1996; 3: 428-435.

141. Gutgesell HP, Pinsky WW, DePuey EG. Thallium-201 myocardial perfusion imaging in infants and children: Value in distinguishing anomalous left coronary artery from congestive cardiomyopathy. Circulation 1980; 61: 659-664.

142. Yamanaka O, Hobbs RE. Coronary artery anomalies in 126,595 patients undergoing coronary arteriography. Cathet Cardiovasc Diagn 1990; 21: 28-40.

143. Almahmeed WA, Haykowski M, Boone J et al. Spontaneous coronary artery dissection in young women. Cathet Cardiovasc Diagn 1996; 37: 201-205.

144. Vavuranakis M, Bush CA, Boudoulas H. Coronary artery fistulas in adults: incidence, angiographic characteristics, natural history. Cathet Cardiovasc Diagn 1995; 35: 116-120.

145. Gascueña-Rubia R, Hernández-Hernández F, Tascón-Pérez JC, Albarrán-González-Trevilla A, Lázaro-Salvador M, Hernández-Simón P. Isquemia miocárdica demostrada secundaria a fistulas coronarias múltiples con drenaje en el ventrículo izquierdo. Rev Esp Cardiol 2000; 53: 748-751.

146. Fuster V, Badimon L, Badimon JJ et al. The pathogenesis of coronary artery disease and the acute coronary syndrome. N Engl J Med 1992; 326: 242-250.

147. Candell Riera J, Armadans L, Simeón CP et al. Comprehensive noninvasive assessment of cardiac involvement in limited systemic sclerosis. Arthritis Rheum 1996; 39: 1138-1145.
148. Zimring H, Fitzgerald RL, Engler RL et al. Intracoronary vs intravenous effects of cocaine on coronary flow and ventricular funtion. Circulation 1994; 89: 1819-1828.
149. Hirzel HO, Senn M, Nuesch K et al. Thallium-201 scintigraphy in complete left bundle branch block. Am J Cardiol 1984; 53: 764-769.
150. Braat SH, Brugada P, Bar FW et al. Thallium-201 exercise scintigraphy and left bundle branch block. Am J Cardiol 1985; 55: 224-226
151. Rothbart RM, Beller GA, Watson DD et al. Diagnostic accuracy and prognostic significance of quantitative thallium-201 scintigraphy in patients with left bundle branch block. Am J Noninvas Cardiol 1987; 1: 197-205.
152. DePuey EG, Guertler-Krawczynska E, Robbins WL. Thallium-201 SPECT in coronary artery disease patients with left bundle branch block. J Nucl Med 1988; 29: 1479-1485.
153. Jazmati B, Sadaniantz A, Emaus SP et al. Exercise thallium-201 imaging in complet left bundle branch block and the prevalence of septal perfusion defects. Am J Cardiol 1991; 67: 46-49.
154. Larcos G, Gibbons RJ, Brown ML et al. Diagnostic accuracy of exercise thallium-201 single-photon emission computed tomography in patients with left bundle branch block. Am J Cardiol 1991; 68: 756-760.
155. Delonca J, Camenzind E, Meier B et al. Limits of thallium-201 exercise scintigraphy to detect coronary disease in patients with complete and permanent bundle branch block: A review of 134 cases. Am Heart J 1992; 123: 1201-1207.
156. Marín-Huerta E, Rodríguez-Padial L, Castro-Beiras JM et al. Thallium-201 exercise scintigraphy in patients having complete left bundle branch block with normal coronary arteries. Int J Cardiol 1987; 16: 43-46.
157. Rockett JF, Wood WC, Moinuddin M, Loveless V, Parrish B. Intravenous dipyridamole thallium-201 SPECT imaging in patients with left bundle branch block. Clin Nucl Med 1990; 15: 401-407.
158. Burns RJ, Galligan R, Wright LM et al. Improved specificity of myocardial thallium-201 single-photon emission computed tomography in patients with left bundle branch block by dipyridamole. Am J Cardiol 1991; 68: 504-508.
159. O'Keefe JH Jr, Bateman TM, Barnhart CS. Adenosine thallium-201 is superior to exercise thallium-201 for detecting coronary artery disease in patients with left budle branch block. J Am Coll Cardiol 1993; 21: 1332-1338.
160. Vaduganathan P, He ZX, Raghavan C et al. Detection of left anterior descending coronary artery stenosis in patients with left bundle branch block: exercise, adenosine or dobutamine imaging? J Am Coll Cardiol 1996; 28: 543-550.
161. Matzer L, Kiat H, Friedman JD et al. A new approach to the assessment of tomographic thallium-201 scintigraphy in patients with left bundle branch block. J Am Coll Cardiol 1991; 17: 1309-1317.
162. Arana R, González JM, Castell J et al. Utilitat de la gammagrafia planar amb tal.li-201 en els malalts amb bloqueig de branca esquerra. Ann Med (Barc) 1993; 79: 138-139.
163. Oller-Martínez G, Candell-Riera J, Rosselló J et al. SPET miocàrdic de perfusió amb esforç (+dipiridamol) i compostos tecneciats en pacients amb bloqueig de branca esquerra. Revista de la Societat Catalana de Cardiologia 2000; 3: 8. (Abstr.).
164. Schulman DS, Francis CK, Black HR et al. Thallium-201 stress imaging in hypertensive patients. Hypertension 1987; 10: 16-21.
165. DePuey EG, Guertler-Krawczynska E, Perkins JV et al. Alterations in myocardial thallium-201 distribution in patients with chronic systemic hypertension undergoing single-photon emission computed tomography. Am J Cardiol 1988; 62: 234-238.
166. Prisant LM, von Dohlen TW, Houghton JL et al. A negative thallium (dipyridamole) stress test excludes significant obstructive epicardial coronary artery disease in hypertensive patients. Am J Hypertens 1992; 5: 71-75.
167. Cecil MP, Pilcher WC, Eisner RL et al. Absence of defects in SPECT thallium-201 myocardial images in patients with systemic hypertension and left ventricular hypertrophy. Am J Cardiol 1994; 74: 43-46.
168. Candell-Riera J, Castell-Conesa J. Exploraciones radioisotópicas en la cardiopatía hipertensiva, in: Iriarte MM ed. Cardiopatía hipertensiva. Barcelona: Harcourt Brace, 1997: 153-168.
169. Tubau JF, Szlachcic, Hollenberg M et al. Usefulness of thallium-201 scintigraphy in predicting the development of angina pectoris in hypertensive patients with left ventricular hypertrophy. Am J Cardiol 1989; 64: 45-49.

170. Meller J, Goldsmith SJ, Rudin A et al. Spectrum of exercise thallium-201 myocardial perfusion imaging in patients with chest pain and normal coronary angiogramas. Am J Cardiol 1979; 43: 717-723.
171. Candell Riera J, Castell Conesa J, Ortega Alcalde D. Estudios radioisotópicos en los pacientes con dolor torácico y coronarias angiográficamente normales. Rev Lat Cardiol 1990; 11: 59-64.
172. Legrand V, Hodgson JM, Bates ER et al. Abnormal coronary flow reserve and abnormal radionuclide exercise test results in patients with normal coronary angiograms. J Am Coll Cardiol 1985; 6: 1245-1253.
173. Marcus ML, White CW. Coronary flow reserve in patients with normal coronary angiograms. J Am Coll Cardiol 1985; 6: 1254-1256.
174. Houghton JL, Frank MJ, Carr AA et al. Relations among impaired coronary flow reserve, left ventricular hypertrophy and thallium perfusion defects in hypertensive patients without obstructive coronary artery disease. J Am Coll Cardiol 1990; 15: 43-51.
175. Iriarte M, Caso R, Murga N et al. Microvascular angina pectoris in hypertensive patients with left ventricular hypertrophy and diagnostic value of exercise thallium-201 scintigraphy. Am J Cardiol 1995; 75: 335-339.
176. Iriarte M, Caso R, Murga N et al. Enalapril-induced regression of hypertensive left ventricular hypertrophy, regional ischemia, and microvascular angina. Am J Cardiol 1995; 75: 850-852.
177. Meller J, Goldsmith SJ, Rudin A et al. Spectrum of exercise thallium myocardial perfusion imaging in patients with chest pain and normal coronary angiograms. Am J Cardiol 1979; 43: 717-723.
178. Maseri A, Parodi O, Severi S et al. Transient trasluminal reduction of myocardial blood flow, demostrated by thallium-201 scintigraphy, as a cause of variant angina. Circulation 1976; 54: 280-285.
179. Berger BC, Abramowitz R, Park CH et al. Abnormal thallium-201 scans in patients with chest pain and angiographically normal coronary arteries. Am J Cardiol 1983; 52: 365-370.
180. Legrand V, Hodgson JM, Bates ER et al. Abnormal coronary flow reserve and abnormal radionuclide exercise test results in patients with normal coronary angiograms. J Am Coll Cardiol 1985; 6: 1245-1253.
181. Kaul S, Newell JB, Chesler DA et al. Quantitative thallium imaging findings in patients with normal coronary angiographic findings and in clinically normal subjects. Am J Cardiol 1986; 57: 509-512.
182. Rosano GM, Kaski JC, Arie S et al. Failure to demostrate myocardial ischaemia in patients with angina and normal coronary arteries. Evaluation by continuous sinous pH monotoring and lactate metabolism. Eur Heart J; 1996; 17: 1175-1180.
183. Rosano GMC, Peters NS, Kaski JC et al. Abnormal uptake and washout of thallium-201 in patients with syndrome X and normal-appearing scans. Am J Cardiol 1995; 75: 400-402.
184. Kaski JC, Rosano JMC, Collins P et al. Cardiac syndrome X: Clinical characteristics and left ventricular function. Long-term follow-up study. J Am Coll Cardiol 1995; 25: 807-814.
185. King MA, Tsui BMW, Pan TS. Attenuation compensation for cardiac single-photon emission computed tomographic imaging: Part 1. Impact of attenuation and methods of estimating attenuation maps. J Nucl Cardiol 1995; 2: 513-524.
186. King MA, Tsui BMW, Pan TS et al. Attenuation compensation for cardiac single-photon emission computed tomographic imaging: Part 2. Attenuation compensation algorithms. J Nucl Cardiol 1996; 3: 55-63.
187. Ficaro EP, Fessler JA, Shreve PD et al. Simultaneous transmission/emission myocardial perfusion tomography. Diagnostic accuracy of attenuation-corrected ^{99m}Tc-sestamibi single-photon emission computed tomography. Circulation 1996; 93: 463-473.
188. Pan TS, King MA, Luo DS et al. Estimation of attenuation maps from scatter and photopeak window single photon-emission computed tomographic images of technetium 99m-labeled sestamibi. J Nucl Cardiol 1997; 4: 42-51.
189. Prvulovich EM, Lonn AHR, Bomanji JB et al. Effect of attenuation correction on myocardial thallium-201 distribution in patients with a low likelihood of coronary artery disease. Eur J Nucl Med 1997; 24: 266-275.
190. Jiménez-Hoyuela JM, McClellan JR, Alavi A et al. Impacto de la corrección de atenuación en la imágen de perfusión miocárdica con SPECT. Rev Esp Cardiol 1998; 51 (Suppl. 1): 26-32.
191. Boonyaprapa S, Ekmachachai M, Thanachaikun N et al. Measurement of left ventricular ejection fraction from gated technetium-99m sestamibi myocardial images. Eur J Nucl Med 1995; 22: 528-531.
192. Williams KA, Taillon LA. Reversible ischemia in severe stress technetium 99m-labeled sestamibi perfusion defects assessed from gated single-photon emission computed tomographic polar map Fourier analysis. J Nucl Cardiol 1995; 2: 199-206.
193. Palmas W, Friedman JD, Diamond GA et al. Incremental value of simultaneous assessment of myocardial function and perfusion with technetium-99m sestamibi for prediction of extent of coronary artery disease. J Am Coll Cardiol 1995; 25: 1024-1031.

194. Williams KA, Taillon LA. Left ventricular function in patients with coronary artery disease assessed by gated tomographic myocardial perfusion images. Comparison with assessment by contrast ventriculography and first-pass radionuclide angiography. J Am Coll Cardiol 1996; 27: 173-181.
195. Germano G, Erel J, Kiat H et al. Quantitative LVEF and qualitative regional function from gated thallium-201 perfusion SPECT. J Nucl Med 1997; 38: 749-754.
196. Maunoury C, Chen CC, Chua KB et al. Quantification of left ventricular function with thallium-201 and technetium-99m.sestamibi myocardial gated SPECT. J Nucl Med 1997; 38: 958-961.
197. Berman DS, Germano G. Evaluation of ventricular ejection fraction, wall motion, wall thickening, and other parameters with gated myocardial perfusion single-photon emission computed tomography. J Nucl Cardiol 1997; 4: S169-171.
198. Ruiz-Salmerón R, Ponce de León E, López A et al. Validación del modelo tridimensional de gated-SPECT con sestamibi para el cálculo de la fracción de eyección ventricular izquierda en pacientes con cardiopatía isquémica. Comparación con la ventriculografía de contraste. Rev Esp Cardiol 1999; 52: 671-80.
199. Yoshioka J, Hasegawa S, Yamaguchi H et al. Left ventricular volumes and ejection fraction calculated from quantitative electrocardiographic-gated 99mTc-tetrofosmin myocardial SPECT. J Nucl Med 1999; 40: 1693-1698.
200. Germano G, Berman DS (1999) Clinical gated cardiac SPECT. Futura Publishing Company, Inc. Armonk, NY.

5. MYOCARDIAL EXERCISE SPET AND WITH PHARMACOLOGIC STIMULATION

JAUME CANDELL-RIERA and CESAR SANTANA-BOADO

1. Influence of exercise parameters on myocardial SPET results

Patients who are referred to the nuclear cardiology department for coronary disease diagnosis constitute a relatively biased population in that, in general, they represent a group in whom the results of a previous stress test had been inconclusive [1-5]. Perfusion scintigraphy is performed, usually, with dynamic exercise and with the same methodology as for a conventional exercise test. The diagnostic efficacy is conditioned, among other factors, by the O_2 consumption (METs) and by the myocardial consumption of O_2 (peak heart rate and the product of heart rate x systolic blood pressure) [6-10].

Some authors have affirmed that insufficient heart rate, generally associated with treatment with beta-blockers, has a small effect on the ^{201}Tl at rest [11] as in stress [12,13]. However, these very optimistic results were obtained in a series of patients with high prevalence of coronary artery disease and with previous myocardial infarction which make the interpretations of these results questionable. What is certain is that in the majority of publications a decrease in the sensitivity of the perfusion scintigraphy is observed when the myocardial consumption of O_2 does not reach optimum values or when the patient is under treatment with beta-blockers [14-23].

Iskandrian et al. [24], using ^{201}Tl single photon emission tomography (SPET), obtained sensitivities of 74%, 88% and 98% for coronary disease of one, two and three vessels respectively, in patients who had reached a peak heart rate ≥85% than the predicted value in the stress test or had a positive electrocardiogram. Conversely, when the patients did not reach 85% of peak predicted heart rate, the sensitivity was significantly lower (52%, 84% and 79%, respectively). For a similar level of heart rate the sensitivity of perfusion scintigraphy is superior to that of the exercise electrocardiogram [25-31]. In exercise electrocardiography a level ≥85% of age-predicted maximal heart rate (220 − age) is considered indicative of a sufficient myocardial O_2 consumption having been reached, but in perfusion scintigraphy there has not, as yet, been established a minimum value of this parameter nor of the product of heart rate x systolic blood pressure, nor of the peak O_2 consumption.

Initial stress studies conducted by us [25-27] demonstrated that perfusion studies might be less demanding for the patient. With the view to establishing the minimum levels of peak heart rate, the heart rate x systolic blood pressure product and the peak consumption of O_2 necessary to obtain an adequate diagnostic accuracy of myocardial perfusion SPET we studied 159 patients [31] with known or suspected coronary

J. Candell-Riera et al. (eds.), Myocardium at Risk and Viable Myocardium, 95–118.
© 2001 *Kluwer Academic Publishers. Printed in the Netherlands.*

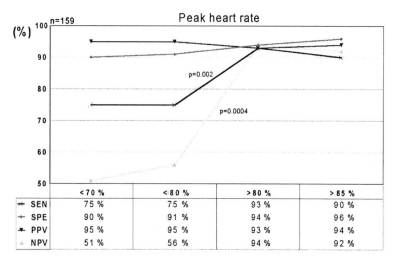

Figure 1. Diagnostic accuracy of myocardial stress SPET with respect to the levels of peak heart rate achieved. The sensitivity and the negative predictive value improve significantly when beyond 80%.

disease and without previous myocardial infarction using perfusion SPET with ^{99m}Tc-MIBI injected in the course of the subjective maximum exercise test. All the patients had a confirmatory coronary angiography.

The results of the study showed that starting from levels >80% of peak heart rate (Figure 1), 18,000 of the product of peak heart rate x maximum systolic pressure product (Figure 2) and 5 METs of maximum consumption of O_2 (Figure 3), the sensitivity of the ^{99m}Tc-MIBI SPET was significantly more elevated than that obtained with lower levels of peak heart rate, of heart rate x systolic blood pressure product and of METs; and similar to that obtained with higher levels of these parameters.

Similarly, the negative predictive value of this test is very low when <80% of peak heart rate (56%), 18,000 of heart rate x systolic blood pressure (52%) and 5 METs (69%) are not reached (Figures 1 to 3). This signifies that before a negative SPET conclusion, the levels of these parameters always need to be assessed since if these levels are not reached there is a large margin of error and a high probability of a false negative.

We believe that the interest of this study lies in that, to-date, there have not been established any minimum levels of induced peak heart rate, of heart rate x systolic blood pressure product and of METs above which the level of physical exercise may be considered sufficient and during which the tracer is injected for the perfusion SPET.

The results indicate that, contrary to conventional exercise electrocardiography in which 85% of predicted heart rate is considered necessary, in perfusion SPET with ^{99m}Tc-MIBI a level of 80% is already adequate. The external work performed and peak heart rate x maximum systolic blood pressure product increase linearly during exercise [32], and we observed as well, in our series of patients, that the levels of 5 METs and 18,000 of peak heart rate x systolic blood pressure product are adequate for

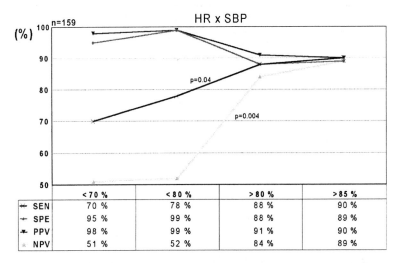

	< 70 %	< 80 %	> 80 %	> 85 %
SEN	70 %	78 %	88 %	90 %
SPE	95 %	99 %	88 %	89 %
PPV	98 %	99 %	91 %	90 %
NPV	51 %	52 %	84 %	89 %

Figure 2. Diagnostic accuracy of myocardial stress SPET with respect to the values of the product peak heart rate and maximum systolic blood pressure achieved. The sensitivity and negative predictive value improve significantly at values beyond 18,000.

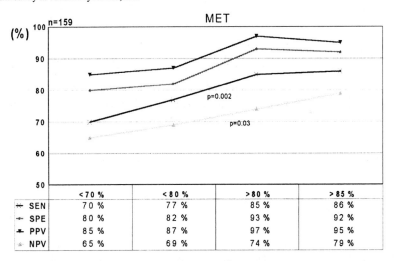

	< 70 %	< 80 %	> 80 %	> 85 %
SEN	70 %	77 %	85 %	86 %
SPE	80 %	82 %	93 %	92 %
PPV	85 %	87 %	97 %	95 %
NPV	65 %	69 %	74 %	79 %

Figure 3. Diagnostic accuracy of myocardial exercise SPET with respect to the values of METs reached. The sensitivity and negative predictive values improve significantly at values beyond 5 METs.

considering as "sufficient" the exercise test that accompanies SPET. If these levels are not reached, it must be remembered that the sensitivity and, more importantly, the negative predictive value of the exploration are sub-optimal.

The evaluation of patients with known or suspected coronary artery disease has shifted to a more elderly and disabled population during the last several years. As this population continues to age, their ability to perform adequate levels of exercise decreases. The clinical rule of thumb is that exercise perfusion imaging is performed in patients who can exercise, vasodilator stressors are given to patients who can not, and inotropic stressors are given to patients in whom vasodilators are contraindicated. Several factors can contribute to a patient's inability to reach a sufficient exercise test, including but not limited to peripheral vascular disease, prior stroke, disabling arthritis and orthopedic problems. Several pharmacologic stressors have been developed to avoid underestimation of perfusion defects [33-35].

2. Alternatives to exercise as a provocation test

2.1. DIPYRIDAMOLE AND ADENOSINE

Intravenous administration of dipyridamole in conjunction with perfusion scintigraphy came into use in 1978 with good results [36-40] in those patients in whom a conventional stress test was not feasible or in whom a dynamic stress test was contra-indicated (abdominal aorta aneurysm, severe arterial hypertension) or in those patients unable to do physical exercise (arterial occlusive disease of the limbs, poor physical capacity, osteo-muscular diseases) or when difficulties existed in the interpretation of the stress electrocardiogram (left bundle branch block, pacemakers) or chronotropic insufficiency.

The intravenous administration of dipyridamole produces a coronary vasodilation via the inhibition of phosphodiesterase and the increment of adenosine monophosphate which diminishes the vascular resistance of the coronary micro-vasculature. The increase in coronary flow in arteries without lesions relative to the stenosed vessels is the basis on which differences in perfusion in the myocardial scintigraphy are detected, as are alterations in ventricular function in radionuclide ventriculography and of contractility defects in echocardiography [41-46]. The scant proportion of patients that present angina and/or ischaemic changes on ECG suggest that an altered distribution in the coronary flow, more than an authentic ischaemic myocardium, may be the cause of the defects observed in perfusion scintigraphy. However, when more sensitive electrocardiographic methods have been utilised, such as thoracic electrocardiographic maps, positive correlations have been obtained between the extent of perfusion defects and the magnitude and extent of the ECG changes, suggesting that the ischaemia is the authentic cause of the reversible perfusion defects caused by the dipyridamole [47]. Other studies, as well, have demonstrated that the extent of perfusion defects is the most important predictive factor for ST segment depression on ECG when adenosine is administered [48].

With the intravenous administration of dipyridamole, slight increases in cardiac output (33%) are produced and of the heart rate (20%-40%) as well as a diminution (4%-10%) of systolic blood pressure [49-51]. The product of the systolic blood pressure x peak heart rate increases by an 11 - 28%. The mean coronary flow can increase between 3 and 5 s its basal level during the administration of dipyridamole and be further increased with isometric exercise and consequent increase in diastolic pressure of the filled coronary artery. The increase in coronary flow with exercise is only 2 to 3 times greater [52-54] with respect to basal.

The most frequently used dose is 0.14 mg/Kg/min over 4 minutes, although in about 1 in 6 patients no maximum vasodilation is produced [55-58]. This can be followed by a supplementary administration of 0.28 mg/Kg. Around 12% of patients with negative echocardiographic tests at the usual dose can respond to 0.84 mg/Kg over 10 minutes [58]. Planar perfusion scintigraphy with ^{201}Tl has resulted in sensitivities similar to the lower doses (0.06 mg/Kg/min. over 4 minutes) and this may have the advantage of producing less undesirable side-effects [59].

The absorption of dipyridamole via the digestion is variable and, hence, the plasma level following oral administration of 300 mg of the drug is unpredictable and necessitates longer periods of supervision of the patient to preclude the possibility of adverse effects. This route of administration was used originally [60-62] but is not employed at present.

Various drugs exert antagonist effects with respect to the action of dipyridamole and can give rise to false negative results. Aminophylline, theophylline and caffeine can block the adenosine receptors and inhibit the vasodilatory action of dipyridamole [63-65].

The appearance of undesirable effects with dipyridamole administration is infrequent: around 30% of patients present angina, 12% ST segment depression, 11% headache and 10% a sensation of giddiness. The administration of sublingual glyceril trinitrate is, in general, sufficient for the treatment of the angina but if it is not eased it may be necessary to recourse to the administration of intravenous aminophylline (doses of up to 250 mg i.v. at a rate of 50 mg/min). Two cases of death in patients with unstable angina have been reported following the oral and intravenous administration of the drug and, hence, the administration of dipyridamole is contra-indicated in patients with angina in the instability phase as well as in patients with chronic obstructive pulmonary disease in whom some cases of respiratory arrest have been described [66, 67].

The results of a multicenter study, conducted in 73,806 patients from 59 hospitals in which 19 countries participated [68] and in whom intravenous dipyridamole was used in conjunction with the studies of myocardial perfusion, highlighted that the risk of serious side-effects is low. There were 6 cases of death from cardiac failure (0.95 x 10,000), 13 non-fatal infarcts (1.76 x 10,000), 6 ventricular arrhythmias (0.95 x 10,000), 9 ischaemic cerebral strokes (1.22 x 10,000) and 9 episodes of severe bronchospasm (1.22 x 10,000).

The values for sensitivity (between 67% and 95%; mean 76%) and of specificity (between 28% and 100%; mean 70%) of myocardial scintigraphy with dipyridamole [69, 70], in general, are lower than that of exercise perfusion scintigraphy and, as such, whenever possible the latter test is recommended. Further, with exercise one can obtain an evaluation of the functional capacity of the patient that with dipyridamole alone is not possible [71].

The vasodilatory effect of dipyridamole is indirect in that the direct mediator of the coronary dilation is the endogenous adenosine. The potent vasodilatory effect of adenosine has been utilised to induce controlled hypotension in patients undergoing surgical repair of intracranial aneurysms. It is for this reason that adenosine [72,73] and adenosine triphosphate (ATP) [74] have been used. The results have been very similar to those of dipyridamole in conjunction with myocardial scintigraphy using

[201]Tl [75] or with combination techniques [76-78]. The protocol of administration consists in the introduction of an intra-venous dose of 140 µg/Kg/min over 5 or 6 minutes followed by the administration of the radionuclide within 3 minutes. The half-life of adenosine is less than 10 seconds and stopping the administration of the drug rapidly reverses secondary side effects. Hence, we prefer to administer dipyridamole such that the infusion pump used for its administration is not fixed and, as we will see later, it is easy to administer while the patient is performing the stress test.

Minor undesirable effects in 81% of cases have been reported in a multicenter study that included 9,000 patients [79] and in whom only one infarct, 7 episodes of severe bronchospasm and one pulmonary oedema were noted as important complications. Two-hundred fifty six cases of first degree atrio-ventricular block, 378 of second degree and 72 of third degree were recorded. All were transitory and resolved spontaneously. There was no case of sustained atrio-ventricular block or death.

2.1.1. Dipyridamole and isometric exercise

Brown et al. [80] reported a study using isometric stress ("handgrip") in conjunction with the intravenous infusion of dipyridamole. They observed that with intra-venous dipyridamole, systemic arterial pressure increased by 8%, heart rate by 23% and coronary flow was 2.4 times above basal value and that these values increased 16%, 34% and 3.3% respectively when isometric stress was added (p<0.02). On the other hand, resistance to the flow in the stenosed regions was augmented by 36% over that which was produced by dipyridamole alone.

This response is attributable to the stimulation by the isometric exercise of the efferent sympathetic nervous system of the coronary arteries producing constriction of the epicardiac arteries and, as well, to the increase in diastolic pressure provoked by the handgrip together with the coronary vasodilation produced by dipyridamole. Associated with the exercise is the diminished splanchnic uptake of the radiotracer thus improving the background signal/activity ratio and, as such, the quality of the image [81,82].

Equally, there are studies that demonstrate that isometric exercise, although producing the effects already described, does not significantly improve the results of dipyridamole alone [83-85].

2.1.2. Dipyridamole followed by dynamic stress

Studies indicating that dynamic exercise following dipyridamole administration improves the results of the test have been described [85-98]. The first publication on this issue was conducted by Walker et al. [85] in 1986 with the administration of oral dipyridamole and the conduct of the stress test one hour later. This study had secondary difficulties due to the variability of absorption of the oral dipyridamole.

The initial studies with intravenous dipyridamole followed by stress were published by Laarman et al. [86,87]. Intravenous dipyridamole was administered followed by a submaximal exercise and planar perfusion study with ^{201}Tl was performed. Various authors [88, 89] have advocated the administration of intravenous dipyridamole prior to dynamic exercise contending that, in combination, the diagnostic efficacy of the test is increased (Table 1) by diminishing background activity and splachnic flow and augmenting the blood flow in the muscles used for the exercise and which improves the heart/background ratio.

TABLE 1. Diagnostic accuracy of myocardial stress scintigraphy performed after the administration of dipyridamole

	SEN (%)	SPE (%)	PPV (%)	NPV (%)
Laarman et al. [86]				
Overall	76	86	94	59
Left anterior descending	82	88	82	88
Left circumflex	48	88	61	81
Right coronary	74	85	78	82
Multivessel	70	92	85	81
Ignaszeweski et al. [95]				
Stenosis >40%	94	53	94	53
Stenosis >70%	95	28	83	59
Left anterior descending	78	65	65	74
Left circumflex	22	92	22	92
Right coronary	71	77	56	87

NPV = Negative predictive value; PPV = Positive predictive value; SEN = sensitivity; SPE = specificity.

The majority of authors have centred their studies on demonstrating that the magnitude of the ischaemia is greater when conducting submaximum stress following the administration of dipyridamole. Stein et al. [98] performed 2 studies with ^{201}Tl in 54 patients (one with dipyridamole alone and the other with dipyridamole followed by submaximum exercise). They found a greater number of ischaemic segments (2.5 vs 1.3; p<0.001) and of true positives (39 vs 30; p<0.001) with the addition of stress to the intravenous administration of dipyridamole.

Other autors [93-95] have further demonstrated that the cardiac image improves with the addition of dipyridamole to the dynamic exercise and that the indices of heart/lung uptake, heart/liver and heart/infra-diaphragmatic tissue improve significantly. Kenneth et al. [96], in a review on the combination of dipyridamole and exercise confirmed its utilisation since it improves the efficiency of the test, decreases the secondary effects and facilitates the evaluation of the patient's response to exercise. This would indicate that prior administration of dipyridamole should be an integral part of the stress test. Hurwitz et al. [99], obtained optimum results with the combination of maximum dynamic exercise subsequent to the infusion of dipyridamole in 600 SPET studies with ^{99m}Tc-MIBI and in 500 planar studies with ^{201}Tl to achieve an improved index of infra-diaphragmatic heart-tissue ratio with this methodology.

2.1.3. Dipyridamole and simultaneous stress in patients without infarction
The simultaneous administration of intra-venous dipyridamole with maximum subjective dynamic exercise is a technique originally developed in the Hospital Universitari Vall d'Hebron [30,100-103] and which retains all the information offered by the ergometric test while, at the same time, evaluating the severity of the coronary artery disease.

Often, when initiating the stress test, neither the level of tachycardia nor the maximum level of oxygen consumption that the patient will reach is known.

However, during the first phase (50 W for 70 Kg represents 5 METs) it becomes evident that the level of stress and of peak heart rate may not be satisfactory. If during the course of the exercise test an optimal heart rate level, a maximum consumption of O_2 without angina and ischaemic changes are not reached, then the administration of intra-venous dipyridamole while the patient continues with the exercise increases the percentage of positives in a manner similar to that obtained with maximum ergometric tests.

Based on the results of our own studies [31] in which we had demonstrated that the diagnostic accuracy of SPET with ^{99m}Tc-MIBI is satisfactory starting at levels of maximum O_2 consumption of 5 METs and of levels of peak heart rate ≥80%, it was decided to adopt a protocol in which dipyridamole was to be administered during the exercise in those patients who do not achieve these criteria. The protocol consists of intravenous administration of dipyridamole (0.16 mg/Kg/min over 4 minutes) to the patient while continuing the exercise with maximum tolerable load up to 3 minutes after the end of the dipyridamole administration (Figure 4). The administration of the drug is discontinued if the patient presents with angina or a depression of the ST segment ≥1mm occurs.

We studied 231 consecutive patients [30] without previous myocardial infarction and in whom SPET with ^{99m}Tc-MIBI was performed within 3 months of the coronary angiography. The patients were divided into 3 groups:

-    Group SUF ET (Sufficient exercise test): 91 patients with a peak heart rate ≥80% of the theoretical maximum for age (220 - age) or appearance ST segment depression ≥1 mm or presentation of angina.
-    Group INSUF ET (Insufficient exercise test): 72 patients with a peak heart rate <80%, an oxygen consumption >5 METs and no depression in ST segment ≥1 mm nor angina.
-    Group INSUF + DIPY (Exercise test insufficient + dipyridamole): 68 patients with a peak heart rate <80%, consumption of O2 <5 METs and without ST segment depression ≥1mm nor angina and in whom intra-venous dipyridamole was administered simultaneously with the exercise.

A greater number of patients in the INSUF ET group (exercise test with peak heart rate <80% but with >5METs) had been receiving treatment with beta-blockers and which was evidently influential in the lower heart rate being reached. The differences are explained by the inclusion criteria to one or other group. On the other hand, the three groups were similar with respect to the presence or absence of coronary disease and in the distribution of the lesions in the arteries (Table 2). The most important point of our study was the confirmation of the hypothesis that the administration of dipyridamole simultaneously with the physical exercise could significantly improve the diagnostic efficiency of the perfusion SPET without loss of important prognostic information from the subjective maximal stress test (Table 3).

With the simultaneous dipyridamole-stress test the sensitivity increased from 71% to 89% (p=0.03) and the negative predictive value increased from 56% to 83% (p=0.002).

As such, a negative result from a SPET with an insufficient stress test does not preclude the possibility that the patient does have coronary disease. When the intravenous dipyridamole is added the situation is clearly improved since the data indicated better results of sensitivity and negative predictive values in the patients in the INSUF ET + DIPY group with respect to those in the INSUF ET group, despite the patients in the former group having achieved a lower level of METs than those of the latter. It needs to be emphasised, as well, that the intravenous administration of dipyridamole was not associated with any serious complication in any patient.

TABLE 2. Exercise test results in patients without previous infarction and sufficient exercise stress test (SUF ET), insufficient (INSUF ET) and insufficient with simultaneous dipyridamole (INSU ET + DIPY) [31]

	SUF ET	INSUF ET	INSUF ET + DIPY
Duration	7.3±2.6	8±2.2	7.6±2.6
Watts	87.8±28	92.3±27	43±26[a]
METs	6.2±1.2	6.1±1.2	3.9±1.3[a]
Peak HR	130±23[b]	106±18	97±20[c]
%HR	80±14[b]	63±9	61±12
SBP	176±26	170±26	157±25[a]
HRxSBP	230±60[d]	181±45	154±48[a]
Angina	34% (31)	0	23% (17)
ST>1mm	39% (42)	0	12% (8)
ST 0.5-1mm	10% (9)	14% (9)	8% (5)

[a] = $p < 0.0001$ vs SUF ET and INSUF ET; [b] = $p < 0.0001$ vs INSUF ET and INSUF ET + DIPY; [c] = $p = 0.01$ vs INSUF ET; [d] = $p = 0.001$ vs INSUF ET.
HR = Heart rate; %HR = Percentage of peak heart rate with respect to the theoretical maximum; SBP = systolic blood pressure; INSUF ET = Insufficient exercise test; INSUF ET + DIPY = Insufficient exercise test + simultaneous dipyridamole; SUF ET = Sufficient ET.

Around 70% of the patients with false negative results had been receiving beta-blockers, which favours lower peak heart rate. As has been described by other authors [14,15,18,19,23], this factor is important from the clinical point of view and highlights the necessity of withdrawing the medication before performing the test when attempting definitive diagnosis or when the severity and extent of the coronary disease is being determined.

TABLE 3. Diagnostic accuracy of myocardial SPET in the three groups of patients

	SEN	SPE	GV	PPV	NPV
SUF ET	93%[a]	94%	93%[b]	96%	89%
INSUF ET	71%	90%	76%	94%	56%
INSUF ET + DIPY	89%[c]	86%	87%	91%	83%[d]

[a] $p = 0.003$ vs INSUF ET; [b] $p = 0.002$ vs INSUF ET; [c] $p = 0.03$ vs INSUF ET; [d] $p = 0.002$ vs INSUF ET.
GV = Global value; INSUF ET = Insufficient exercise test; INSUF ET + DIPY = Insufficient exercise test + simultaneous dipyridamol ; NPV = Negative predictive value; PPV = Positive predicitve value; SEN = Sensitivity; SPE = Specificity; SUF ET = Sufficient exercise test.

The diagnostic accuracy of simultaneous exercise + dipyridamole is similar to that with maximum exercise tests [104-107] and with dipyridamole + maximum subjective exercise [81,83,87,89,90,95].
   In the diagnosis of vessel disease of the three groups (Table 4), the same tendency is maintained as that observed in the overall analysis for the right coronary artery and left anterior descending coronary artery. The best results were obtained, again, in

those groups SUF ET and SUF ET+DIPY and the worst for the left circumflex coronary artery in the INSUF ET group.

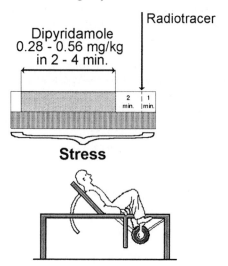

Figure 4. Scheme of the protocol for the administration of dipyridamole during the course of the stress test.

TABLE 4. Diagnostic accuracy of myocardial SPET for each of the arteries in the three groups of patients

	SEN	SPE	GV	PPV	NPV
Left anterior descending					
SUF ET	82%[a]	88%[b]	85%[c]	8%	85%[d]
INSUF ET	56%	79%	68%	79%	59%
INSUF ET + DIPY	78%[e]	86%[f]	82%[b]	85%	79%[b]
Left circumflex					
SUF ET	54%	95%	79%	86%	77%
INSUF ET	43%	96%	78%	83%	77%
INSUF ET + DIPY	52%	98%	81%	93%	77%
Right coronary					
SUF ET	81%[f]	90%	86%	87%	84%
INSUF ET	65%	86%	78%	74%	80%
INSUF ET + DIPY	89%[f]	80%	83%	74%	92%[g]

[a] $p = 0.02$ vs INSUF ET; [b] $p = 0\ 0.001$ vs INSUF ET; [c] $p = 0.0001$ vs INSUF ET;
[d] $p = 0.03$ vs INSUF ET; [e] $p = 0.05$ vs INSUF ET; [f] $p = 0.01$ vs INSUF ET; [g] $p = 0.04$ vs INSUF ET.
GV = Global value; NPV = Negative predictive value; PPV = Positive predictive value; INSUF ET = Insufficient exercise test; INSUF ET + DIPY = Insufficient exercise test + simultaneous dipyridamole. SEN = Sensitivity; SPE = Specificity; SUF ET: Sufficient exercise test.

With the objective of demonstrating that the simultaneous administration of dipyridamole with the physical exercise test increases the extent of the ischaemia in the perfusion scintigraphy, we studied a series of 20 patients with documented coronary disease. We performed two stress tests of identical characteristics separated by a one week interval and quantified the extent of overall ischaemia as well as by regions in all of the left ventricle applying our own methodology of polar map (Plate5.1).

Essentially, we demonstrated that the extent of ischaemia (difference in uptake at rest and stress >10%) was significantly greater for each of the four regions studied (anterior-septal, apical, inferior and lateral) as well as at the overall level of extent of ischaemia of the left ventricle (Table 5).

TABLE 5. Percentage of extent of ischaemia in each region in the 20 patients who performed an exercise stress test alone (EXERCISE) and an exercise stress test with simultaneous dipyridamole (ET + DIPY)

	EXERCISE		ET + DIPY
Antero-septal	6% ± 8	P = 0.003	15% ± 15
Inferior	10% ± 12	P = 0.003	18% ± 18
Lateral	7% ± 8	P = 0.006	20% ± 19
Apical	10% ± 15	P = 0.02	21% ± 29
Overall	10% ± 10	P = 0.0003	17% ± 14

These results coincide with those of Daou et al. [108] who encountered a greater number of reversible segments in patients that performed exercise-only test or with dipyridamole added compared to those in whom only dipyridamole was administered.

The vasodilation produced by dipyridamole, which can be three or more times greater than that produced by exercise, explains the increment in flow to the regions normally perfused compared to the ischemic ones [86-108]. Further, as indicated by other authors [86-99] the addition of dipyridamole to the physical exercise reduces undesirable secondary effects of the drug which, in the absence of contra-indications such as bronchial asthma and unstable ischaemia, are very rare [66-68].

Daou et al. [108], in a series of 397 patients, observed that, compared to dipyridamole administration alone, simultaneous exercise improved the indices heart/liver and heart/abdomen (p<0.001), diminished the undesirable effects and increased the sensitivity of the test. The basic conclusions were that: 1. The addition of exercise increases the tolerance to dipyridamole, 2. The quality of the image is better in the combination of exercise with dipyridamole, 3. The sensitivity of the combination is superior to that of dipyridamole alone and similar to the maximum exercise, and 4. Prognostic information obtained from the exercise test is not lost.

Pennell et al. [109] studied the addition of submaximal exercise to the pharmacologic stress induced by adenosine and obtained better results when adenosine was infused simultaneously with the submaximum exercise; better heart/background ratio and lower incidence of extra-cardiac effects produced by the adenosine (43% less, p<0.0001). These authors concluded that the addition of dynamic exercise to the adenosine infusion improves the detection of diseased coronaries and produces a lower percentage of secondary effects due to the drug.

We believe that these results indicate that the systematic administration of intravenous dipyridamole is to be recommended during the stress test for all those patients who do not have the capacity to reach sufficient levels of myocardium consumption of oxygen or of maximum oxygen consumption. In this way, there is no loss of electrocardiographic clinical information derived from the performance of a subjective maximum stress test and can optimise the results of the perfusion SPET.

2.1.4. Dipyridamole and simultaneous stress in patients with previous infarction
The demonstration of residual ischaemia, whether at a distance or in the same region of the infarct, is of considerable post-infarct prognostic value [110-114]. However, the accuracy of perfusion scintigraphy in the diagnosis of multivessel disease is not optimal neither in patients without [115-117] nor in those with [118-121] previous infarction.

To demonstrate that the sensitivity of ^{99m}Tc-MIBI SPET in combination with the simultaneous administration of dipyridamole during the exercise is superior to the stress test on its own (when insufficient) in the diagnosis of multivessel disease (ischaemia at distance) and of patentcy of the infarct-related vessel (residual ischaemia in the infarct region) in patients with previous infarction, we designed a study that consisted in the application of the same protocol of dipyridamole with simultaneous stress as used in the patients without previous infarction [122].

We included 209 patients who had had a myocardial infarction and documented coronary angiography and who, based on the results of the stress test (and with the same criteria as those patients without infarction) were classified into three groups:
-   Group SUF ET   (Sufficient exercise test): 107 patients with a peak heart rate $\geq$80% of the theoretical maximum for age (220 - age) or that presented with angina or depression of the ST segment (horizontal or descending) $\geq$1mm.
-   Group INSUF ET (Insufficient exercise test): 55 patients with a peak heart rate <80%, a consumption of O_2 >5METs and that did not present with angina or depression in ST segment $\geq$1mm.
-   Group INSUF ET + DIPY (Insufficient exercise test + dipyridamole): 47 patients with a peak heart rate <80%, consumption of O_2 <5 METs and without angina nor depression in the ST segment $\geq$1mm and in whom intra-venous dipyridamole was administered simultaneously with the exercise.

The variable considered as true positive of multivessel disease (ischaemia at distance) was reversible perfusion defects in whichever region not corresponding to that of the infarct when there was a stenosis >50% in the corresponding coronary artery. The variable considered as true positive of patency of the infarct-related artery (peri-infarct residual ischaemia) was defects with a degree of reversibility of uptake in the region of the infarction and the corresponding artery ·· ' being occluded (Plate 5.2).

Table 6 summarises the results of the conventional stress test and the treatment that the patients were following at the time of the   ometr   est. The patients of the INSUF ET + DIPY reached a lower myocardial O_2 consumption and a lower maximum oxygen consumption expressed in METs.

The sensitivity, specificity, positive predictive and negative predictive values of the SPET for the diagnosis of multivessel disease in the different groups of patients are presented in Table 7. The sensitivity for the diagnosis of multivessel disease in the SUF ET and INSUF ET + DIPY groups was significantly greater than that of the INSUF ET group. In 51% of patients in Group 1 and 48% of Group 3 there was reversibility in the same region of the infarct. These percentages were significantly greater compared to the INSUF ET group, both globally as well as for each of the coronary arteries (Figure 5).

TABLE 6. Exercise test results in patients with previous myocardial infarction and sufficient exercise test, insufficient exercise and insufficient exercise + simultaneous dipyridamole.

	SUF ET (n = 107)	INSUF ET (n = 55)	INSUF ET + DIPY (n = 47)
Duration (min)	7 ± 2	6.9 ± 2	5.8 ± 2
Watts	81 ± 28	91 ± 25	42 ± 23[a]
METs	5.6 ± 1	5.9 ± 1	3.9 ± 1[a]
Peak HR	118 ± 22	106 ± 15	93 ± 21[a]
%HR	73 ± 13	66 ± 9	59 ± 12[b]
SBP	163 ± 26	161 ± 25	154 ± 22
HR x SBP	19200 ± 5400	17300 ± 4300	14000 ± 4200[a]
ST (mm)	0.99 ±0.9[c]	0.1 ± 0.2	0.3 ± 0.5[d]
ST >1mm	56 (52%)	-	9 (19%)
Angina	50 (46%)	-	12 (25%)

[a] p=0.0001 vs SUF ET and INSUF ET; [b] p=0.006 vs SUF ET and INSUF ET; [c] p= 0.0001 vs SUF ET and INSUF ET; [d] p= 0.01 vs INSUF ET.
HR = Heart rate; %HR = Percentage of peak heart rate with respect to the theoretical maximum; INSUF ET = Insufficient exercise test; INSUF ET + DIPY = Insufficient exercise test + simultaneous dipyridamole; SBP = Systolic blood pressure; SUF ET = Sufficient exercise test.

As will be discussed in Chapter 6, the sensitivity of perfusion scintigraphy for the diagnosis of multivessel disease is not optimal especially if the exercise test is submaximum and if the planar technique is used to obtain the scintigraphic images [118-121]. Haber et al. [121] obtained very low values of sensitivity (35%) in a series of 88 patients with acute myocardial infarction and who had planar scintigraphy ^{201}Tl performed prior to discharge from hospital.

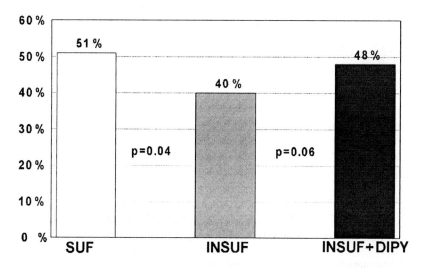

Figure 5. Percentage of patients with reversible patterns of ^{99m}Tc-MIBI in the same region of the infarct following sufficient exercise test (SUF ET), insufficient (INSUF ET) and insufficient plus simulataneous dipyridamole (INSUF ET + DIPY).

TABLE 7. Results of myocardial SPET for the diagnosis of multivessel disease in the three groups of patients with previous myocardial infarction

	SEN	SPE	PPV	NPV
SUF ET	80%[a]	61%	81%	49%
INSUF ET	59%	74%	80%	51%
INSUF ET + DIPY	76%[b]	67%	79%	53%

[a] p = 0.009 vs INSUF ET; [b] p= 0.02 vs INSUF ET.
INSUF ET = Insufficient exercise test; INSUF ET + DIPY = Insufficient exercise test + simultaneous dipyridamole; SEN = Sensitivity; SPE = Specificity, SUF ET = Sufficient exercise test;;NPV = Negative predictive value; PPV = Positive predictive value

The low sensitivity of myocardial perfusion scintigraphy in the diagnosis of multivessel disease is due, in part, to that the exploration preferentially detects the most severe defects in relation to the better-perfused regions that, in the case of patients with multivessel disease, may not be normal. It has been demonstrated, in patients without [4] and with [121] previous infarction, that significant ST segment depression significantly increases the sensitivity of SPET. Taken together, the reversible defects at distance together with ST segment depression in a series of patients of Haber et al. [121], the sensitivity increased to 58% albeit with a decrease of specificity which went from 87% to 78%. Other factors that can explain this decrease in sensitivity is that, in many cases following an infarct, tests of submaximal stress are indicated and with which maximum consumption of O_2 and myocardial consumption of O_2 are much lower and, hence, the effectiveness of the test as well.

The results from our own studies indicate that the sensitivity of the SPET in the diagnosis of multivessel disease in patients with previous infarction is low (59%) when the stress test is insufficient. Now, the administration of dipyridamole during the course of the exercise in these cases provides significant improvement in the sensitivity (76%) and reach values similar to those in patients who perform a sufficient test (80%). The use of SPET and of the combined techniques in our study undoubtedly contribute to obtaining of better sensitivity values compared to that described previously by others [110,111,113,118-121].

TABLE 8. Results of the myocardial SPET for the diagnosis of patency of the infarct related artery in the three groups of patients with previous myocardial infarction

	SEN	SPE	PPV	NPV
SUF ET	87%[a]	17%	52%	56%
INSUF ET	68%	39%	39%	68%
INSUF ET + DIPY	82%[b]	23%	42%	65%

[a] p=0.003 vs INSUF ET; [b] p=0.005 vs INSUF ET.
INSUF ET = Insufficienr exercise test; INSUF ET + DIPY = Insufficient exercise test + simulataneous dipyridamole; PPV = Positive predicitive value; NPV = Negative predicitive value; SEN = Sensitivity; SPE = Specificity; SUF ET = Sufficient exercise test

Table 8 summarises the results obtained in the diagnosis of patency of the infarct-related artery. In the patients in the Groups SUF ET and INSUF ET + DIPY, sensitivity was significantly higher than that of the patients in Group INSUF ET. No differences in the specificity and predictive values were observed between the three groups of patients.

The prognosis of patients that had presented with infarction is better if recanalisation of the infarct-related artery exists [123-126]. The permeability of the infarct-related artery can beneficially influence ventricular remodeling [127], the development of a more stable electro-physiologic substrate [128] and the increase in the extent of viable myocardium [129]. On the other hand the presence of increased residual ischaemia is encouraged and, as such, the possibility of ischaemic complications during the follow-up as well [130]. The reversibility of the scintigraphic uptake in the same region suggests residual ischaemia in the region and which could be due to the patency of the infarct-related artery and/or to the presence of collateral circulation. Indeed, in our series, the values of specificity in the diagnosis of permeability of the infarct-related artery were very low (17% - 39%) and strengthens the hypothesis that different grades of collateral circulation exist in the presence of occluded arteries.

In our series, the sensitivity of the ^{99m}Tc-MIBI for the diagnosis of the patency of the infarct-related artery was satisfactory (87%) if the stress test had been sufficient. This sensitivity was much lower (68%) in those patients with insufficient test and, again, improved when dipyridamole was administered to those patients that performed an insufficient stress test (82%).

We believe that our results indicate that intravenous administration of dipyridamole be recommended during the stress test in patients with previous infarction and who do not have the capacity to achieve levels of sufficiency of maximum oxygen consumption nor of maximal myocardial oxygen consumption. In this way, the clinical and electrocardiographic information derived from the performance of subjective maximum stress test is not lost and can optimise the results of the perfusion SPET in the diagnosis of multivessel disease and of the permeability of the infarct-related artery.

2.2. OTHER PHARMACOLOGIC AGENTS

Other drugs, apart from dipyridamole and adenosine, have been used with the objective of reproducing the event, from the clinical, electrocardiographic, echocardiographic and isotopic point of view, but the results obtained have not been as good. Among these drugs are angiotensin [131, 132], phenylephrine [133], pitressin [134] and ergonovine [135]. With the exception of the last of these, that can induce coronary vasospasm, for which reason, they are rarely used.

Ergonovine has been used as a provocation test [136-144] with the objective of reproducing coronary vasospasm in those patients with suspected Prinzmetal's angina. It is administered as bolus of 0.0125, 0.025, 0.05, 0.1, 0.3, and 0.4 mg with intervals of 5 minutes and the vasospastic response is evaluated in the form of elevation of the ST segment in the ECG, defect of perfusion in scintigraphy and direct visualisation of the coronary spasm on the coronary angiography. Although this type of test has been used in patients admitted to the coronary unit as well as in ambulatory patients, the possibility that persistent spasm can be induced and which may necessitate the administration of intracoronary nitroglycerine, make it unwise for this test to be employed in the catheterization laboratory.

The purpose for the administration of other vasoconstrictive drugs [131-134] is to increase the demand for oxygen following the increase of the post-load. However, despite an increase in the systolic and diastolic pressures, heart rate practically does not alter and, hence, the peak heart rate x maximal systolic blood pressure product is low, as is the sensitivity of the test as well.

Beta-stimulant drugs such as isoproterenol (at doses of 1-2 µg/min) [145], epinephrine (progressive doses of 0.03, 0.06, 012, 0.18, 0.24 and 0.30 µg/Kg every 5 minutes) [146], dopamine (progressive doses of 2.5 µg/Kg/min every 5 minutes up to a maximum dose of 15 µg/Kg/min) [147] and, above all, dobutamine (progressive doses 5 µg/Kg/min in intervals of 5 minutes up to a maximum dose of 20-40 µg/Kg/min) [148,149] have been used as alternatives in the performance of the conventional stress test. In general these drugs produce an increment in the myocardial contractility and of the myocardial frequency. Epinephrine and dopamine, at the appropriate doses, can produce alpha-adrenergic stimulation which adds vasoconstrictive activity to the usual activities of the drugs. In general, these drugs do not greatly alter (isoproterenol) or increase (epinephrine, dopamine, dobutamine) systolic pressure while diastolic pressure can diminish (isoproterenol, epinephrine) or increase (dopamine, dobutamine). Isoproterenol and dobutamine can produce a coronary vasodilatatory effect and, hence, increase the coronary flow in the healthy coronary arteries. As such then, in those patients with coronary disease the phenomenon of coronary steal can present and is similar to that described with dipyridamole.

Whatever provocation test is used, it is necessary to constantly maintain a correct electrocardiographic and haemodynamic monitorisation of the patient since it is not infrequent that supraventricular and/or ventricular arrhythmias can be induced during the administration of these drugs. The intra-venous administration of 5 mg

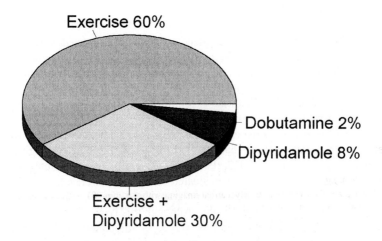

Figure 6. Percentage of patients in the Hospital General Universitari Vall d'Hebron who had performed an exercise test, an insufficient exercise test with simultaneous dipyridamole, dipyridamole at rest and with dobutamine.

propranolol should be sufficient to counteract this effect and, hence, the possible appearance of signs of persistent ischaemias.

The administration of dobutamine [150-153] or of arbutamine [154,155] together with the performance of perfusion scintigraphy have been employed recently for the diagnosis of coronary disease, although the use of these drugs is preferable in combination with tests directed towards the evaluation of ventricular contractility such as electrocardiography and radionuclide ventriculography.

In the nuclear cardiography laboratory of the Hospital General Universitari Vall d'Hebron, 60% of the patients perform exercise alone as a manoeuvre of provocation, 30% perform a stress test insufficient with simultaneous dipyridamole, 8% have dipyridamole administered at rest and only 2% have had dobutamine administered because of contra-indications to dipyridamole (Figure 6).

References

1. Candell-Riera J, Ortega D, Alijarde M, et al. Gammagrafía miocárdica con Tl^{201}: sensibilidad, especificidad y valor predictivo. Med Clín (Barc) 1984; 82: 656-660.
2. Candell-Riera J, Castell J, Ortega D et al. Diagnostic accuracy of radionuclide techniques in patients with equivocal electrocardiographic exercise testing. Eur Heart J 1990; 11: 980-989.
3. Candell-Riera J, Bardají A, Castell-Conesa J, Jurado JA, Magriñá J. IV. La cardiología nuclear en la cardiopatía isquémica crónica. Rev Esp Cardiol 1997; 50: 83-91.
4. Castell J, Santana-Boado C, Candell-Riera J et al. La tomogammagrafía miocárdica y el ECG de esfuerzo en el diagnóstico de la enfermedad coronaria multivaso. Rev Esp Cardiol 1997; 50: 635-642.
5. Santana-Boado C, Candell-Riera J, Castell J et al. Diagnostic accuracy of ^{99m}Tc-isonitrile SPET in women and in men. J Nucl Med 1998; 39: 751-755.
6. Amsterdam EA, Price JE, Berman D et al. (1977) Exercise testing in the indirect assessment of myocardial oxygen consumption: application for evaluation of mechanisms and therapy of angina pectoris, in Amsterdam EA, Wilmore JH and DeMaria AN (eds.), Exercise in cardiovascular health and disease, Yorke Medical Books, New York, pp. 218-233.
7. Naughton J (1988) Clinical and physiological adaptations to multistage exercise tests, in Naughton J (ed.), Exercise testing. Physiological, biomechanical and clinical principles, Futura Publishing Company, New York, pp. 63-94.
8. Fletcher GF, Balady G, Froelicher VF et al. Exercise standards. A statement for healthcare professionals from the American Heart Association. Circulation 1995; 91: 580-615.
9. Gibbons RJ, Balady GJ, Beaseley JW et al. ACC/AHH guidelines for exercise testing. J Am Coll Cardiol 1997; 30: 260-315.
10. Gerson MC (1987) Test accuracy, test selection, and test result interpretation in chronic coronary artery disease, in Gerson MC (ed.), Cardiac nuclear medicine, McGraw-Hill Book Company, New York, pp. 309-347.
11. Kaul S, Newell JB, Chesler DA et al. Quantitative thallium imaging findings in patients with normal coronary angiographic findings and in clinically normal subjects. Am J Cardiol 1986; 57: 509-512.
12. McCarthy DM, Blood DK, Sciacca RR et al. Single dose myocardial perfusion imaging with thallium-201: application in patients with nondiagnostic electrocardiographic stress tests. Am J Cardiol 1979; 43; 899-906.
13. Hamilton GW, Narahara KA, Yee H et al. Myocardial imaging with thallium-201: effect of cardiac drugs on myocardial images and absolute tissue distribution. J Nucl Med 1978; 19: 10-16.
14. Brown KA, Rowen M. Impact of antianginal medications, peak heart rate and stress level on the prognostic value of a normal exercise myocardial perfusion imaging study. J Nucl Med 1993; 34: 1467-1471.
15. Steele P, Sklar J, Kirch D et al. Thallium-201 myocardial imaging during maximal and submaximal exercise: comparison of submaximal exercise with propranolol. Am Heart J 1983; 106: 1353-1357.

16. Young DZ, Guiney TE, McKusick KA et al. Unmasking potential myocardial ischemia with dipyridamole thallium imaging in patients with normal submaximal exercise thallium test. Am J Noninvas Cardiol 1987; 1: 11-14.
17. Heller GV, Ahmed I, Tilkemeier PL et al. Influence of exercise intensity on the presence, distribution and size of thallium-201 defects. Am Heart J 1992; 123: 909-916.
18. Hockings B, Saltissi S, Croft DN et al. Effect of beta adrenergic blockade on thallium-201 myocardial perfusion imaging. Br Heart J 1983; 49: 83-89.
19. Martin GJ, Henkin RE, Scanlon PJ. Beta blockers and the sensitivity of the thallium treadmill test. Chest 1987; 92: 486-487.
20. Massie BM, Wisneski J, Kramer B et al. Comparison of myocardial thallium-201 clearance after maximal and submaximal exercise: implications for diagnosis of coronary artery disease: concise comunication. J Nucl Med 1982; 23: 381-385.
21. Kaul S, Chesler DA, Pohost GM et al. Influence of peak exercise heart rate on normal thallium-201 myocardial clearance. J Nucl Med 1986; 27: 26-30.
22. Nordrehaug JE, Danielsen R, Vik-Mo H. Effects of heart rate on myocardial thallium-201 uptake and clearance. J Nucl Med 1989; 30: 1972-1976.
23. Oosterhuis WP, Breeman A, Niemeyer MG et al. Patients with a normal exercise thallium-201 myocardial scintigram: always a good prognosis ?. Eur J Nucl Med 1993; 20: 151-158.
24. Iskandrian AS, Heo J, Kong B et al. The effect of exercise level on the ability of thallium-201 tomographic imaging in detecting coronary artery disease: analysis of 461 patients. J Am Coll Cardiol 1989; 14: 1477-1486.
25. Candell-Riera J (1994) Prognostic evaluation and follow-up of chronic coronary artery disease, in Candell-Riera J and Ortega-Alcalde D (eds.), Nuclear Cardiology in everyday practice, Kluwer Academic Publishers, Dordrecht, pp. 216-240.
26. Castell J, Fraile M, Candell J et al. El rendimiento diagnóstico de la gammmagrafía de esfuerzo con talio y la "mayoría silenciosa". Rev Esp Cardiol 1988; 41: 12-19.
27. Santana-Boado C, Candell-Riera J, Castell-Conesa J et al. Diagnóstico de la enfermedad coronaria mediante la tomogammagrafía de esfuerzo con isonitrilos-tecnecio-99m. Med Clín (Barc.) 1995; 105: 201-204.
28. Beller GA, Zaret BL. Contributions of nuclear cardiology to diagnosis and prognosis of patients with coronary artery disease. Circulation 2000; 101: 1465-1478.
29. Fraile M, Santana-Boado C, Candell-Riera J et al. Exercise SPET ^{99m}Tc-MIBI in diagnosis of coronary artery disease in patients with equivocal electrocardiographic exercise testing. J Nucl Cardiol 1995; 10: P01-039. (Abstr.).
30. Candell-Riera J, Santana-Boado C, Castell-Conesa J et al. Simultaneous dipyridamole /maximal subjective exercise with ^{99m}Tc-MIBI SPECT. Improved diagnostic yield in coronary artery disease. J Am Coll Cardiol 1997; 29: 531-536.
31. Santana-Boado C, Candell-Riera J, Castell J et al. Importancia de los parámetros ergométricos en los resultados de la tomogammagrafía de perfusión miocárdica. Med Clin (Barc) 1997; 109: 406-409.
32. Rutheford JD, Braunwald E (1992) Chronic ischemic heart disease, in Braunwald E (ed.), Heart Disease, W. B. Saunders Company, Philadelphia, pp. 1292-1364.
33. White MP. Pharmacologic stress testing: understanding the options. J Nucl Cardiol 1999; 6: 672-675.
34. Travin MI, Wexler JP. Pharmacological stress testing. Semin Nucl Med 1999; 29: 298-318.
35. Hashimoto A, Palmer EL, Scott JA et al. Complications of exercise and pharmacologic stress tests: differences in younger and elderly patients. J Nucl Cardiol 1999; 6: 612-619.
36. Gould KL, Westcott RJ, Albro PC et al. Noninvasive assessment of coronary stenoses by myocardial imaging during pharmacologic coronary vasodilatation. II. Clinical methodology and feasibility. Am J Cardiol 1978; 41: 279-287.
37. Albro PC, Gould KL, Westcott RJ et al. Noninvasive assessment of coronary stenoses by myocardial imaging during pharmacologic coronary vasodilatation. III. Clinical trial. Am J Cardiol 1978; 42: 751-760.
38. Gould KL. Noninvasive assessment of coronary stenoses by myocardial imaging during pharmacologic coronary vasodilatation. IV. Limits of detection of stenosis with idealized experimental cross-sectional myocardial imaging. Am J Cardiol 1978; 42: 761-768.
39. Ranhosky A, Kempthorne-Rawson J. Intravenous dipyridamole thallium imaging study group. The safety of intravenous dipiridamole thallium myocardial perfusion imaging. Circulation 1990; 81: 1205-1209.

40. Del Rio A, Castro Beiras JM, Asin Cardiel E et al. Talio-201 dipiridamol. Valor diagnóstico en la enfermedad coronaria. Rev Esp Cardiol 1984; 37: 90-94.
41. Hendel RC, Layden JJ, Leppo JA. Prognostic value of dipyridamole thallium scintigraphy for evaluation of ischemic heart disease. J Am Coll Cardiol 1990; 15: 109-116.
42. Picano E. Dipyridamole-echocardiography test: historical background and physiologic basis. Eur Heart J 1989; 10: 365-376.
43. Leppo JA. Dipyridamole-thallium imaging: The lazy man's stress test. J Nucl Med 1989; 30: 291-287.
44. Beller GA. Dipyridamole thallium-201 scintigraphy: an excellent alternative to exercise scintigraphy. J Am Coll Cardiol 1989; 14: 1642-1644.
45. Beller GA. Dipyridamole thallium 201 imaging. How safe is it?. Circulation 1990; 81: 1425-1427.
46. Wackers FJ. Pharmacologic stress with dipyridamole: how lazy can one be?. J Nucl Med 1990; 30: 1024-1027.
47. Galli M, Marcassa C, Bosimini E, Zoccarato O, Comazzi F, Giannuzzi P. ECG-manifest and ECG-silent dipyridamole technetium-99m sestamibi SPET perfusion defects in patients with ischaemic heart disease. Eur J Nucl Med 1997; 24: 160-169.
48. Amanullah AM, Aasa M. Significance of ST segment depression during adenosine-induced coronary hyperemia in angina pectoris and correlation with angiographic, scintigraphic, hemodynamic, and echocardiographic variables. Int J Cardiol 1995; 48: 167-176.
49. Josephson MA, Brown BG, Hecht HS et al. Noninvasive detection and localization of coronary stenoses in patients: Comparison of resting dipyridamole and exercise thallium-201 myocardial perfusion imaging. Am Heart J 1982; 103: 1008-1018.
50. Schelbert HR, Wisenberg G, Phelps ME et al. Noninvasive assessment of coronary stenoses by myocardial imaging during coronary vasodilation. V. Detection of 47% diameter coronary stenosis with intravenous nitrogen-13 ammonia and emission-computed tomography in intact dogs. Am J Cardiol 1979; 43: 200-208.
51. Leppo J, Boucher CA, Okada RD et al. Serial thallium-201 myocardial imaging after dipyridamole infusion: Diagnostic utility in detecting coronary stenoses and relationship to regional wall motion. Circulation 1982; 66: 649-657.
52. Iskandrian AS, Verani MS (1996) Exercise perfusion imaging in coronary artery disease: Physiology and diagnosis, in Iskandrian AS and Verani MS (eds.), Nuclear cardiac imaging: principles and applications. F.A. Davis Company, Philadelphia, pp. 73-143.
53. Sorensen S, Groves B, Chaudhuri T. Regional myocardial blood flow and hemodynamics in man after intravenous dipyridamole. Circulation 1980; 62 (Suppl. III): III-9 (Abstr.).
54. Wilson RF, Laughlin DE, Ackell PH et al. Transluminal, subselective measurement of coronary artery blood flow velocity and vasodilator reserve in man. Circulation 1985; 72: 82-92.
55. Okada RD, Dai Y, Boucher CA, Pohost GM. Serial thallium-201 imaging after dipyridamole for coronary disease detection: Quantitative analysis using myocardial clearance. Am Heart J 1984; 107: 475-485.
56. Hayne MP, Gould FL, Gerson MC (1991) Methods alternative to dynamic leg exercise for detecting chronic coronary artery disease, in Gerson MC (ed.), Cardiac Nuclear Medicine, pp. 273-298.
57. Rockectt JF, Magill HL, Lovelless VS et al. Intravenous Dipyridamole thallium SPECT imaging. Methodology, applications, and interpretations. Clin Nucl Med 1990; 15: 712-725.
58. Picano E, Lattanzi F, Masini M et al. High dose dipyridamole echocardiography test in effort angina pectoris. J Am Coll Cardiol 1986; 8: 848-854.
59. Martínez-Martínez A, Vázquez R, Sánchez A et al. Estudio prospectivo con talio-201 y dipiridamol a dosis bajas como test diagnóstico incruento predictor de lesiones coronarias. Rev Esp Cardiol 1984; 37: 418-424.
60. Loeb HS, Danoviz J, Miller A et al. Effects of oral dipyridamole on coronary dynamics and myocardial metabolism at rest and during pacing-induced angina in patients with coronary artery disease. Am Heart J 1983; 105: 906-910.
61. Segall GM, Davis MJ. Variability of serum drug level following a single oral dose of dipyridamole. J Nucl Med 1988; 29: 1662-1667.
62. Iskandrian AS, Verani MS (1996) Pharmacologic stress testing and other alternative techniques in the diagnosis of coronary artery disease, in Iskandrian AS and Verani MS (eds.), Nuclear cardiac imaging: principles and applications. F.A. Davis Company, Philadelphia, pp. 219-241.
63. Smits P, Boekema P, de Andreu R et al. Evidence for an antagonism between caffeine and adenosine in the human cardiovascular system. J Cardiovasc Pharmacol 1987; 10: 136-143.

64. Fredholm BB, Persson CGA. Xanthine derivates as adenosine receptor antagonists. Eur J Pharmacol 1982; 81: 673-676.
65. Alfonso S. Inhibition of coronary vasodilating action of dipyridamole and adenosine by aminophylline in the dog. Circ Res 1970; 26: 743-752.
66. Holgate ST, Mann JS, Cushley MJ. Adenosine as a bronchoconstrictor mediator in asthma and its antagonism by methylxanthines. J Allergy Clin Immunol 1984; 74: 302-306.
67. Taviot B, Pavheco Y, Coppere B et al. Bronchospasm induced in an asthmatic by the injection of adenosine. Presse Med 1986; 15: 1103-1117.
68. Lette J, Tatum JL, Fraser S et al. Safety of dipyridamole testing in 73,806 patiens: The Multicenter Dipyridamole Safety Study. J Nucl Cardiol 1995; 2: 3-17.
69. Miller DD, Younis LT, Chaitman BR, Stratmann H. Diagnostic accuracy of dipyridamole technetium 99m-labeled sestamibi myocardial tomography for detection of coronary artery disease. J Nucl Cardiol 1997; 4: 18-24.
70. He ZX, Iskandrian AS, Gupta NC, Verani MS. Assessing coronary artery disease with dipyridamole technetium-99m-tetrofosmin SPECT: A multicenter trial. J Nucl Med 1997; 38: 44-48.
71. Primeau M, Taillefer R, Essiambre R et al. Tecnetium 99m SESTAMIBI myocardial perfusion imaging: comparison between treadmill, dipyridamole and trans-oesophageal atrial pacing "stress" tests in normal subjects. Eur J Nucl Med 1991; 18: 247-251.
72. Verani MS, Mahmarian JJ, Hixson JB et al. Diagnosis of coronary artery disease by controlled coronary vasodilation with adenosine and thallium-201 scintigraphy in patients unable to exercise. Circulation 1990; 82: 80-87.
73. Lee J, Chae SC, Kyubo L et al. Biokinetics of thallium-201 in normal subjects: Comparison between adenosine, dipyridamole, dobutamine and exercise. J Nucl Med 1994; 35: 535-541.
74. Miyagawa M, Kumano S, Sekiya M et al. Thallium-201 myocardial tomography with intravenous infusion of adenosine triphosphate in diagnosis of coronary artery disease. J Am Coll Cardiol 1995; 26: 1196-1201.
75. Taillefer R, Amyot R, Turpin S, Lambert R, Pilon C, Jarry M. Comparison between dipyridamole and adenosine as pharmacologic coronary vasodilators in detection of coronary artery disease with thallium 201 imaging. J Nucl Cardiol 1996; 3: 204-211.
76. Nicolai E, Cuocolo A, Pace L et al. Adenosine coronary vasodilation quantitative technetium 99m methoxy isobutyl isonitrile myocardial tomography in the identification and localization of coronary artery disease. J Nucl Cardiol 1996; 3: 9-17.
77. Cuocolo A, Sullo P, Pace L et al. Adenosine coronary vasodilation in coronary artery disease: Technetium-99m tetrofosmin myocardial tomography versus echocardiography. J Nucl Med 1997; 38: 1089-1094.
78. Amanullah AM; Berman DS, Kiat H, Friedman JD. Usefulness of hemodynamic changes during adenosine infusion in predicting the diagnostic accuracy of adenosine technetium-99m sestamibi single-photon emission computed tomography (SPECT). Am J Cardiol 1997; 79: 1319-1322.
79. Cerqueira MD, Verani MS, Schwaiger M, Heo J, Iskandrian AS. Safety profile of adenosine stress perfusion imaging: Results from the adenoscan multicenter trial registry. J Am Coll Cardiol 1994; 23: 384-389.
80. Brown BG, Josephson MA, Peterson RB et al. Intravenous dipyridamole combined with isometric handgrip for near maximal acute increase in coronary flow in patients with coronary artery disease. Am J Cardiol 1981; 48: 1077-1085.
81. Huikuri HV, Korhonen UR, Airaksinen J et al. Comparison of dipyridamole-handgrip test and bicycle exercise test for thallium tomographic imaging. Am J Cardiol 1988; 61: 264-268.
82. Iskandrian AS, Verani MS, Heo J. Pharmacologic stress testing: Mechanism of action, hemodynamic responses, and results in detection of coronary artery disease. J Nucl Cardiol 1994; 1: 94-111.
83. Laarman GJ (1988) Thallium-201 myocardial scintigraphy after dipyridamole infusion, in Laarman GJ (ed.), Utrecht, pp. 27-117.
84. Rossen JD, Simonetti I, Marcus ML et al. Coronary dilation with standard dose dipyridamole and dipyridamole combined with handgrip. Circulation 1989; 79: 566-572.
85. Walker PR, James MA, Wilde PRH et al. Dipyridamole combined with exercise for thallium-201 myocardial imaging. Br Heart J 1986; 55: 321-329.
86. Laarman GJ, Verzijlbergen FJ, Ascoop CA. Ischemic ST segment changes after dipyridamole infusion. Int J Cardiol 1987; 14: 384-386.
87. Laarman GJ, Bruschke AVG, Verzijlbergen FJ et al. Efficacy of intravenous dipyridamole with exercise in thallium-201 myocardial perfusion scintigraphy. Eur Heart J 1988; 9: 1206-1214.

88. Freidrich L. Myocardial ^{201}Tl washout after combined dipyridamole submaximal exercise stress: Reference values from different groups. Eur J Nucl Med 1989; 15: 81-86.

89. Laarman GJ, Bruschke AVG, Verzijlbergen JF et al. Thallium-201 scintigraphy after dipyridamole infusion with low level exercise. II. Quantitative analysis vs visual analysis. Eur Heart J 1990; 11: 162-172.

90. Laarman GJ, Serruys PW, Verzijlbergen JF et al. Thallium-201 scintigraphy after dipyridamole infusion with low-level exercise. III. Clinical significance and additional diagnostic value of ST segment depression and angina pectoris during the test. Eur Heart J 1990; 11: 705-711.

91. Casale PN, Guiney TE, Strauss HW et al. Simultaneous low level treadmill exercise and intravenous dipyridamole stress thallium imaging. Am J Cardiol 1988; 62: 799-802.

92. Verzijlbergen JF, Vermeersch PHMJ, Laarman GJ et al. Inadequate exercise leads to suboptimal imaging. Thallium-201 myocardial perfusion imaging after dipyridamole combined with low-level exercise unmasks ischemia in symptomatic patients with non-diagnostic thallium-201 scans who exercise submaximally. J Nucl Med 1991; 32: 2071-2078.

93. Stren S, Greenberg D, Corne R. Effect of exercise supplementation on Dipyridamole thallium-201 Imaging Quality. J Nucl Med 1991; 32: 1559-1564.

94. Stren S, Greenberg D, Corne R. Quantification of walking exercise improvement of dipiridamole thallium-201 image quality. J Nucl Med 1992; 33: 2061-2066.

95. Ignaszewski AP, McCormick LX, Heslip PG et al. Safety and clinical utility of combined intravenous dipyridamole/symptom-limited exercise stress test with thallium-201 imaging in patients with known or suspected coronary artery disease. J Nucl Med 1993; 34: 2053-2061.

96. Kenneth AB. Exercise-Dipyridamole myocardial perfusion imaging: the circle is now complete. J Nucl Med 1993; 34: 2061-2063.

97. Marten-Jan C, Verzijlbergen JF, Van der Wall EE et al. Head-to-head comparison between technetium-99-sestamibi and thallium-201 tomographic imaging for the detection of coronary disease using combined dipyridamole-exercise stress. J Nucl Cardiol 1994; 5: 787-791.

98. Stein L, Burt R, Oppenheim B et al. Symptom-limited arm exercise increases detection of ischemia during dipyridamole tomographic thallium stress testing in patients with coronary artery disease. Am J Cardiol 1995; 75: 568-572.

99. Hurwitz GA, Saddy S, O'Donoghue et al. The VEX-Test for myocardial scintigrafhy wiht thallium-201 and sestamibi: effect on abdominal background activity. J Nucl Med 1995; 36: 914-920.

100. Candell-Riera J (1992) Pruebas de esfuerzo y de provocación, in Candell-Riera J and Ortega-Alcalde D (eds.), Cardiología Nuclear, Doyma S.A., Barcelona, pp. 44-64.

101. García-Burillo A, Santana-Boado C, Castell-Conesa J et al. Simultaneous Dipyridamole/Exercise SPET ^{99m}Tc-MIBI in the diagnosis of coronary artery disease in patiens with low peak heart rate. J Nucl Cardiol 1995; 10: P1-40 (Abstr).

102. Santana-Boado C, Candell-Riera J, Castell-Conesa J et al. Test simultáneo esfuerzo/dipiridamol asociado a la tomogammafría con tecnecio 99mTc-MIBI en el estudio de la enfermedad arterial coronaria. Rev Esp Cardiol 1995; 48: 88 (Abstr).

103. Santana-Boado C, Candell-Riera J, Castell-Conesa J et al. Tomogammafría de perfusió amb isonotrils-99mTc i esforç+dipiridamol simultani per a l'estudi de la cardiopatia isquèmica. Rev Catalana Cardiol 1995; 1: 30 (Abstr).

104. Van Train KF, García EV, Maddahi J et al. Multicenter trial validation for quantitative analysis of same-day rest-stress technetium-99m-sestamibi myocardial tomogramas. J Nucl Med 1994; 35: 609-618.

105. Van Train KF, Garcia EV, Cooked AJ (1995) Quantitative analysis of SPECT myocardial perfusion, in De Puey EG, Berman DS and Garcia EV(eds.), Cardiac SPECT Imaging, Raven Press, New York, pp. 49-74.

106. Berman DS, Kiat H, Germano G et al. (1995) ^{99m}Tc-Sestamibi SPECT in cardiac SPECT imaging, in De Puey EG, Berman DS and Garcia EV (eds.), Cardiac SPECT imaging, Raven Press, New York, pp. 121-146.

107. Fintel DJ, Links JM, Brinker JA et al. Improved diagnostic performance of exercise thallium-201 single photon emission computed tomography over planar imaging in the diagnosis of coronary artery disease: a receiver operating characteristic analysis. J Am Coll Cardiol 1989; 13: 600-612.

108. Daou D, Le Guludec D, Faraggi M et al. Nonlimited exercise test combined with high-dose dipyridamole for thallium-201 myocardial single-photon emission computed tomography in coronary artery disease. Am J Cardiol 1995; 76: 753-758.

109. Pennell DJ, Mavrogeni SI, Forbat SM et al. Adenosine combined with dynamic exercise for myocardial perfusion imaging. J Am Coll Cardiol 1995; 25: 1300-1309.
110. Gibson RS, Beller GA, Gheorghiade M et al. The prevalence and clinical significance of residual myocardial ischemia 2 weeks after uncomplicated non-Q wave infarction: a prospective natural history study. Circulation 1986; 73: 1186-1198.
111. Brown KA, Weiss RM, Clements JP, Wackers FJ. Uselfulness of residual ischemic myocardium within prior infarct zone for identifying patients at high risk late after acute myocardial infarction. Am J Cardiol 1987; 60: 15-19.
112. Candell-Riera J, Permanyer-Miralda G, Castell J et al. Uncomplicated first myocardial infarction: Strategy for comprehensive prognostic studies. J Am Coll Cardiol 1991; 18: 1207-1219.
113. Gimple LW, Beller GA. Assessing prognosis after acute myocardial infarction in the thrombolytic era. J Nucl Cardiol 1994: 1: 198-209.
114. Olona M, Candell-Riera J, Permanyer-Miralda G et al. Strategies for prognostic assessment of uncomplicated first myocardial infarction: A 5-years follow up study. J Am Coll Cardiol 1995; 25: 815-822.
115. Christian TF, Miller TD, Bailey KR, Gibbons RJ. Noninvasive identification of severe coronary artery disease using exercise tomographic thallium-201 imaging. Am J Cardiol 1992; 70: 14-20.
116. Iskandrian AS, Heo J, Lemlek J, Ogilby JD. Identification of high risk patients with left main and three-vessel coronary artery disease using stepwise discriminant analysis of clinical, exercise, and tomographic thallium data. Am Heart J 1993; 125: 221-225.
117. Candell-Riera J (1994) Diagnosis of coronary artery disease, in Candell-Riera J and Ortega-Alcalde D (eds.), Nuclear Cardiology in everyday practice, Kluwer Academic Publishers, Dordrecht, pp. 187-215.
118. Dunn RF, Freedman B, Bailey IK, Uren R, Kelly DT. Noninvasive prediction of multivessel disease after myocardial infarction. Circulation; 1980; 62: 726-734.
119. Patterson RE, Horowitz SF, Eng C et al. Can noninvasive exercise test criteria identify patients with left main or 3-vessel coronary disease after a first myocardial infarction? Am J Cardiol 1983; 51: 361-372.
120. Abraham RD, Freedman D, Dunn RF et al. Prediction of multivessel coronary artery disease and prognosis early after acute myocardial infarction by exercise electrocardiography and thallium-201 myocardial perfusion scanning. Am J Cardiol 1986; 58: 423-427.
121. Haber HL, Beller GA, Watson DD, Gimple LW. Exercise thallium-201 scintigraphy after thrombolytic therapy with or without angioplasty for acute myocardial infarction. Am J Cardiol 1993; 71: 1257-1261.
122. Candell-Riera J, Santana-Boado C, Castell-Conesa J et al. Dipyridamole administration at the end of an insufficient exercise Tc-99m MIBI SPECT improves detection of multivessel coronary artery disease in patients with previous myocardial infarction. Am J Cardiol 2000; 85: 532-535.
123. ISIS-2 (Second International Study of Infarct Survival) Collaborative Group. Randomized trial of intravenous streptokinase, oral aspirin, both, or neither among 17,187 cases of suspected acute myocardial infarction: ISIS-2. Lancet 1988; 2: 349-360.
124. Kennedy JW, Ritchie JL, Davis KB, Stadius ML, Maynard C, Fritz J. The Western Washington randomized trial of intracoronary streptokinase in acute myocardial infarction: a 12-month follow-up report. N Engl J Med 1985; 312: 1073-1078.
125. Galvani M, Ottani F, Ferrini D, Sorbello F, Rusticali F. Patency of the infarct-related artery and left ventricular function as the major determinants of survival after Q-wave acute myocardial infarction. Am J Cardiol 1993; 71: 1-7.
126. McCully RB, ElZeky F, Van Der Zwaag R, Ramanathan KB, Sullivan JM. Impact of patency of the left anterior descending coronary artery on long-term survival. Am J Cardiol 1995; 76: 250-254.
127. Lamas GA, Vaughan DE, Pfeffer MA. Left ventricular thrombus formation after first anterior wall acute myocardial infarction. Am J Cardiol 1988; 62: 31-35.
128. Gang ES, Lew AS, Hong M, Wang FZ, Siebert CA, Peter T. Decreased incidence of ventricular late potentials after successful thrombolytic therapy for acute myocardial infarction. N Engl J Med 1989; 321: 712-716.
129. Kim CB, Braunwald E. Potential benefits of late reperfusion of infacted myocardium. The open artery hypothesis. Circulation 1993; 88: 2426-2436.
130. DiCarli MF, Asgarzadie F, Schelbert HR et al. Quantitative relation between myocardial viability and improvement in heart failure symptoms after revascularization in patients with ischemic cardiomyopathy. Circulation 1995; 92: 3436-3444.

131. Payne RM, Horowitz LD, Mullins CM. Comparison of isometric exercise and angiotensin infusion as stress test for evaluation of left ventricular function. Am J Cardiol 1973; 31: 428-435.
132. Ross J, Braunwald E. The study of left-ventricular function in man by increasing resistance to ventricular ejection with angiotensin. Circulation 1964; 29: 739-749.
133. Watkins J, Slutski R, Tubau J; Karliner J. Scintigraphic study of relation between left ventricular peak systolic pressure and end-systolic volume in patients with coronary artery disease and normal subjects. Br Heart J 1982; 48: 39-47.
134. Ruskin A. Pitressin test of coronary insufficiency. Am Heart J 1947; 36: 569-579.
135. Stein I. Observations on the action of ergonovine on the coronary circulation and its use in the diagnosis of coronary artery insufficiency. Am Heart J 1949; 37: 36-45.
136. Fuller CM, Raizner AE, Chahine RA et al. Exercise-induced coronary arterial spasm: Angiographic demonstration, documentation of ischemia by myocardial scintigraphy and results of pharmacologic intervention. Am J Cardiol 1980; 46: 500-506.
137. Waters DD, Théroux P, Szlachcic J et al. Ergonovine testing in a Coronary Care Unit. Am J Cardiol 1980; 46: 922-930.
138. Waters DD, Szlachcic J, Théroux P, Dauwe F, Mizgala HF. Ergonovine testing to detect spontaneous remissions of variant angina during long-term treatment with calcium antagonist drugs. Am J Cardiol 1981; 47: 179-184.
139. Waters DD, Théroux P, Slachcic J, Dauwe F. Provocative testing with ergonovine to assess the efficacy of treatment with nifedipine, diltiazem and verapamil in variant angina. Am J Cardiol 1981; 48: 123-130.
140. Ginsburg R, Lamb IH, Bristow MR, Schroeder JS, Harrison DC. Application and safety of outpatient ergonovine testing in accurately detecting coronary spasm in patients with possible variant angina. Am Heart J 1981; 102: 698-702.
141. DiCarlo LA, Botvinick EH, Canhasi BS, Schwartz AS, Chatterjee K. Value of noninvasive assessment of patients with atypical chest pain and suspected coronary spasm using ergonovine infusion and thallium-201 scintigraphy. Am J Cardiol 1984; 54: 744-748.
142. Kronenber MW, Robertson RM, Born ML, Steckley RA, Robertson D, Friesinger GC. Thallium-201 uptake in variant angina: Probable demonstration of myocardial reactive hyperemia in man. Circulation 1982; 66: 1332-1338.
143. Yano H, Hiasa Y, Aihara T, Nakaya Y, Mori H. Inverted U wave in ergonovine-induced vasospastic angina. Clin Cardiol 1987; 10: 633-639.
144. Kugiyama K, Yasue H, Okumura K et al. Simultaneous multivessel coronary artery spasm demonstrated by quantitative analysis of thallium-201 single photon emission computed tomography. Am J Cardiol 1987; 60: 1009-1014.
145. Combs DT, Martin CM. Evaluation of isoproterenol as a method of stress testing. Am Heart J 1974; 87: 711-715.
146. Schechter E, Wilson MF, Kong YS. Physiologic responses to epinephrine infusion: the basis for a new stress test for coronary artery disease. Am Heart J 1983; 105: 554-560.
147. Wisenberg G, Zawadowski AG, Gebhardt VA et al. Dopamine: its potential for inducing left ventricular dysfunction. J Am Coll Cardiol 1985; 6: 84-92.
148. Mason JR, Palac RT, Freeman ML et al. Thallium scintigraphy during dobutamine infusion: nonexercise-dependent screening test for coronary disease. Am Heart J 1984; 107: 481-485.
149. Coma-Canella I. Sensitivity and specificity of dobutamine-electrocardiography test to detect multivessel disease after acute myocardial infarction. Eur Heart J 1990; 11: 249-257.
150. Voth E, Baer FM, Theissen P, Schneider CA, Sechtem U, Schicha H. Dobutamine ^{99m}Tc-MIBI single-photon emission tomography: non-exercise-dependent detection of haemodynamically significant coronary artery stenoses. Eur J Nucl Med 1994; 21: 537-544.
151. Dakik HA, Vempathy H, Verani MS. Tolerance, hemodynamic changes, and safety of dobutamine stress perfusion imaging. J Nucl Cardiol 1996; 3: 410-414.
152. Elhendy A, Geleijnse ML, Roelandt JRTC et al. Dobutamine-induced hypoperfusion without transient wall motion abnormalities: Less severe ischemia or less severe stress? J Am Coll Cardiol 1996; 27: 323-329.
153. Geleijnse ML, Elhendy A, Van Domburg RT et al. Prognostic significance of systolic blood pressure changes during dobutamine-atropine stress technetium-99m sestamibi perfusion scintigraphy in patients with chest pain and known or suspected coronary artery disease. Am J Cardiol 1997; 79: 1031-1035.

154. Kiat H, Iskandrian AS, Villegas BJ, Starling MR, Berman DS. Arbutamine stress thallium-201 single-photon emission computed tomography using a computerized closed-loop delivery system. Multicenter trial for evaluation of safety and diagnostic accuracy. J Am Coll Cardiol 1995; 26: 1159-1167.
155. Khattar RS, Senior R, Joseph D, Lahiri A. Comparison of arbutamine stress 99mTc-labeled sestamibi single-photon emission computed tomographic imaging and echocardiography for detection of the extent and severity of coronary artery disease and inducible ischemia. J Nucl Cardiol 1997; 4: 211-216.

6. MYOCARDIUM IN JEOPARDY

JAUME CANDELL-RIERA and CESAR SANTANA-BOADO

1. Detection of the culprit lesion

Over the past few years the evaluation of coronary artery disease has been, essentially, anatomical and based on the coronary angiography. Recently, greater emphasis has been placed on knowledge of the functional repercussions of a particular coronary stenosis and which may be investigated using perfusion gammagraphy; both procedures, however, may be considered complementary in the assessment of the severity of coronary disease [1].

The coronary angiograph provides information on the anatomical state of the coronary tree and, specifically, on the large epicardial arteries, while perfusion SPET facilitates the evaluation of the grade of ischaemia that a particular stenosis produces [1,2]. In the Hospital General Universitari Vall d'Hebron, approximately half of the perfusion SPET studies were indicated following the results of the coronary angiography. It provides the clinician, apart from the anatomical status, a functional evaluation before a decision is taken on patient therapy.

In a study conducted in our centre [2] the contribution of both studies to the therapeutic decision taken by the cardiologist was analysed. In 85% of the cases the results of both explorations were concordant with respect to the severity of the disease and, in consequence, with respect to the clinical attitude adopted (conservative or revascularisation). Figure 1 shows the indications of the perfusion SPET as a

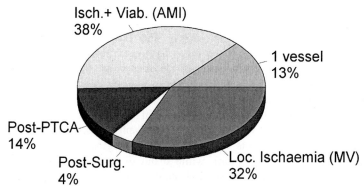

Figure 1. Indications for myocardial SPET as a complement to coronary angiography in the Hospital General Universitari Vall d'Hebron.
Loc. Ischaemia (MV): Localisation of the ischaemia in pacients with multivessel disease, Isch.+Viab. (AMI): Evaluation of ischaemia and viability in patients with prior infarction, Post-PTCA: Evaluation post-angioplasty, Post-Surg.: Evaluation post-surgery, 1 vessel: Functional repercusion of one vessel stenosis.

J. Candell-Riera et al. (eds.), Myocardium at Risk and Viable Myocardium, 119–144.
© 2001 *Kluwer Academic Publishers. Printed in the Netherlands.*

complement to the coronary angiography in this series of patients.

Myocardial perfusion scintigraphy is of considerable use in the procedural indications of partial revascularisation in patients with chronic coronary artery disease [3-6]. In these cases the purpose is to detect the coronary stenosis that provokes the ischaemia and is termed the "culprit lesion". This term is used as being synonymous with the coronary lesion responsible for the patient's ischaemic symptoms [7,8].

Some authors have relied on coronary angiography [8] and others on perfusion scintigraphy [7] to detect the culprit lesion before proceeding to partial revascularisation. The first option occurs, generally, in patients with unstable angina and the latter in stabilised patients.

Wohlgelernter et al. [8] performed coronary angioplasty of the culprit lesion in 27 patients with unstable angina and multivessel disease based on the morphological aspect of the coronary lesion (intraluminal defect, excentric stenosis, subtotal occlusion) observed in the arteriography. Conversely, Breissblatt et al. [7], in a series of 85 patients with multivessel disease and with stable angina, used stress perfusion SPET with ^{201}Tl to identify the culprit lesion on which to perform angioplasty. Only in 6 patients were they unable to detect the culprit lesion using perfusion scintigraphy and, in these cases, the decision was based on the coronary angiography.

Joye et al. [9] demonstrated that the assessment of myocardial ischaemia using perfusion scintigraphy had a good correlation with the reserve coronary flow as determined by Doppler in patients with intermediate coronary stenosis (between 40% and 70%). Hence, in those cases in whom the visual or quantitative assessment of the coronary angiography is not optimum [10-18], perfusion SPET is of considerable use in the assessment of the severity of the ischaemia.

With a view to evaluating the degree of concordance between coronary angiography and scintigraphy in the diagnosis of the culprit lesion, we studied 93 patients with multivessel disease without antecedents of infarct using stress-rest SPET with ^{99m}Tc-MIBI in addition to coronary angiography. "Scintigraphic culprit lesions" were those that produced perfusion defects of high severity and "coronariographic culprit lesions" those with high grade of severity of stenosis. Anterior and septal defects were assigned to the left anterior descending artery, inferior defects to the right coronary, and lateral defects to the circumflex.

Concordance between the coronary angiography and the scintigraphy for the diagnosis of the culprit lesion was 84% and this was higher for the right coronary (91%) and the anterior descending (79%) than for the circumflex (62%). In the 16% of cases in whom no concordance was found between the perfusion SPET and the coronary angiography, this discordance corresponded to problems of the SPET assignment of the ischaemia to the region of the right coronary artery or to the circumflex. Thus, 2 out of 3 cases with coronary angiography culprit lesions of the right coronary artery had been defects of perfusion in the region attributed to the circumflex coronary artery (lateral region), while 6 out of 8 cases with coronary angiography culprit lesion of the circumflex had been perfusion defects in the inferior region.

Twelve of the 17 discrepant cases had triple vessel disease with a similar severity of stenosis in at least two out of the three affected arteries. It is known that some false negative results from perfusion scintigraphy occur especially in patients with triple vessel disease, because homogeneous myocardial ischaemia may exist in these patients and not be detected by scintigraphy. Also, the visual assessment (including quantitation) of the coronary angiography is not always optimum [10-23].

2. Myocardial ischaemia and the occluded artery

Correlation between perfusion scintigraphy and coronary angiography in the assessment of myocardium in jeopardy is not optimum since various factors can influence the results of both explorations [24]. Among these influences are the methods employed for the quantitation of the scintigraphy [25-27] and of the coronary angiography [28-31], the presence of collateral circulation [32-34], the type of stress used to provoke the ischaemia [35,36], the levels of maximum O_2 consumption and of the myocardial O_2 consumption reached during the test [37] and the treatment that the patient had received [38,39].

The extreme case of culprit lesion, from the coronary angiographic point of view, is the occluded artery. Occluded arteries are frequently observed in coronary angiographic studies of patients without previous myocardial infarction. Together with different grades of severity of uptake defects in regions corresponding to the occluded arteries, it highlights the disparity that can exist between a basic anatomical test (coronary angiography), and a functional test (myocardial perfusion scintigraphy).

In our hospital we conducted a study whose purpose was to quantitatively evaluate, in patients without previous infarction, the reversible perfusion defects in the regions dependent on the occluded coronary arteries [40]. We selected 149 patients with demonstrated coronary artery disease and without previous infarction. We performed a SPECT perfusion study with ^{99m}Tc-MIBI and a coronary angiography within an interval no greater than 3 months of the isotopic study. The patients were divided into two groups, with respect to the coronary stenosis in the mayor/major/ greater epicardial arteries:

- Group 1: 95 patients (64%) with no occluded coronary artery and with at least one coronary artery with stenosis between 50% and 99%.
- Group 2: 54 patients (36%) with at least one coronary stenosis of 100%.

In all the patients we performed a limited stress test for symptoms using bicycle. Of these patients, 50 who had an insufficient stress test had intravenous dipyridamole (0.14 mg/kg/min) administered simultaneously with the excercise test and which was prolonged with the maximum load tolerable to the patient [36].

In addition to a subjective quantification of the reversible defects, a special program of quantification of the reversibility of the perfusion defects over the polar maps was applied and which generated a map of the "rest minus stress difference" or "reversibility" [36]. Each map was divided into the following regions: anterior-septal, apical, inferior and lateral (Figure 2). With this map the site and extent of the regions was assessed with respect to a difference in uptake between rest and stress >10% i.e. the reversibility of the defect in the two groups. In the 54 patients of Group 2, the results of good and poor collateral circulation were compared. The presence of collateral circulation in the patients with 100% stenosis was assessed with the following criteria [32-34]: Grade 0 = without evidence of collaterals; Grade 1 =

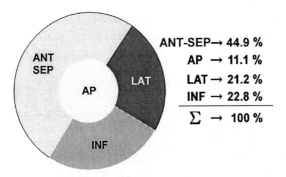

ANT-SEP→ 44.9 %

AP → 11.1 %

LAT → 21.2 %

INF → 22.8 %

Σ → 100 %

Figure 2. Polar map with the percentage territory corresponding to each region.

visible collaterals but without epicardial vessel filling; Grade 2 = partial filling of the epicardial vessel; Grade 3 = complete filling of the epicardial vessel.

The results of the visual analysis of the scintigraphy for each of the major epicardial arteries are presented in Table 1. While no scintigraphy was normal in the patients with descending anterior and right coronary arteries occluded, in the half of the cases with occluded circumflex no reversible defects were observed. The patients with occluded left anterior coronary artery showed a higher percentage of moderate and severe perfusion defects (50% vs 16% and 25% vs 6%, respectively; p<0.001) with respect to those patients with stenosis between 50% and 90%. The patients with occlusion of the right coronary artery showed a higher percentage of severe perfusion defects (56% vs 6%; p>0.001) with respect to the patients with stenosis between 50% and 99%. No significant differences were observed for the circumflex.

TABLE 1. Results of the visual analysis of the SPET in the regions corresponding to the arteries with stenosis between 50% and 90% and the occluded arteries.

LEFT ANTERIOR DESCENDING			
	Stenosis 50%-99% n: 105		Stenosis 100% n: 20
Normal	37 (35%)	p= 0.001	0
Mild Defect	45 (43%)	p= 0.13	5 (25%)
Moderate Defect	17 (16%)	p< 0.001	10 (50%)
Severe Defect	6 (6%)	p< 0.001	5 (25%)
RIGHT CORONARY			
	Stenosis 50%-99% n: 70		Stenosis 100% n: 27
Normal	18 (26%)	p= 0.003	0
Mild Defect	35 (50%)	p= 0.01	6 (22%)
Moderate Defect	13 (19%)	p= 0.68	6 (22%)
Severe Defect	4 (6%)	p< 0.001	15 (56%)
CIRCUMFLEX			
	Stenosis 50%-99% n: 61		Stenosis 100% n: 22
Normal	30 (49%)	p= 0.94	11 (50%)
Mild Defect	22 (36%)	p= 0.12	4 (18%)
Moderate Defect	7 (11%)	p= 0.20	5 (23%)
Severe Defect	2 (3%)	p= 0.27	2 (9%)

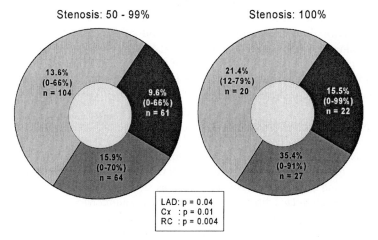

Figure 3. Minimum, maximum and mean values of the extent of ischaemia in the regions corresponding to arteries stenosed between 50% and 99% and occluded arteries.
RC: Right coronary, CX: Circumflex, LAD: Left anterior descending.

The degree of reversibility in the regions corresponding to the occluded arteries was significantly greater to that of the arteries with stenosis between 50% and 90%, both for the anterior descending coronary artery as well as for the right and the circumflex (Figure 3). The range of the reversibility in the regions corresponding to the occluded arteries was very wide for each of the three coronary arteries. The range of the reversibility in the regions corresponding to the occluded arteries with good collateral circulation was less (albeit not reaching statistical significance) than that of the occluded arteries with bad collateral circulation (Figure 4).

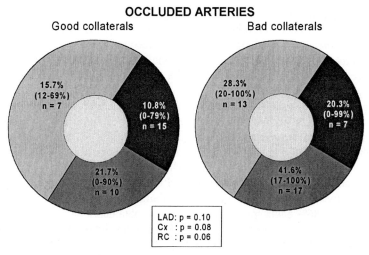

Figure 4. Minimum, maximum and mean values of the extent of ischaemia in the regions corresponding to occluded arteries with good and bad collateral circulation.
CX: Circumflex, LAD: Left anterior descending, RC: Right coronary.

From these results one can conclude that in patients without infarction: 1) occlusions of the left anterior descending coronary artery and of the right coronary artery invariably produce reversible defects (as assessed by the ^{99m}Tc-MIBI SPET) while occlusions of the circumflex do so in only half of the cases; 2) the extent of ischaemia is greater in the regions dependent on an occluded coronary artery, and even more so in the absence of good collateral circulation.

3. Diagnosis of multivessel disease

The diagnosis of the multivessel disease using perfusion scintigraphy is based principally on the detection of reversible defects of perfusion in more than one coronary region and on other indirect signs such as slow washout of ^{201}Tl, transitory ischaemic left ventricular dilation and post-stress pulmonary uptake of the radionuclide.

Pollock et al. [41], in a series of 383 patients studied with^{201}Tl, observed that the probability of multivessel disease was >80% in those patients with more than one ischaemic territory, with ischaemic depression on the ECG and >58 years of age. This probability was <5% when the scintigraphy with ^{201}Tl and the exercise ECG was not pathological and the age of the patient was <58 years. In a series of 688 consecutive patients, Christian et al. [42] observed that the magnitude of the ST segment depression and the extent of the perfusion defects were the most significant, independent predictors in the diagnosis of multivessel disease. Iskandrian et al. [43], in a series of 834 patients studied with stress SPET with ^{201}Tl , the three independent predictor variables of left main stenosis and triple vessel disease were the depression of the ST segment, the heart rate frequency and the number of defects observed in the SPET.

Gewirtz et al. [44] observed that a slow thallium clearance in zones with apparently normal post-stress uptake was useful in identifying patients with triple vessel disease which could, occasionally, present segmental defects in post-stress perfusion scintigraphy. Similar results were obtained by Bateman et al. [45] with submaximal stress tests. Nevertheless, it needs to be taken into account that a clear relationship exists between the cardiac heart rate attained and the clearance level of ^{201}Tl. Thus, a slow clearance of ^{201}Tl may be observed in the submaximal stress test without it signifying myocardial ischaemia [46].

In a series of 105 consecutive patients with suspected coronary artery disease, Maddahi et al. [47] observed that, although the specificity of abnormal responses of arterial pressure, electrocardiogram and visual analysis of the ^{201}Tl were high (98%, 88% and 96%, respectively) in diagnosing left main stenosis or triple vessel disease, the sensitivity was very low (14%, 45% and 16%, respectively). However, when the data derived from the arterial blood pressure and electrocardiogram were combined with the quantitative analysis of the regional distribution and of the clearance of the ^{201}Tl, a sensitivity of 86% and a specificity of 76% was obtained.

The presence of pulmonary post-stress ^{201}Tl uptake is an index of left ventricular dysfunction and/or multivessel disease [48-52]. Its assessment can be visual or quantitative and needs to be performed early after the exercise since, as has been demonstrated, a diminution of the pulmonary activity occurs within 18 minutes after the stress and, as such, the sensitivity of this sign diminishes [47]. A relationship between maximum pulmonary activity and myocardial activity of the segment with maximum uptake >0.55 is indicative of the presence of severe coronary disease [51].

Another sign of severity in perfusion scintigraphy that is related to the presence of post-stress ventricular dysfunction is ischaemic dilation of the left ventricle. Manno et al. [53] observed that a ratio of the thickness of the ventricular wall to the diameter of the cavity (measured in the left anterior oblique projection) of <0.7 was associated with an ejection fraction < 49% and large ventricular volumes. Weiss et al. [54] observed that post-stress left ventricular area to rest ratio >1.12 indicated the possibility of critical stenosis in 2 or 3 vessels. This criterion, in their series, had a sensitivity of 60% and a specificity of 95% for the diagnosis of the critical multivessel disease. These values were significantly greater to other markers of severity such as defects in multiple territories and/or abnormalities in ^{201}Tl clearance.

Combining these supplementary perfusion scintigraphy indicators of severe ischaemia with the signs of severity in the stress electrocardiogram improves the results of either test considered separately [55,56]. In practice, perfusion scintigraphy with ^{201}Tl is almost always used together with the conventional stress test. Using both severity criteria (electrocardiography and scintigraphy) Canhasi et al. [57] obtained a positive predictive value for the diagnosis of multivessel disease of 93% and a negative predictive value of 97%.

To investigate the diagnostic performance of myocardial SPET with ^{99m}Tc-MIBI in the prediction of multivessel disease, we studied 231 consecutive patients without previous infarct (104 with multivessel disease) for whom we had coronary angiograms [58]. The SPET was considered positive for multivessel disease on the basis of 2 criteria: one visual and consisted of observation of reversible perfusion defects in more than one coronary region (Plate 6.1) and the other quantitative and consisted of developing a scoring scale proportional to the extent and severity of the post-stress defects (maximum score: 65) [24] (Figure 5). The cut-off point that best discriminated between one vessel and multivessel disease (score 20/65) was determined using logistic regression analysis. ST segment depression of >1 mm (horizontal or descending) on exercise ECG was considered positive for multivessel disease.

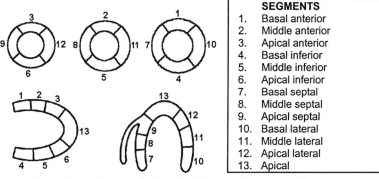

Figure 5. Myocardial SPET score used at the Hospital General Universitari Vall d'Hebron [24].

Results showed that stress myocardial SPET had a higher sensitivity than the exercise test in the diagnosis of multivessel disease although the results were not optimum (65% vs 34%; p<0.0001). For both tests, the specificity (87% and 87%) and negative predictive value (76% vs 72%) were acceptable and similar for both studies. This has been observed by several authors [59,60].

Bivariate analysis showed significant differences between the patients with single vessel and those with multivessel disease in four parameters: decrease in ST>1mm (p<0.01), decrease in ST corrected for heart rate (p<0.005), reversible defects in more than one region (p<0.009) and scintigraphic score (p<0.002). With multivariate analysis we could determine that the patients with a score >20 had a probability of 84% of having multivessel disease.

These results improve slightly when combined with the criterion of ST segment depression >1mm. When both criteria were combined the probability of presenting with multivessel disease was 90% while that of not fulfilling either of the two was 16%. When this same analysis was performed while adding to the series those individuals without coronary stenosis, the probability of multivessel disease in a patient with a score <20 and with a negative stress test was <5%.

It seems clear that SPET is a technique sufficient for the detection of the ischaemic regions but not to identify all the stenosed coronary arteries. What needs to be taken into account is the co-existence of stenosis in the different coronary arteries that could induce signs of myocardial ischaemia necessitating interruption of the stress test when hypoperfusion is only evident in the most critically threatened territory while, as yet, no significant defects are apparent in other regions and which would have required a higher stress to show-up as hypo-uptake on the perfusion images.

As such, using perfusion SPET with ^{99m}Tc-MIBI, the detection of reversible defects in more than one coronary region or the score of severity and extent of these defects together with the signs of severe ischaemia in the ECG, are the criteria that best predict the presence of multivessel disease. When the combined techniques are employed, analysis of the clearance of the radionucleide is not a valuable parameter since the phenomenon of redistribution as observed with ^{201}Tl, is practically non-existent. Increase in post-stress pulmonary uptake, as well, has been demonstrated to be an indicator of severity and the SPET investigation with ^{201}Tl [61], despite being very effective with the combined technique (Plate 6.2), is a parameter that is not usually systematically quantified in the tomographic studies. Transitory ischaemic dilation of the left ventricle, whether after physical stress [62] or after the administration of dipyridamole [63], is another sign that has been described in studies using SPET. However, its value is relative when it is taken into account that, with the combination techniques, post-stress detection is not performed immediately following the exercise.

4. Clandestine ischaemia, silent ischaemia and angina

It had been establish during the 70s, using exercise ECG [64] and Holter [65], that angina does not always accompany myocardial ischaemia. The ischaemia detected in exercise ECG or in Holter and without anginal pain had been termed "silent". In the

80s studies attempting to assess the prognostic value of silent [66] ischaemia were performed. In the 90s investigations were directed towards the evaluation of different therapies for the reduction of silent ischaemia [67-69] while, at the same time, improving the precision of the techniques in the diagnosis of this asymptomatic ischaemia [70-73]

Among the techniques are those that evaluate myocardial perfusion [70,72] and those that evaluate myocardial function: echocardiography [72-74] and radionuclide ventriculography [71]. These are more sensitive than ECG since the detection of ischaemia is earlier. For example, using continuous monitoring of ventricular function with radionuclide ventriculography, it has been demonstrated that the appearance of systolic dysfunction precedes the appearance of pain in episodes of symptomatic ischaemia by 30-90 seconds [75].

Owing to the greater sensitivity of perfusion SPET compared to exercise electrocardiography [76], it is not infrequently observed that patients show unquestionable perfusion defects but without ischaemic changes in the ECG and without angina. To define this situation, the terms of clandestine ischemia [77-79] or truly silent ischemia [80] have been coined.

Several studies (using Holter ECG monitoring [81,82], coronary angiography [70,82-87], radionuclide ventriculography [71,83,84], perfusion gammagraphy [70,72,82,86] and stress echocardiography [73,74]) have compared the alterations of contractile function, the extent of ischaemia and the coronary lesions in patients that present with episodes of silent ischaemia relative to those with episodes of angina.

In monitored patients with unstable angina, the more severe episodes of ischaemia in the ECG produce, in general, more symptomology than those episodes of lesser duration. Similarly, in the stress test as in the Holter, ischaemic changes in the ECG are observed prior to the appearance of angina. Nevertheless, the relationship between the angina and the extent of perfusion defects during the stress is not so evident. Gasparetti et al. [70] and Hecht et al. [80] did not encounter any relationship between the appearance of angina and the extent of the perfusion defects with [201]Tl. Klein et al. [82], on the other hand, demonstrated a certain relationship between the extent of the reversibility of the scintigraphy perfusion defects and the anginal symptomatology.

From the metabolic viewpoint, the extent of the relatively hypo-perfused myocardium may not necessarily reflect the quantity of ischaemic tissue. In this sense, the techniques of evaluating contractile function (echocardiography, radionuclide ventriculography) can show better correlation between the severity of the disorder and the appearance of angina. Although this has been observed in some studies [74,84], in others there have not been differences between the episodes that result in angina and those that show-up only as electrocardiographic changes of ischaemia [71,73,83,88]. Radionuclide stress ventriculography has demonstrated that abnormalities in ventricular function precede the electrocardiographic changes suggestive of ischaemia and angina [77,78]. These studies re-affirm that the sensitivity of the clinical criteria and electrocardiography in the diagnosis of myocardial ischaemia is limited and that it is possible, with non-invasive methods, to detect myocardial ischaemia in the absence of ST segment decrease in the ECG and of angina (clandestine ischaemia).

On the other hand, with perfusion scintigraphy studies, it is relatively frequent to detect reversible defects without the patient having presented signs of ischaemia on the ECG or angina during the ergometric provocation test. Despite this, assessment of clandestine ischaemia using perfusion scintigraphy has attracted slight attention in the clinical literature [79]. There have not been any studies assessing the extent of the ischaemic defects in treated patients with demonstrated coronary artery disease with clandestine ischaemia compared to those patients with silent ischaemia and those that present with angina.

With this in mind, we studied a series of 85 consecutive patients with coronary disease without prior infarct and who were under treatment. In these patients we performed a maximum stress test and a perfusion SPET with ^{99m}Tc-MIBI. The patients were divided into three groups according to clinical presentation: angina during the stress test (angina group); decrease in ST segment >1mm without angina (silent ischaemia group); and reversible perfusion defect without decrease in ST segment >1mm nor angina during the stress test (clandestine ischaemia group).

Assessment of myocardial uptake was by consensus of expert observers without knowledge of the coronary angiography results. The SPET was divided into 13 segments each being scored from 1 to 5 according to the severity of the ischaemia (maximum score = 65) [24] (Figure 5). The extent of the ischaemia (uptake at rest - uptake at stress >10%) was assessed for each group and in each of the regions of the polar map of the left ventricle with respect to the affected artery. The anterior and septal regions were assigned to the left anterior descending, the lower region to the right coronary and the lateral region to the circumflex.

The SPET and catheterisation results in the three groups are summarised in Table 2. There were no significant differences between the three groups of patients with respect to the percentage of patients with light and moderate defects. However, the percentage of severe defects (11% vs 39%; p = 0.004) and the SPET score of the patients with clandestine ischaemia was less that that of the patients with silent ischaemia (25 ± 8 vs 32 ± 9; p = 0.008). Significant differences were observed between these patients and those with angina. The coronary angiography, as well, showed lower scores in the group with clandestine ischaemia. When the extent of the perfusion defects for each of the regions according to the artery affected were compared (Figure 6), those patients with clandestine ischaemia showed a lower extent of ischaemia in all the regions, albeit these differences did not reach statistical significance.

As such then, treated patients with coronary disease that have clandestine ischaemia in stress SPET with ^{99m}Tc-MIBI, show less severity of ischaemia and coronary lesions than patients with silent ischaemia.

Williams et al. [79] observed, in a group of 38 patients with coronary disease (19 with prior stress angina, 18 with prior revascularisation surgery, 14 with prior infarct and 5 with prior angioplasty), that clandestine ischaemia (detected using SPET with ^{201}Tl or with stress radionuclide ventriculography) was more frequent when the stress tests were performed using bicycle (82%) than with the treadmill (42%). Myocardial O_2 consumption was greater when the former was modality is employed and, hence, for which reason the number of patients that presented with symptoms or changes in the ECG, as well, was greater. In our series, the percentage of patients with clandestine ischaemia was 53% (45/85) but the characteristics of the patients were totally different in that patients with infarction and those revascularised had been

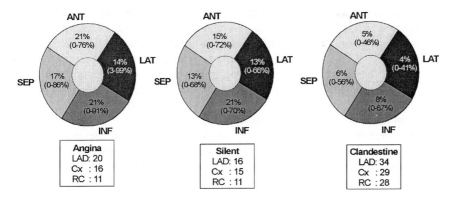

Figure 6. Extent of the ischaemia in each region and with respect to the affected artery in patients with angina, silent ischaemia and clandestine ischaemia during the stress test performed while under treatment. ANT: Anterior, RC: Right Coronary, CX: Circumflex, INF: Inferior, LAD: Anterior Descending, LAT: Lateral, SEP: Septal.

excluded. However, we had used the ergometric bicycle and it could be possible that this percentage would have been lower had the treadmill been employed.

TABLE 2. Results of ^{99m}Tc-MIBI SPET and coronary angiography in patients with angina, silent ischaemia and clandestine ischaemia.

SPET	ANGINA	SILENT	CLANDESTINE
Number	22	18	45
Mild defects	7 (32%)	5 (28%)	20 (44%)
Moderate defects	9 (41%)	6 (33%)	20 (44%)
Severe defects	6 (27%)	7 (39%)	5 (11%) [a]
SPET score	27 ± 8	32 ± 9	25 ± 8 [b]

CATHETERISATION	ANGINA	SILENT	CLANDESTINE
LVEF (%)	57 ± 13	59 ± 8	56 ± 9
1 vessel	5 (23%)	1 (6%)	16 (35%)
2 vessels	9 (41%)	10 (56%)	12 (27%)
3 vessels	8 (36%)	7 (39%)	17 (38%)
Coronary angiography score	27 ± 8	30 ± 7	24 ± 8 [c]

[a]: p = 0.004 vs SILENT, [b]: p = 0.008 vs SILENT, [c]: p = 0.008 vs SILENT,
LVEF: Left ventricular ejection fraction

5. Quantification of jeopardised myocardium

Classification of the extent of coronary disease as single, double and triple vessel disease has been very useful in assessing the prognosis of the patient with coronary artery disease and for the selection of patients for revascularisation [89-91]. However, this criterion is too simple and does not take into account the limitations such as, right or left dominance. In 10% of patients the left system is dominant and, in these cases, irrigation of the territory by the right coronary may be insignificant. Another example is the difference in distribution such as that contributed by the anterior descending artery. In some cases the artery has a very short course without reaching the apex while, in other cases, the inferior-apical part may be reached by the anterior descending artery after it has branched into a long diagonal that irrigates the lateral wall as well as the septals and, as such, irrigating two thirds of the septum [92]. Due to these differences, several systems have been designed for scoring the coronary angiography [93-99] although not with the intent of assessing the extent of the ischaemia as has been adopted for perfusion SPET.

The term "myocardium in jeopardy" is usually used to define the extent of the myocardium threatened by all the stenosed coronary arteries although, it refers to the quantity of the myocardium that could be infarcted by occlusion only of the most stenosed coronary artery [92].

The anatomy-function correlation of coronary lesions is not optimum [93] and it is becoming increasingly apparent that the therapeutic management of the diseased artery necessitates a complementary functional documentation such as a conventional stress test or a perfusion scintigraphy [100-103]. The latter test provides more precise information regarding the localisation, extent and severity of the ischaemia which, in some cases, is vital [104].

Independent of the methodology and interpretation (visual or quantitative) of the explorations, the effects of exercise on the myocardium have to be taken into account. As has been explained in the previous chapter, the treatment that the patient followed and the type of stress performed can influence the result of the SPET.

Different SPET scores have been used to assess the jeopardised myocardium and to establish the patient's prognosis. It is customary to quantify the uptake of the radiotracer in stress [104,105] or the difference in uptake between stress and rest (reversibility) [106-108] but, in the case of the ^{201}Tl, it is possible to quantify the clearance as well [109].

Correlations between different quantitative SPET methods for the assessment of the extent of the perfusion defects have been very acceptable, as has been demonstrated by the results of Ceriani et al. [110]. Three quantitative methods for the assessment of myocardium-at-risk with ^{99m}Tc-MIBI SPET were compared. The first was a planimetric method applied to the polar map by Verani et al. [111] and the other two were the methods validated by Tamaki et al. [112] and O'Connor et al. [113].

In our hospital we evaluated the correlation between the coronary angiography and perfusion SPET in the quantification of the jeopardised myocardium. We studied 159 patients with coronary artery disease without previous infarction [114] and in whom we performed a stress-rest SPET with ^{99m}Tc-MIBI within an interval of <3 months of the haemodynamic study.

The scoring system for the SPET was our own (as described above) and which assessed the number of segments affected as well as the grade of perfusion defect (maximum score: 65) [24] (Figure 5).

For the quantification of the myocardium-at-risk, three different coronary angiography scores were evaluated:

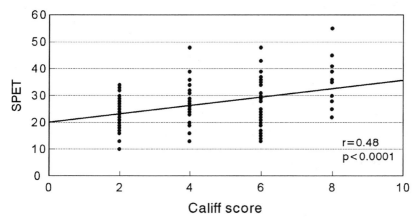

	Site of stenosis
LAD	Left anterior descending
DIAG	Diagonal
SEPT	Septal
LCx	Left circumflex
OM	Obtuse marginal
RCA	Right coronary artery

Stenosis score	
0	< 75%
2	≥ 75%

Figure 7. Califf coronary angiography [94] score and its correlation with the SPET score.

1. Califf scoring [94]: In the "Califf scoring", the coronary circulation was divided into 6 coronary segments and a score of 2 points for each stenosis >75% (maximum score: 12) was assigned to each segment (Figure 7).
2. Gensini scoring [95,96]: In the modified "Gensini scoring", 11 coronary segments were assessed and assigned to each was a score as a function of the grade of each stenosis (maximum score: 72) (Figure 8).
3. Our own scoring: The coronary tree was divided into three segments, scoring each between 1 and 5 as a function of the severity of stenosis while taking into account the presence of collateral circulation (subtracting one point) in the cases of coronary occlusion (maximum score: 65) (Figure 9).

The correlations between the SPET score and the different coronary angiography scores for the myocardium at risk were significant, although not optimal. The correlations improved with increasing complexity of the scoring system (r = 0.48 for the Califf method, r = 0.59 for the modified Gensini and r = 0.65 for our method) (Figures 7 to 9).

These results are in accord with those of other authors who, similarly, had observed a poor correlation between the extent of the myocardium-at-risk and the SPET and the severity of the coronary stenosis [115-119]. Haronian et al. [116] observed, using injection of ^{99m}Tc-MIBI during balloon inflation in the course of angioplasty, that the area-at-risk (as estimated by coronary angiography) did not correlate satisfactorily with the quantification of the hypo-perfused area in the tomogammagraphy. Coronary angiography can underestimate the role of the collateral circulation. Indeed, in our series of patients, the best correlation was observed with our own coronary

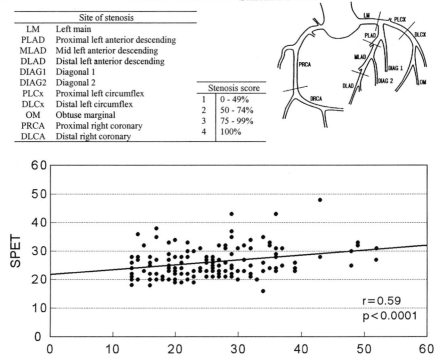

Site of stenosis	
LM	Left main
PLAD	Proximal left anterior descending
MLAD	Mid left anterior descending
DLAD	Distal left anterior descending
DIAG1	Diagonal 1
DIAG2	Diagonal 2
PLCx	Proximal left circumflex
DLCx	Distal left circumflex
OM	Obtuse marginal
PRCA	Proximal right coronary
DLCA	Distal right coronary

Stenosis score	
1	0 - 49%
2	50 - 74%
3	75 - 99%
4	100%

Figure 8. Gensini coronary angiography score [95,96] and its correlation with the SPET score.

angiographic scoring which was the only one that took into account the collateral circulation in those cases which had occluded coronary arteries.

Since it is known that it is not necessarily the most stenosed artery that would invariably be responsible for the future infarct [119-121], it would be more logical to use the term "myocardium in jeopardy" to define the extent of the myocardium that could infarct from the occlusion of the coronary artery with the most severe lesion [122]. In our series, the best correlation (r = 0.85) between the myocardium-at-risk as evaluated with the SPET and that determined by the coronary angiography (our own scoring) was obtained by considering only the culprit lesion (Figure 10). This is not unexpected when it is taken into account that perfusion SPET does not facilitate an absolute quantification of the coronary flow but provides information only on the most hypo-perfused region with respect to the least hypo-perfused.

In conclusion, the correlation between coronary angiography and SPET in the evaluation of the myocardium at risk is not optimum when the intention is to quantify territories threatened by all stenosed coronary arteries but it does clearly improve the assessment of the myocardium at risk resulting specifically from the culprit lesion.

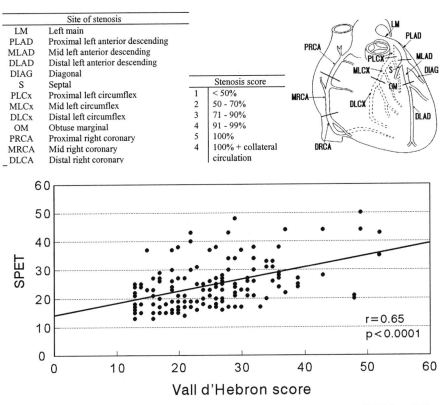

	Site of stenosis
LM	Left main
PLAD	Proximal left anterior descending
MLAD	Mid left anterior descending
DLAD	Distal left anterior descending
DIAG	Diagonal
S	Septal
PLCx	Proximal left circumflex
MLCx	Mid left circumflex
DLCx	Distal left circumflex
OM	Obtuse marginal
PRCA	Proximal right coronary
MRCA	Mid right coronary
DLCA	Distal right coronary

	Stenosis score
1	< 50%
2	50 - 70%
3	71 - 90%
4	91 - 99%
5	100%
4	100% + collateral circulation

r = 0.65
p < 0.0001

Figure 9. Coronary angiography score used at the Hospital General Universitari Vall d'Hebron [24] and its correlation with the SPET score.

6. Prognostic value of SPET

Up to this point we have described the complementary roles of perfusion SPET and coronary angiography and it is evident that if they do not offer improved management of patients with coronary artery disease, then there would be little sense in recommending their use. However, several studies have put forward the proposal that perfusion scintigraphy increases the prognostic value as do conventional exercise test and coronary angiography in the patients without [123-137] and with prior myocardial infarction [137-140]. This applies to the use of stress as a provocation manoeuvre but also to the use of dipyridamole [141], adenosine [142] and dobutamine [143-146] as well.

Machecourt et al. [146] in a 33 ± 10 months of follow-up of 1926 patients who had had a myocardial SPET with [201]Tl (1121 with exercise and 805 with dipyridamole), observed a mortality rate of 0.42% per year in patients with a negative test and of 2.1% in those in whom the results of the test had been considered abnormal. Further,

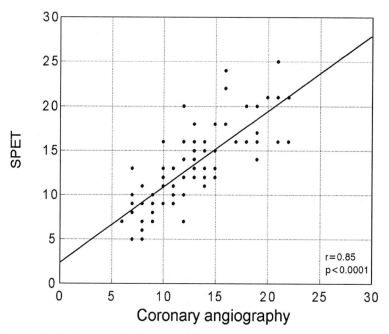

Figure 10. Correlation between the SPET score and the coronary angiography of the myocardium at risk [24] corresponding to the culprit lession alone.

they observed a significant relationship between the number of abnormal segments and mortality (p<0.02).

Iskandrian et al. [147] investigated the increase in prognostic value of stress SPET with ^{201}Tl in 316 patients in a follow-up of 28 months. Bivariate analysis demonstrated that exercise level, extent of coronary disease, ejection fraction and possitivity of the ^{201}Tl were the variables with significant prognostic value while the extent of the perfusion defects was the variable with the greatest predictive power. Further, the information obtained with ^{201}Tl-SPET significantly increased the prognostic value of the cardiac catheterisation (p<0.01). In another study [124] from the same group in which the follow-up was over 29 months (316 patients with and 121 without coronary artery disease), the predictive power for complications (infarction and death) of the score derived from the ^{201}Tl stress SPET was significantly greater than the score obtained from the data of the conventional stress and improved, as well, the predictive power of catheterisation.

Stratmann et al. [148] followed-up over 13±5 months 521 patients investigated with stress ^{99m}Tc-MIBI SPET (short protocol) and observed that not only the extent of the post-stress but also the reversible defects were independent predictors of infarction and death of cardiac origin.

Our experience, as well, furthers these conclusions, as well. In our hospital we investigated the prognosis of medically treated patients with clandestine myocardial ischaemia compared to those with silent myocardial ischaemia and those with angina pectoris in a series of 120 patients without previous myocardial infarction. All patients underwent a symptom-limited exercise on a bicycle ergometer, myocardial

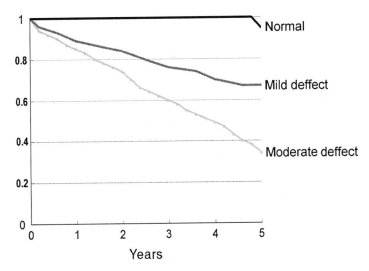

Figure 11. Survival curves free of severe complications (death, infarction and/or re-vascularisation) in those patients with normal myocardial stress SPET, with reversible mild defects and with moderate or severe reversible defects.

perfusion ^{99m}Tc-MIBI SPET and coronary angiography. They were classified into 3 groups (angina group, 34 patients; silent group, 20 patients; and the clandestine group, 58 patients). During the follow-up (mean 3.6 years, range 6 months to 5.5 years) 9 patients died (5%), another 9 (5%) suffered a non-fatal infarct and 53 (32%) were revascularised (30 by PTCA and 27 by surgery). Only angina and severe reversible SPET defects were predictive for cardiac events: death + myocardial infarction + revascularization [149,150] (Figure 11).

Although some authors [151] have recommended routine cardiac catheterisation and coronary arteriography in all patients after acute myocardial infarction, reports [152-155] that compared outcomes of patients assigned to routine coronary arteriography with those of patients assigned to conservative management without routine coronary arteriography have not found differences in the rates of death, nonfatal infarction, or myocardial revascularisation procedures. Based on previous studies [138,139] carried out in our hospital, cardiac catheterisation is not routinely performed after a first uncomplicated myocardial infarction.

The detection of residual ischemia is the most relevant prognostic factor after a first uncomplicated myocardial infarction in the thrombolytic era. However, the number of patients with silent ischaemia, either detected by exercise ECG, stress echo or SPET, is lower at the present time. In order to evaluate the prognostic value of stress echo and gated single photon emission computed tomography after a first uncomplicated acute myocardial infarction we prospectively studied 103 consecutive patients aged <70 years with a first acute myocardial infarction with predischarge maximal subjective exercise echo and gated SPET with ^{99m}Tc-tetrofosmin [156]. During a 12-month follow up period, 2 patients died, 9 developed cardiac failure and 29 (28%) developed ischaemic complications (4 reinfarction and 25 angina). Predictive variables for cardiac failure in multivariate analysis was ejection fraction evaluated by echo (OR:8.5, p=0.016) or by gated SPECT (OR:10.7, p=0.009), and for ischaemic complications were <5 METs in exercise test (OR:5.2, p=0.007) and >15% ischaemic extent in the polar map (OR:3.6, p=0.04) of SPECT. We concluded that exercise echocardiography and ^{99m}Tc-tetrofosmin gated SPET were predictive for cardiac failure but SPECT was the only test with predictive power for ischaemic complications (Figure 12). In this study none of the stress-echo parameters was predictive of ischaemic complications. This observation is discordant with respect to the results of other series in which ischaemia dectected by exercise echo was predictive of ischaemic complications [157-160] but confirms the opinion of Brown [161] that, after a revision of the two largest studies [162,163] of post-myocardial risk stratification with stress echocardiography, found no significant prognostic value of echocardiographically-defined ischaemia.

In line of other studies that have observed a higher sensitivity of radionuclide techniques for the detection of multivessel disease [164,165] and post-infarction complications [166,167], in our series gated SPET was more sensitive for the detection of residual ischemia. Only in 20% of patients new contractility alterations at least in one segment were detected with echo after exercise stress test, whereas reversible defects were observed in a 48% of the patients with SPECT. Low peak heart rate in exercise test, attributed to treatment with betablockers, could accentuate the lower sensitivity of exercise echo. It is not surprising, then, that SPET was more predictive of ischaemic complications during the follow up.

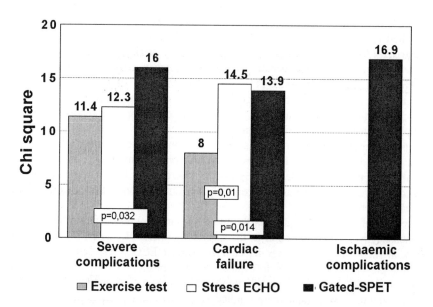

Figure 12. Bar grahs ilustrate incremental prognostic value (depicted by χ^2 value on y axis) of exercise test, exercise ECHO and gated-SPET for severe complications, cardiac failure and ischaemic complications, after uncomplicated first myocardial infarction.

References

1. Steinberg EP, Klag MJ, Bakal CW et al. Exercise thallium scans: patterns of use and impact on management of patients with known or suspected coronary artery disease. Am J Cardiol 1987; 59: 50-55.
2. Palet-Balart J, Candell-Riera J, Castell-Conesa J et al. La tomogammagrafía de perfusión y la coronariografía como exploraciones complementarias en la decisión terapéutica de pacientes con cardiopatía isquémica. Rev Esp Cardiol 1994; 47: 796-802.
3. Gibson RS, Watson DD, Taylor GJ et al. Prospective assessment of regional myocardial perfusion before and after coronary revascularization surgery by quantitative thallium-201 scintigraphy. J Am Coll Cardiol 1983; 1: 804-815.
4. Lim YL, Okada RD, Chesler DA et al. A new approach to quantitation of exercise thallium-201 scintigraphy before and after an intervention: Application to define the impact of coronary angioplasty on regional myocardial perfusion. Am Heart J 1984; 108: 917-925.
5. Ritchie JL, Narahara KA, Trobaugh GB et al. Thallium-201 myocardial imaging before and after coronary revascularization. Assessment of regional myocardial blood flow and graft patency. Circulation 1977; 56: 830-836.
6. Rasmussen SL, Nielsen SL, Amtorp O et al. 201-thallium imaging as an indicator of graft patency after coronary artery bypass surgery. Eur Heart J 1984; 5: 494-499.
7. Breisblatt WM, Barnes JV, Weiland F et al. Incomplete revascularization in multivessel percutaneous transluminal coronary angioplasty: The role for stress thallium-201 imaging. J Am Coll Cardiol 1988; 11: 1183-1190.
8. Wohlgelernter D, Cleman M, Highman HA et al. Percutaneous transluminal coronary angioplasty of the "culprit lesion" for management of unstable angina pectoris in patients with multivessel coronary artery disease. Am J Cardiol 1986; 58: 460-464.
9. Joye JD, Schulman DS, Lasorda D et al. Intracoronary doppler guide wire versus stress single-photon emission computed tomographic thallium-201 imaging in assessment of intermediate coronary stenoses. J Am Coll Cardiol 1994; 24: 904-907.
10. White CW, Wright CB, Doty DB et al. Does visual interpretation of the coronary arteriogram predict the physiologic importance of a coronary stenosis? N Engl J Med 1984; 310: 819-824.
11. Trask N, Califf RM, Conley MJ et al. Accuracy and interobserver variability of coronary cineangiography: a comparison with postmortem evaluation. J Am Coll Cardiol 1984; 3: 1145-1154.
12. Kleiman NS, Rodriguez AR, Raizner AE. Interobserver variability in grading of coronary arterial narrowings using the American College of Cardiology / American Heart Association grading criteria. Am J Cardiol 1992; 69: 413-415.
13. Gurley JC, Nissen SE, Booth DC et al. Influence of operator- and patient-dependent variables on the suitability of automated quantitative coronary arteriography for routine clinical use. J Am Coll Cardiol 1992; 19: 1237-1243.
14. Legrand V, Mancini GBJ, Le Free MT et al. Clinical value of digital radiographic coronary quantification: comparison with visual assessment and coronary flow reserve. Eur Heart J 1992; 13: 95-101.
15. Danchin N, Juilliere Y, Foley D et al. Visual versus quantitative assessment of the severity of coronary artery stenoses: can the angiographer's eye be reeducated?. Am Heart J 1993; 126: 594-600.
16. Leung WH, Alderman EL, Lee TC, Stadius ML. Quantitative arteriography of apparently normal coronary segments with nearby or distant disease presence of occult, nonvisualized atherosclerosis. J Am Coll Cardiol 1995; 25: 311-317.
17. Di Carli M, Czernin J, Hoh CK et al. Relation among stenosis severity, myocardial blood flow, and flow reserve in patients with coronary artery disease. Circulation 1995; 91: 1944-1951.
18. Keane D, Haase J, Slager CJ et al. Comparative validation of quantitative coronary agiography systems. Results and implications from a multicenter study using a standardized approach. Circulation 1995; 91: 2174-2183.
19. Beauman GJ, Vogel RA. Accuracy of individual and panel visual interpretations of coronary arteriograms: Implications for clinical decisions. J Am Coll Cardiol 1990; 16: 108-113.
20. DeRouen T, Murray J, Owen W. Variability in the analysis of coronary angiograms. Circulation 1977; 55: 324-328.
21. Klein JL, Boccuzzi SJ, Treasure CB et al. Performance standards and edge detection with computerized quantitative coronary arteriography. Am J Cardiol 1996; 77: 815-822.

22. Heller LI, Cates C, Popma J et al. Intracoronary Doppler assessment of moderate coronary artery disease. Comparison with ^{201}Tl imaging and coronary angiography. Circulation 1997; 96: 484-490.

23. Ozaki Y, Violaris AG, Kobayashi T et al. Comparison of coronary luminal quantification obtained from intracoronary ultrasound and both geometric and videodensitometric quantitative angiography before and after balloon angioplasty and directional atherectomy. Circulation 1997; 96: 491-499.

24. Candell-Riera J, Santana-Boado C, Castell-Conesa J et al. Culprit lesion and jeopardized myocardium: Correlation between coronary angiography and single photon emission computed tomography. Clin Cardiol 1997; 20: 345-350.

25. Castell-Conesa J (1994) Methods for quantifying myocardial perfusion, in Candell-Riera J and Ortega-Alcalde D (eds.), Nuclear Cardiology in everyday practice, Kluwer Academic Publishers, Dordrecht, pp. 88-108.

26. Maddahi J, Van Train K, Prigent F et al. Quantitative single photon emission computed thallium-201 tomography for detection and localization of coronary artery disease: Optimization and prospective validation of a new technique. J Am Coll Cardiol 1989; 14: 1689-1699.

27. Van Train KF, Garcia EV, Cooked AJ (1995) Quantitative analysis of SPECT myocardial perfusion, in De Puey EG, Berman DS and Garcia EV (eds.), Cardiac SPECT Imaging, Raven Press, New York, pp. 49-74.

28. Gibson CM, Cannon CP, Daley WL et al. TIMI frame count. A quantitative method of assessing coronary artery flow. Circulation 1996; 93: 879-888.

29. Bartúnek J, Sys SU, Heyndrickx GR et al. Quantitative coronary angiography in predicting functional significance of stenoses in an unselected patient cohort. J Am Coll Cardiol 1995; 26: 328-334.

30. Arnese M, Salustri A, Fioretti PM et al. Quantitative angiographic measurements of isolated left anterior descending coronary artery stenosis. Correlation with exercise echocardiography and technetium-99m 2-methoxy isobutyl isonitrile single-photon emission tomography. J Am Coll Cardiol 1995; 25: 1486-1491.

31. Mancini GB, Simin SB, McGillen MJ et al. Automated quantitative coronary arteriography: Morphologic and physiologic validation in vivo of rapid digital angiographic method. Circulation 1987; 75: 452-460.

32. Rentrop KP, Cohen M, Blanke H, Phillips RA. Changes in collateral channel filling immediately after controlled coronary artery occlusion by an angioplasty balloon in human subjects. J Am Coll Cardiol 1985; 5: 587-592.

33. Rentrop KP, Feit F, Sherman W, Thornton JC. Serial angiographic assessment of coronary artery obstruction and collateral flow in acute myocardial infarction. Report from the Second Mount Sinai-New York University Reperfusion Trial. Circulation 1989; 80: 1166-1175.

34. Pijls NH, Bech JW, El Gamal MIH et al. Quantification of recruitable coronary collateral blood flow in conscious humans and its potential to predict future ischemic events. J Am Coll Cardiol 1995; 25: 1522-1528.

35. Candell-Riera J, (1994) Stress testing, in Candell-Riera J and Ortega-Alcalde D (eds.), Nuclear Cardiology in everyday practice. Kluwer Academic Publishers, Dordrecht, pp. 43-66.

36. Candell-Riera J, Santana-Boado C, Castell-Conesa J et al. Simultaneous dipyridamole/maximal subjective exercise with ^{99m}Tc-MIBI SPECT: Improved diagnostic yield in coronary artery disease. J Am Coll Cardiol 1997; 29: 531-536.

37. Santana-Boado C, Candell-Riera J, Castell-Conesa J et al. Importancia de los parámetros ergométricos en los resultados de la tomogammagrafía de perfusión miocárdica. Med Clín (Barc.) 1997; 109: 406-409.

38. Hockings B, Saltissi S, Croft DN, Webb-Peploe MM. Effect of beta adrenergic blockade on thallium-201 myocardial perfusion imaging. Br Heart J 1983; 49: 83-89.

39. Martin GJ, Henkin RE, Scanlon PJ. Beta blockers and the sensitivity of the thallium treadmill test. Chest 1987; 92: 486-487.

40. Santana-Boado C, Candell-Riera J, Aguadé-Bruix S et al. Cuantificación de la isquemia miocárdica en regiones dependientes de arterias coronarias ocluidas de pacientes sin infarto previo. Rev Esp Cardiol 1998; 51: 388-395.

41. Pollock SC, Abbot RD, Boucher CA et al. A model to predict multivessel coronary artery disease from the exercise thallium-201 stress test. Am J Med 1991; 90: 345-352.

42. Christian TF, Miller TD, Bailey KR et al. Noninvasive identification of severe coronary artery disease using exercise tomographic thallium-201 imaging. Am J Cardiol 1992; 70: 14-20.

43. Iskandrian AS, Heo J, Lemlek J et al. Identification of high risk patients with left main and three-vessel coronary artery disease using stepwise discriminant analysis of clinical, exercise, and tomographic thallium data. Am Heart J 1993; 125: 221-225.

44. Gewirtz H, Paladino W, Sullivan M et al. Value and limitations of myocardial thallium washout rate in the noninvasive diagnosis of patients with triple-vessel coronary artery disease. Am Heart J 1983; 106: 681-686.

45. Bateman TM, Maddahi J, Gray RJ et al. Diffuse slow washout of myocardial thallium-201: A new scintigraphic indicator of extensive coronary artery disease. J Am Coll Cardiol 1984; 4: 55-64.

46. Nordrehaug JE, Danielsen R, Vik-Mo H. Effects of heart rate on myocardial thallium-201 uptake and clearance. J Nucl Med 1989; 30: 1972-1976.

47. Maddahi J, Abdulla A, García EV et al. Noninvasive identification of left main and triple vessel coronary artery disease: Improved accuracy using quantitative analysis of regional myocardial stress distribution and washout of thallium-201. J Am Coll Cardiol 1986; 7: 53-60.

48. Rothendler JA, Boucher CA, Strauss W et al. Decrease in the ability to detect elevated lung thallium due to delay in commencing imaging after exercise. Am Heart J 1985; 110: 830-835.

49. Brown KA, McKay R, Heller GV et al. Hemodynamic determinants of thallium-201 lung uptake in patients during atrial pacing stress. Am Heart J 1986; 111: 103-107.

50. Gill JB, Ruddy TD, Newell JB et al. Prognostic importance of thallium uptake by the lungs during exercise in coronary artery disease. N Engl J Med 1987; 317: 1485-1489.

51. Kaul S, Finkelstein DM, Homma S et al. Superiority of quantitative exercise thallium-201 variables in determining long-term prognosis in ambulatory patients with chest pain: A comparison with cardiac catheterization. J Am Coll Cardiol 1988; 12: 25-34.

52. Levy R, Rozanski A, Berman DS et al. Analysis of the degree of pulmonary thallium washout after exercise in patients with coronary artery disease. J Am Coll Cardiol 1983; 2: 719-728.

53. Manno B, Hakki A, Kane SA et al. Usefulness of left ventricular wall thickness-to-diameter ratio in thallium-201 scintigraphy. Cath Cardiovasc Diag 1983; 9: 483-491.

54. Weiss AT, Berman DS, Lew AS et al. Transient ischemic dilation of the left ventricle on stress thallium-201 scintigraphy: A marker of severe and extensive coronary artery disease. J Am Coll Cardiol 1987; 9: 752-759.

55. Forslund L, Hjemdahl P, Held C et al. Prognostic implications of results from exercise testing in patients with chronic stable angina pectoris treated with metoprolol or verapamil. A report from The angina Prognosis Study in Stockholm (APSIS). Eur Heart J 2000; 21: 901-910.

56. Kwowk JMF, Christian TF, Miller TD, Hodge DO, Gibbons RJ. Identification of severe coronary artery disease in patients with a single abnormal coronary territory on exercise thallium-201 imaging. J Am Coll Cardiol 2000; 35: 335-344.

57. Canhasi B, Dae M, Botvinick E et al. Interaction of "supplementary" scintigraphic indicators of ischemia and stress electrocardiography in the diagnosis of multivessel coronary disease. J Am Coll Cardiol 1985; 6: 581-588.

58. Castell-Conesa J, Santana-Boado C, Candell-Riera J et al. La tomogammagrafía miocárdica de esfuerzo en el diagnóstico de la enfermedad coronaria multivaso. Rev Esp Cardiol 1997; 50: 635-642.

59. Iskandrian AS, Verani MS (1996) Exercise perfusion imaging in coronary artery disease: Physiology and diagnosis, in Iskandrian AS and Verani MS (eds.), Nuclear cardiac imaging, F.A. Davis Company, Philadelphia, pp. 73-143.

60. Detrano R, Gianrossi R, Mulvihill D et al. Exercise-induced ST depression in the diagnosis of coronary artery disease: A metaanalisis. J Am Coll Cardiol 1989; 14: 1501-1508.

61. Morise AP. An incremental evaluation of the diagnostic value of thallium single-photon emission computed tomographic imaging and lung/heart ratio concerning both the presence and extent of coronary artery disease. J Nucl Cardiol 1995; 2: 238-245.

62. Mazzanti M, Germano G, Kiat H et al. Identification of severe and extensive coronary artery disease by automatic measurement of transient ischemic dilation of the left ventricle in dual-isotope myocardial perfusion SPECT. J Am Coll Cardiol 1996; 27: 1612-1620.

63. McClellan JR, Travin MI, Herman SD et al. Prognostic importance of scintigraphic left ventricular cavity dilation during intravenous dipyridamole technetium-99m sestamibi myocardial tomographic imaging in predicting coronary events. Am J Cardiol 1997; 79: 600-605.

64. Lindsey H Jr, Cohn PF. "Silent" myocardial ischemia during and after exercise testing in patients with coronary artery disease. Am Heart J 1978; 95: 441-447.

65. Deanfield JE, Maseri A, Selwyn AP et al. Myocardial ischemia during daily life in patients with stable angina: its relation to symptoms and heart rate changes. Lancet 1983; 2: 753-758.

66. Cohn PF. Silent myocardial ischemia. Ann Intern Med 1988; 109: 312-317.
67. Frishman WH, Teicher M. Antianginal drug therapy for silent myocardial ischemia. Am Heart J 1987; 114: 140-147.
68. Pepine C, Cohn PF, Deedwania PC, Gibson R, Gottlieb S, Hill J. The pronostic and economic implications of a strategy to detect and treat asymptomatic ischemia: The Atenolol Silent Ischemia Trial (ASIST) protocol. Clin Cardiol 1991; 14: 457-461.
69. ACIP investigators. Asymptomatic Cardiac Ischemia Pilot Study (ACIP). Am J Cardiol 1992; 70: 744-747.
70. Gasparetti CM, Burwell LR, Beller GA. Prevalence of and variables associated with silent myocardial ischemia on exercise thallium-201 stress testing. J Am Coll Cardiol 1990; 16: 115-123.
71. Vassiliadis IV, Machac J, O'Hara M, Sezhiyan T, Horowitz SF. Exercise-induced myocardial dysfunction in patients with coronary artery disease with and without angina. Am Heart J 1991; 121: 1403-1408.
72. Travin MI, Flores AR, Boucher CA, Newell JB, LaRaia PJ. Silent versus symptomatic ischemia during a thallium-201 exercise test. Am J Cardiol 1991; 68: 1600-1608.
73. Marwick TH, Nemec JJ, Torelli J, Salcedo EE, Stewart WJ. Extent and severity of abnormal left ventricular wall motion detected by exercise echocardiography during painful and silent ischemia. Am J Cardiol 1992; 69: 1483-1484.
74. Nihoyannopoulos P, Marsonis A, Joshi J, Athanassopoulos G, Oakley CM. Magnitude of myocardial dysfunction is greater in painful than in painless myocardial ischemia: an exercise echocardiographic study. J Am Coll Cardiol 1995; 25: 1507-1512.
75. Tamaki N, Yasuda T, Moore R et al. Continous monitoring of left ventricular function by an ambulatory radionuclide detector in patients with coronary artery disease. J Am Coll Cardiol 1988; 12: 669-679.
76. Candell-Riera J (1994) Diagnosis of coronary artery disease, in Candell-Riera J and Ortega-Alcalde D (eds.), Nuclear cardiology in everyday practice, Kluwer Academic Publishers, Dordrecht, pp.187-215.
77. Williams KA, Taillon LA, Carter JE. Asymptomatic and electrically silent myocardial ischemia during upright leg cycle ergometry and treadmill exercise (clandestine myocardial ischemia). Am J Cardiol 1993; 72: 1114-1120.
78. Upton MT, Rerych SK, Newman GE, Port S, Cobb FR, Jones RH. Detecting abnormalities in left ventricular function during exercise before angina and ST-segment depression. Circulation 1980; 62: 341-349.
79. Williams KA, Sherwood DS, Fisher KM. The frequency of asymptomatic and electrically silent exercise-induced regional myocardial ischemia during first-pass radionuclide angiography with upright bicycle ergometry. J Nucl Med 1992; 33: 359-364.
80. Hecht HS, BeBord L, Sotomayor N, Shaw R, Ryan C. Truly silent ischemia and the relationship of chest pain and ST segment changes to the amount of ischemic myocardium: evaluation by supine bicycle stress echocardiography. J Am Coll Cardiol 1994; 23: 369-376.
81. Chierchia S, Lazzari M, Freedman B, Brunelli C, Maseri A. Impairment of myocardial perfusion and function during painless myocardial ischemia. J Am Coll Cardiol 1983; 1: 924-930.
82. Klein J, Chao SY, Berman DS, Rozanski A. Is "silent" myocardial ischemia really as severe as symptomatic ischemia? The analytical effect of patient selection biases. Circulation 1994; 89: 1958-1966.
83. Cohn PF, Brown EJ, Wynne J, Holman BL, Atkins HL. Global and regional left ventricular ejection fraction abnormalities during exercise in patients with silent myocardial ischemia. J Am Coll Cardiol 1983; 1: 931-933.
84. Iskandrian AS, Hakki A. Left ventricular function in patients with coronary heart disease in the presence or absence of angina pectoris during exercise radionuclide ventriculography. Am J Cardiol 1984; 53: 1239-1243.
85. Ouyang P, Shapiro EP, Chandra NC, Gottlieb SH, Chew PH, Gottlieb SO. An angiographic and functional comparison of patients with silent and symptomatic treadmill ischemia early after myocardial infarction. Am J Cardiol 1987; 59: 730-734.
86. Hecht HS, Shaw RE, Bruce T, Myler RK. Silent ischemia: evaluation by exercise and redistribution tomographic thallium-201 myocardial imaging. J Am Coll Cardiol 1989; 14: 895-900.
87. Mark DB, Hlatky MA, Califf RM et al. Painless exercise ST deviation on the treadmill: long-term prognosis. J Am Coll Cardiol 1989; 14: 885-892.

88. Mahmarian JJ, Pratt CM, Cocanougher MK, Verani MS. Altered myocardial perfusion in patients with angina pectoris or silent ischemia during exercise as assessed by quantitative thallium-201 single-photon emission tomography. Circulation 1990; 82: 1305-1315.

89. Bruschke AVG, Proudfit WL, Sones FM. Progress study of 590 consecutive nonsurgical cases of coronary disease followed 5 - 9 years. I. Arteriographic correlations. Circulation 1973; 47: 1147-1153.

90. Humphries JO, Kuller L, Ross RS et al. Natural history of ischemic heart disease in relation to arteriographic findings. A twelve year study of 224 patients. Circulation 1974; 49: 489-497.

91. Burggraf GW, Parker JO. Prognosis in coronary artery disease. Angiographic, hemodynamic, and clinical factors. Circulation 1975; 51: 146-156.

92. Hutter AM. Is there a left main equivalent? Circulation 1980; 62: 207-211.

93. Folland ED, Vogel RA, Hartigan P et al. Relation between coronary artery stenosis assessed by visual, caliper, and computer methods and exercise capacity in patients with single-vessel coronary artery disease. Circulation 1994; 89: 2005-2014.

94. Califf RM, Phillips HR, Hindman MC et al. Prognostic value of a coronary artery jeopardy score. J Am Coll Cardiol 1985; 5: 1055-1063.

95. Marwick T, D'Hondt AM, Baudhuin T et al. Optimal use of dobutamine stress for the detection and evaluation of coronary artery disease: Combination with echocardiography or scintigraphy, or both? J Am Coll Cardiol 1993; 22: 159-167.

96. Austen WG, Edwards JE, Frye RL et al. A reporting system on patients evaluated for coronary artery disease. Report of the Ad Hoc Committee for grading of coronary artery disease, Council on Cardiovascular Surgery, American Heart Association. Circulation 1975; 51 (suppl 51): 5-40.

97. Leaman DM, Brower RW, Meester GT et al. Coronary artery atherosclerosis: severity of the disease, severity of angina pectoris and compromised left ventricular function. Circulation 1981; 63: 285-292.

98. Favaloro RG. Computerized tabulation of cine coronary angiograms. Circulation 1990; 81: 1992-2003.

99. Ellis SG, Cowley MJ, DiSciascio et al. Determinants of 2-year outcome after coronary angioplasty in patients with multivessel disease on the basis of comprehensive preprocedural evaluation. Implications for patient selection. Circulation 1991; 83: 1905-1914.

100. Weyner DA, Ryan TJ, McCabe CH et al. The role of exercise testing in identifying patients with improved survival after coronary artery bypass surgery. J Am Coll Cardiol 1986; 8: 741-748.

101. Plotnick GD. Coronary artery bypass surgery to prolong life?: Less anatomy/more physiology. J Am Coll Cardiol 1986; 8: 749-751.

102. Mahmarian JJ, Pratt CM, Boyce TM et al. The variable extent of jeopardized myocardium in patients with single vessel coronary artery disease: quantification by thallium-201 single photon emission computed tomography. J Am Coll Cardiol 1991; 17: 355-362.

103. Iskandrian AS. Relation between functional and anatomic descriptors of coronary artery disease. J Am Coll Cardiol 1991; 17: 363-364.

104. Ritchie JL, Bateman TM, Bonow RO et al. Guidelines for clinical use of cardiac radionuclide imaging. A report of the American Heart Association/American College of Cardiology Task Force on assessment of diagnostic and therapeutic cardiovascular procedures, Committee on Radionuclide imaging, developed in collaboration with the American Society of Nuclear Cardiology. Circulation 1995; 91: 1278-1303.

105. Wackers FJTh, Russo DJ, Russo D et al. Prognostic significance of normal quantitative planar thallium-201 stress scintigrafhy in patients wiht chest pain. J Am Coll Cardiol 1985; 6: 27-30.

106. Santana-Boado C, Candell-Riera J, Castell-Conesa J et al. Lesión culpable y miocardio en riesgo. Correlación entre la coronariografía y la tomogammagrafía de perfusión con tecnecio-99m-MIBI. Rev Esp Cardiol 1995; 48: 89. (Abstr.).

107. Van Train KF, Berman DS, Garcia EV et al. Quantitative analysis of stress thallium-201 myocardial scintigrams: a multicenter trial. J Nucl Med 1986; 27:17-25.

108. Pereztol O, Batista L, Senra L et al. Valor del análisis cuantitativo de la perfusión miocárdica empleando ^{201}Tl SPECT en la enfermedad coronaria multivaso. Rev Esp Med Nucl 1995; 14: 18-22.

109. Garcia E, Maddahi J, Berman D et al. Space/time quantitation of thallium-201 myocardial scintigraphy. J Nucl Med 1981; 22: 309-317.

110. Ceriani L, Verna E, Giovanella L et al. Assessment of myocardial area at risk by technetium-99 sestamibi during coronary artery occlusion: comparison between three tomographic methods of quantification. Eur J Nucl Med 1996; 23: 31-39.

111. Verani MS, Jeoroundi MO, Mahamarian JJ et al. Quantification of myocardial infartion during coronary occlusion and myocardial salvage after reperfusion using cardiac imaging wiht technetium-99m hexaquis-2-methoxyisobutil isonitrile. J Am Coll Cardiol 1988; 12: 1573-1581.
112. Tamaki S, Nakajima H, Murakami T et al. Estimation of infarct size by myocardial emission computed tomography with thallium 201 and its relation to creatine kinase-MB release after myocardial infarction in man. Circulation 1982; 66: 994-1001.
113. O'Connor MK, Hammel T, Gibbsons RJ. In vitro validation of a simple tomographic technique for estimation of percentage myocardium at risk using methoxyisobutil isonitrile technetium 99m (sestamibi). Eur J Nucl Med 1990; 16: 69-76.
114. Beller GA (1995) Detection of coronary artery disease, in G.A. Beller (ed.), Clinical Nuclear Cardiology, W. B. Saunders Company, Philadelphia, pp. 82-136.
115. Herrington DM, Siebes M, Sokol DK et al. Variability in measures of coronary lumen dimensions using quantitative coronary angiography. J Am Coll Cardiol 1993; 22: 1068-1074.
116. Haronian HL, Remetz MS, Sinusas AJ et al. Myocardial risk area defined by technetium-99m sestamibi imaging during percutaneous transluminal coronary angioplasty: comparison with coronary angiography. J Am Coll Cardiol 1993; 22: 1033-1043.
117. Beller GA (1995) Radionuclide evaluation of coronary bypass surgery and percutaneous trasluminal coronary angioplasty, in Beller GA (ed.), Clinical Nuclear Cardiology, W. B. Saunders Company, pp. 337-372.
118. Candell-Riera J, de la Hera JM, Santana-Boado C et al. Eficacia diagnóstica de la tomogammagrafía miocárdica en la detección de reestenosis coronaria postangioplastia. Rev Esp Cardiol 1998; 51: 648-654.
119. Carballo J, Candell-Riera J, Aguadé-Bruix S et al. Eficacia de la tomogammagrafía miocárdica en la valoración de la permeabilidad de los injertos aortocoronarios. Rev Esp Cardiol 2000; 53: 611-616.
120. Little WC, Constantinescu M, Applegate RJ et al. Can coronary angiography predict the site of a subsequent myocardial infarction in patients with mild- to-moderate coronary artery disease? Circulation 1988; 78: 1157-1166.
121. Ambrose JA, Tannenbaum MA, Alexopoulos D et al. Angiographic progression of coronary artery disease and the development of myocardial infarction. J Am Coll Cardiol 1988; 12: 56-62.
122. Giroud D, Li JM, Urban P et al. Relation of the site of acute myocardial infarction to the most severe coronary arterial stenosis at prior angiography. Am J Cardiol 1992; 69: 729-732.
123. Beller GA. Myocardial perfusion imaging with thallium-201. J Nucl Med 1994; 35: 674-680.
124. Iskandrian AS, Johnson J, Le TT, Wasserleben V, Cave V, Heo J. Comparison of the treadmill exercise score and single-photon emission computed tomographic thallium imaging in risk assessment. J Nucl Cardiol 1994; 1: 144-149.
125. Petretta M, Cuocolo A, Carpinelli A et al. Prognostic value of myocardial hypoperfusion indexes in patients with suspected or known coronary artery disease. J Nucl Cardiol 1994; 1: 325-337.
126. Raiker K, Sinusas AJ, Wackers FJT, Zaret BL. One-year prognosis of patients with normal planar or single-photon emission computed tomographic technetium 99m-labeled sestamibi exercise imaging. J Nucl Cardiol 1994; 1: 449-456.
127. Gibbons RJ. Role of nuclear cardiology for determining management of patients with stable coronary artery disease. J Nucl Cardiol 1994; 1: S118-130.
128. Bateman TM, O'Keefe JH, Dong VM, Barnhart C, Ligon RW. Coronary angiographic rates after stress single-photon emission computed tomographic scintigraphy. J Nucl Cardiol 1995; 2: 217-223.
129. Berman DS, Hachamovitch R, Kiat H et al. Incremental value of prognostic testing in patients with known or suspected ischemic heart disease: A basis for optimal utilization of exercise technetium-99m sestamibi myocardial perfusion single-photon emission computed tomography. J Am Coll Cardiol 1995; 26: 639-647.
130. Marie PY, Danchin N, Durand JF et al. Long-term prediction of major ischemic events by exercise thallium-201 single photon emission computed tomography. Incremental prognostic value compared with clinical, exercise testing, catheterization and radionuclide angiographic data. J Am Coll Cardiol 1995; 26: 879-886.
131. Stratmann HG, Younis LT, Wittry MD, Amato M, Miller DD. Exercise technetium-99m myocardial tomography for the risk stratification of men with medically treated unstable angina pectoris. Am J Cardiol 1995; 76: 236-240.Nallamothu N, Pancholy SB, Lee KR, Heo J, Iskandrian AS. Impact on exercise single-photon emission computed tomographic thallium imaging on patient management and outcome. J Nucl Cardiol 1995; 2: 334-338.

132. Blumenthal RS, Becker DM, Moy TF, Coresh J, Wilder LB, Becker LC. Exercise thallium tomography predicts future clinically manifest coronary heart disease in a high-risk assymptomatic population. Circulation 1996; 93: 915-923.
133. Hachamovitch R, Berman DS, Kiat H et al. Exercise myocardial perfusion SPECT in patients without known coronary artery disease. Incremental prognostic value and use in risk stratification. Circulation 1996; 93: 905-914.
134. Bateman TM, O'Keefe JH, Williams ME. Incremental value of myocardial perfusion scintigraphy in prognosis and outcomes of patients with coronary artery disease. Current Opinion in Cardiology 1996; 11: 613-620.
135. Pavin D, Delonca J, Siegenthaler M, Doat M, Rutishauser W, Righetti A. Long-term (10 years) prognostic value of a normal thallium-201 myocardial exercise scintigraphy in patients with coronary artery disease documented by angiography. Eur Heart J 1997; 18: 69-77.
136. Beller GA, Zaret BL. Contributions of nuclear cardiology to diagnosis and prognosis of patients with coronary artery disease. Circulation 2000; 101: 1465-1478.
137. Boyne TS, Koplan BA, Parsons WJ, Smith WH, Watson DD, Beller GA. Predicting adverse outcome with exercise SPECT technetium-99m sestamibi imaging in patients with suspected or known coronary artery disease. Am J Cardiol 1997; 79: 270-274.
138. Candell-Riera J, Permanyer-Miralda G, Castell J et al. Uncomplicated first myocardial infarction: Strategy for comprehensive prognostic studies. J Am Coll Cardiol 1991; 18: 1207 - 1219.
139. Olona M, Candell-Riera J, Permanyer-Miralda G et al. Strategies for prognostic assessment of uncomplicated first myocardial infarction: A 5-years follow up study. J Am Coll Cardiol 1995; 25: 815-822.
140. Gimple LW, Beller GA. Assessing prognosis after acute myocardial infarction in the thrombolytic era. J Nucl Cardiol 1994; 1: 198-209.
141. Di Bello V, Gori E, Bellina CR et al. Incremental diagnostic value of dipyridamole echocardiography and exercise thallium 201 scintigraphy in the assessment of presence and extent of coronary artery disease. J Nucl Cardiol 1994; 1: 372-381.
142. Kamal AM, Fattah AA, Pancholy S et al. Prognostic value of adenosine single-photon emission computed tomographic thallium imaging in medically treated patients with angiographic evidence of coronary artery disease. J Nucl Cardiol 1994; 1: 254-261.
143. Geleijnse ML, Elhendy A, Van Domburg RT et al. Prognostic value of dobutamine-atropine stress technetium-99m sestamibi perfusion scintigraphy in patients with chest pain. J Am Coll Cardiol 1996; 28: 447-454.
144. Di Bello V, Bellina CR, Gori E et al. Incremental diagnostic value of dobutamine stress echocardiography and dobutamine scintigraphy (technetium 99m-labeled sestamibi single-photon emission computed tomography) for assessment of presence and extent of coronary artery diasease. J Nucl Cardiol 1996; 3: 212-220.
145. Senior R, Raval U, Lahiri A. Prognostic value of stress dobutamine technetium-99m sestamibi single-photon emission computed tomography (SPECT) in patients with suspected coronary artery disease. Am J Cardiol 1996; 78: 1092-1096.
146. Machecourt J, Longère P, Fagret D et al. Prognostic value of thallium-201 single-photon emission computed tomographic myocardial perfusion imaging according to extent of myocardial defect. Study in 1,926 patients with a follow-up at 33 months. J Am Coll Cardiol 1994; 23: 1090-1106.
147. Iskandrian A, Chae S, Hea J, Stanberry C, Wasserleben V, Cave V. Independent and incremental prognostic value of exercise in single-photon emission computed tomography (SPECT) thallium imaging in coronary artery disease. J Am Coll Cardiol 1993; 22: 665-670.
148. Stratmann HG, Williams GA, Wittry MD, Chaitman BR, Miller DD. Exercise technetium-99m sestamibi tomography for cardiac risk stratification of patients with stable chest pain. Circulation 1994; 89: 30: 441-449.
149. Candell-Riera J, Santana-Boado C, Bermejo B et al. Prognosis of clandestine myocardial ischemia, silent myocardial ischemia and angina pectoris in medically treated patients. Am J Cardiol 1998; 82: 1333-1338.
150. Santana-Boado C, Figueras J, Candell-Riera J et al. Pronóstico de los pacientes con angina y con isquemia silente en la tomogammagrafía de esfuerzo con ^{99m}Tc-MIBI. Rev Esp Cardiol 1998; 51: 297-301.
151. Kulick DL, Rahimtoola SH. Risk stratification in survivors of acute myocardial infarction: routine cardiac catheterization and angiography is a reasonable approach in most patients. Am Heart J 1991; 121: 641-656.

152. Rouleau JL, Moyé LA, Pfeffer MA et al. for the SAVE investigators. A comparison of management patterns after acute myocardial infarction in Canada and the United States. N Engl J Med 1993; 328: 779-784.

153. Every NR, Larson EB, Litwin PE et al. for the Myocardial Infarction Triage and Intervention Project Investigators. The association between on-site cardiac catheterization facilities and the use of coronary angiography after acute myocardial infarction. N Engl J Med 1993; 329: 546-551.

154. Marrugat J, Sanz G, Masiá R et al. for the RESCATE investigators. Six-month outcome in patients with myocardial infarction initially admitted to tertiary and nontertiary hospitals. J Am Coll Cardiol 1997; 30: 1187-1192.

155. Boden WE, O'Rourke RA, Crawford MH et al. for the Veterans Affairs Non-Q-Wave Infarction Strategies in Hospital (VANQWISH) Trial Investigators. Outcomes in patients with acute non-Q-wave myocardial infarction randomly assigned to an invasive as compared with a conservative management strategy. N Engl J Med 1998; 338: 1785-1792.

156. Candell-Riera J, Llevadot J, Santana C et al. Prognostic assessment of uncomplicated first myocardial infarction by exercise echocardiography and ^{99m}Tc-tetrofosmin gated SPECT. J Nucl Cardiol (in press).

157. Jaarsma W, Visser CA, Kupper AJF, Res JCJ, Van Eenige MJV, Roos JP. Usefulness of two-dimensional exercise echocardiography shortly after myocardial infarction. Am J Cardiol 1986; 57: 86-90.

158. Applegate RJ, Dell'Italia LJ, Crawford MH. Usefulness of two-dimensional echocardiography during low-level exercise testing early after uncomplicated acute myocardial infarction. Am J Cardiol 1987; 60: 10-14.

159. Quintana M, Lindvall K, Ryden L, Brolund F. Prognostic value of predischarge exercise stress echocardiography after acute myocardial infarction. Am J Cardiol 1995; 76: 1115-1121.

160. González-Alujas T, Armada E, Alijarde M et al. Valor pronóstico de la ecocardiografía de esfuerzo postinfarto agudo de miocardio antes del alta hospitalaria. Rev Esp Cardiol 1998; 51: 21-26.

161. Brown KA. Do stress echocardiography and myocardial perfusion imaging have the same ability to identify the low-risk patient with known or suspected coronary artery disease? Am J Cardiol 1998; 81:1050-1053.

162. Poldermans D, Fioretti PM, Boersma E et al.. Dobutamine-atropine stress echocardiography and clinical data for predicting late cardiac events with suspected coronary artery disease. Am J Med 1994; 97: 119-125.

163. Sicari R, Picano E, Landi P et al. Prognostic value of dobutamine-atropine stress echocardiography early after acute myocardial infarction. J Am Coll Cardiol 1997; 29: 254-260.

164. Khattar RS, Basu SK, Raval U, Senior R, Lahiri A. Prognostic value of predischarge exercise testing, ejection fraction, and ventricular ectopic activity in acute myocardial infarction treated with streptokinase. Am J Cardiol 1996; 78: 136-141.

165. Pozzoli MMA, Fioretti PM, Salustri A, Reijs AEM; Roelandt JRTC. Exercise echocardiography and technetium-99m MIBI single-photon emission computed tomography in the detection of coronary artery disease. Am J Cardiol 1991; 67: 350-355.

166. O'Keefe JH, Barnhart CS, Bateman TM. Comparison of stress echocardiography and stress myocardial perfusion scintigraphy for diagnosing coronary artery disease and assessing its severity. Am J Cardiol 1995;75:25D-34D.

167. Zanco P, Zampiero A, Favero A et al. Prognostic evaluation of patients after myocardial infarction: Incremental value of sestamibi single-photon emission computed tomography and echocardiography. J Nucl Cardiol 1997; 4: 117-124.

7. STUNNED MYOCARDIUM AND HIBERNATING MYOCARDIUM: PATHOPHYSIOLOGY

DAVID GARCIA-DORADO and JORDI SOLER-SOLER

The first observations on the effects of decreased blood flow on myocardial contractility were made by Tennant and Wigers in 1935 in coronary occlusion experiments [1]. The relationships between the duration and severity of the ischaemia and their functional, biochemical and structural consequences have been established much more recently only when sophisticated technology became available for application in laboratory animals. It became clear, subsequently, that myocardial ischaemia rapidly causes (in seconds) severe contractile dysfunction [2] and that restoration of coronary flow is capable of reversing this effect in a manner that clearly depends on the period of duration of the ischaemia. If sufficiently brief, the contractile recovery is total but, beyond a certain time limit, reperfusion does not prevent necrosis of parts of the ischaemic myocardium and this is progressively greater the more protracted the ischaemia [3-5] and the contractile recovery is incomplete or none. A simple model was established and widely accepted in which the ischaemia would be accompanied by severe contractile dysfunction and reperfusion by contractile recovery that is assumed to be complete and more or less immediate; at least that which produced myocardial necrosis. Contractile dysfunction and necrosis would be consequences of progressive deterioration of the cellular energy status produced by the protracted anaerobic metabolism

However, experimental observations do not fit well within this model. In the first place, the contractile failure caused by the coronary occlusion is produced too rapidly in that the concentration of ATP, the principal cellular energy reserve, is still practically normal [6]. In the second place, as already observed by Heyndrickx et al. [7] in 1975, the functional recovery following a coronary occlusion of 15 minutes would require up to 12 hours. Subsequently, it was shown that this delay in recovery could be produced despite an energy recovery that is practically immediate [8]. The term stunned myocardium was coined by Braunwald and Kloner in 1982 to describe the post-ischaemic, transitory, prolonged contractile dysfunction with conserved coronary flow and in the absence of irreversible myocardial damage [9].

A commonly accepted implication of the initial model of the pathophysiology of ischaemic contractile dysfunction was that of a relationship, more or less linear, between the severity of the ischaemia and the grade of dysfunction. Severe dysfunction would indicate the existence of very significant metabolic alterations and, in particular, of a drop in the concentration of the cytosolic ATP incompatible with long-term cellular survival. However, relatively recent observations have demonstrated that the severe and chronic contractile dysfunction of some patients with chronic coronary artery disease can disappear when the coronary flow is

145

J. Candell-Riera et al. (eds.), Myocardium at Risk and Viable Myocardium, 145–163.
© 2001 *Kluwer Academic Publishers. Printed in the Netherlands.*

normalised by revascularisation surgery. Rahimtoola, in 1985, introduced the term "hibernation" to describe this reversible chronic contractile dysfunction [10,11]. It has been demonstrated more recently that the myocardium is capable, under certain circumstances, of decreasing its consumption of ATP, decreasing its contraction by adaptation to the rate of synthesis and to maintain the energy levels within normal limits [12-14] when coronary flow is reduced.

The stunned and the hibernating myocardium both constitute, then, situations of ischaemic dysfunction, the first with conserved coronary flow and following a brief ischaemic period and the other during a state of persistent hypoperfusion in which contractile failure occurs despite the cellular energy status being normal. Both phenomena have awakened a great deal of interest because of their considerable clinical potential. To know whether the abnormalities of ventricular contraction in a patient are due to the presence of necrotic areas or to the presence of potentially-reversible contractile dysfunction has obvious prognostic and therapeutic implications. However, the stunned and the hibernating myocardium are being seen as extraordinarily complex phenomena whose molecular mechanisms continue to be incompletely understood despite the weight of research over the last decade. In this present chapter we summarise the mechanisms thought to be responsible for the stunned and the hibernated myocardium and of the possible diagnostic and therapeutic implications that both phenomena have in the diagnosis and treatment of patients with coronary artery disease.

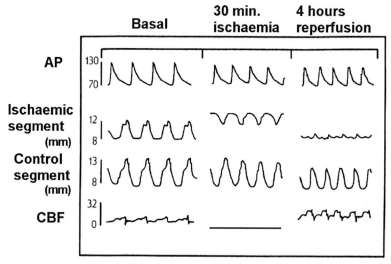

Figure 1. Original tracing obtained in an experiment of coronary occlusion (48 minutes) and reperfusion in the porcine model and in which the absence of systolic shortening is demonstrated in the reperfused segment reperfused 30 minutes after the restoration of flow. The histological analysis performed at the end of the experiment demonstrated that only 10% of the reperfused myocardium suffered necrosis and it would appear that its dysfunction was due, essentially, to stunning. The curves show the variations in the distance between two piezoelectric mycocristals implanted in the territory of the left anterior descending coronary artery (ischaemic segment). Note: in the territory of the left anterior descending, the systolic shortening is substituted by expansion (dyskinesis) that persists during the reperfusion.
AP: aortic pressure, CBF: coronary blood flow

1. Myocardial stunning

The term "stunned myocardium" describes the contractile dysfunction that occurs following a period of ischaemia and which resolves spontaneously [9]. The severity and duration of the post-ischaemic contractile dysfunction depends, essentially, on the severity of the ischaemic insult that triggers it. However, the relationships between the two variables have not been completely defined in the different experimental situations and species. Coronary occlusions of 5 minutes are enough to result in a a clear reduction of regional systolic shortening that can persist for hours. After 30 minutes of severe ischaemia the contractile dysfunction can become severely depressed over a period of days in the absence of myocardial necrosis (Figure 1). The time course of recovery is progressive and slow. In various experimental models it has been observed that, after a partial recovery of the contractile activity during the first few minutes of reperfusion, a rapid contractile deterioration occurs which is resolved very slowly and progressively. Strikingly, the inotropic reserve of the stunned myocardium is, at all times, normal [15-20] (Figure 2).

However, it is important to highlight that the zones of stunned myocardium frequently coexist with others of necrosed myocardium in the reperfused territory and that the necrosed zones can have a very undefined geometry such that the dead and the stunned myocardium are encountered firmly intertwined [20] (Plate7.1).

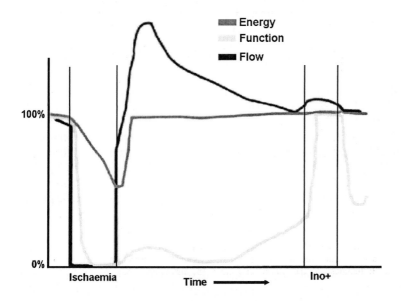

Figure 2. Pathophysiology scheme of stunned myocardium. Note: the dissociation between the rapid recovery of cellular energy status (energy) and the slow recovery of contractile function (function). Normalisation occurs during inotropic stimulation (ino+) without deterioration of biochemical and cellular energy status.

1.1. STRUCTURAL AND BIOCHEMICAL CHARACTERISATION OF STUNNED MYOCARDIUM

Using histology and/or magnetic resonance techniques, cellular and interstitial oedema can be observed in the stunned myocardium [21] in the first few moments of reperfusion and ultrastructural analyses reveal decreases in the glycogen granules in the myocites. These anomalies disappear much earlier than the complete recovery of contractile function. It is to be concluded, therefore, that contractile dysfunction of the stunned myocardium can occur in the absence of histological or ultrastructural abnormalities [22].

The most outstanding biochemical characteristic of the stunned myocardium is, indeed, the absence of significant abnormalities; in clear contrast to the severity of the functional abnormalities encountered. During myocardial ischaemia the cellular energy state deteriorates rapidly with decreasing cellular pH and, if sufficiently prolonged, elevations in the concentrations of Na^+ and Ca^{2+} [3,23-27]. Numerous studies have demonstrated that the cellular energy load, as measured by the concentrations of the high energy compounds (CP, ATP) and the free energy of dissociation, normalises almost immediately following the restoration of oxygenation [8,28-33]. The cytosolic concentrations of Na^+ as well as the pH of the reperfused myocites normalise rapidly as a result of the activation of an efficient system of transporters and exchangers in the sarcolema, the sarcoplasmic reticulum and the mitochondria. The Na^+ / H^+ exchange, the co-transport of $Na^+CO_3H^-$ and the ATPase Na^+/K^+ system performs a fundamental role in this process [27,34]. The behaviour of the cytosolic concentration of Ca^{2+} is one of the principal determinants of survival or death of the myocites during reperfusion [35,36]. This behaviour depends, essentially, on the efficacy of the uptake of Ca^{2+} by the sarcoplasmic reticulum mediated by the corresponding ATPase and of the magnitude of the incorporation of external Ca^{2+} from the Na^+/Ca^{2+} exchange and, as well in part, from the Ca^{2+} channels. In viable myocites the cytosolic concentrations of Ca^{2+} can transiently increase to restore the oxygen load but decrease very rapidly during the first minutes of reperfusion and, following a period of oscillation of variable frequency and amplitude, reach normal diastolic values [36-39]. Conversely, the inflammatory response and the cytokine-mediated changes (those that stimulate the accumulation of neutrophils and platelets in the reperfused myocardium and the induction of specific enzymes in different cell types, including the myocites) appear various hours after the restoration of blood flow and would seem unable to explain the post-ischaemic contractile dysfunction. It would appear, then, that there are no gross (but perhaps subtle) biochemical alterations that are consistently associated with the stunned myocardium.

1.2. CAUSAL MECHANISMS

Results from different experimental models, despite a few discrepancies probably related with methodological aspects, indicate that the contractile dysfunction of the stunned myocardium is due, essentially, to a decrease in the sensitivity of contractile proteins to Ca^{2+} [16,40-44]). Studies conducted in different *in vitro* models agree on the normality of temporary elevations of systolic Ca^{2+} concentrations that occur during systole together with a shift in the relationship between the concentration of Ca^{2+} and the contractile force i.e. a decrease in the force developed for a given level of Ca^{2+} but without diminution in the maximal force at adequately-elevated concentrations of Ca^{2+} [18,45]. The data obtained in studies *in vivo* are less consistent with respect to the normality of the temporary elevations and the preservation of the maximum force activated by Ca^{2+} in the stunned myocardium. These recent studies have demonstrated that the Ca^{2+} ATPase of the sarcoplasmic reticulum can be damaged during ischaemia-reperfusion [46]. The diminished amplitude of the systolic increase of the cytosolic Ca^{2+} by inadequate liberation from the sarcoplasmic reticulum could contribute to the contractile dysfunction of the stunned myocardium. However, this possibility has not been demonstrated [47,48] whether in the manipulations that increase the availability of cytosolic Ca^{2+} such as post-extrasystolic potentiation, adrenergic stimulation or the increase in extracellular calcium facilitating the recruitment of the inotropic reserve in the stunned myocardium.

The molecular bases of the decrease in the sensitivity of the myofilaments to Ca^{2+} have not been completely clarified. Recent studies have demonstrated that these could be due to changes in the myofilaments themselves [41]. These changes may consist of proteolytic degradation or in conformational changes without breakdown such as those induced by modifications of the phosphorylation state [41,49]. It has been demonstrated that troponin I shows a particular sensitivity to proteolytic degradation as a consequence of the activation of the Ca^{2+} dependent calpain protease over the first few minutes of reperfusion and that the inhibition of calpain or the attenuation of Ca^{2+} entry during reperfusion are capable of attenuating the proteolysis of troponin I and of the stunning [41].

During reperfusion, considerable amounts of free radicals of oxygen are generated from different cellular and extracellular sources whose relative importance varies in different species [50-56]. Evidence that oxygen free radicals are implicated in the genesis of the stunned myocardium, based on the protector effect of anti-free-radical substances, is quite solid [57]. Nevertheless, the mechanism by which it is effected has only recently begun to be partially understood [49]. Oxygen free radicals are capable of interfering in the control of cytosolic Ca^{2+}, of the Ca^{2+}ATPase of the sarcoplasmic reticulum, of directly oxidising proteins essential for contraction, in particular the creatine kinase [58] and to acting on fundamental kinases among which is protein kinase C that, in turn, modifies the phosphorylation status of the contractile proteins [49].

Finally, post-ischaemic dysfunction can be modulated by cellular interactions that take place in the reperfused myocardium. Liberation of free radicals from neutrophils occurs hours following the commencement of reperfusion [59,60] and is generally admitted to not participating in the genesis of the stunned myocardium. Nevertheless, it is possible that substances liberated from the endothelial cells modulate contractile dysfunction of the reperfused myocardium [61]. The increased synthesis of prostacyclin, probably stimulated by the bradykines, appears to have a protective effect against stunning [62-65] and the liberation from the endothelium of a factor that inhibits the natural non-subsidiary contractility has been recently described [61].

1.3. ROLE OF VASCULAR STUNNING

Multiple microvascular abnormalities have been described in the stunned myocardium including oedema and contraction of the endothelial cells, capillary obstruction by accumulation of polymorphonuclear leukocytes and abnormalities of nitric oxide (NO) homeostasis the last of which is of particular interest. The production of NO by the endothelial cells is very diminished during ischaemia and the levels of NO are not detectable during the first few seconds of reperfusion due, in greater part, to the consumption of NO in the reaction with oxygen free radicals (O_2^-) for which there is a great affinity. Nevertheless, over the subsequent hours, the concentration of NO increases to levels very much greater than normal as a result of the NO synthase induced in endothelial cells, myocites and macrophages. As a result of these and other changes, microvascular function presents with marked abnormalities, essentially a loss of capacity for rapid modulation of the coronary terminal resistance. This phenomenon is called vascular or endothelial stunning [66-69]. It should be emphasised, however, that contractility in the stunned myocardium occurs in the presence of normal regional myocardial flow or is increased by the reactive hyperaemia that follows ischaemia [70] so it would seem that vascular stunning is not implicated in the temporary post-ischaemic dysfunction.

TABLE 1. Clinical situations in which stunned myocardium could be produced

High probability of significant stunning
Cardiac surgery with extra-corporeal circulation
Coronary surgery without cardiac arrest
Cardiac transplant
Acute myocardial infarction with early reperfusion (spontaneous or therapeutic)
Following spontaneous cardiac arrest
Lower probability of significant stunning
Coronary angioplasty
Unstable angina
Prinzmetal angina
Stable exertional angina
Other situations of transient myocardial ischaemia

1.4. CLINICAL IMPLICATIONS

The formal demonstration of stunned myocardium as a cause of contractile dysfunction in the human heart was made difficult by the existing technical limitations that were unable to demonstrate a decrease concomitant with myocardial flow. However, this being demonstrable in all experimental species studied without exception [71], albeit with different intensities, allows the assumption with reasonable certitude that it occurs in man as well [72] and is confirmed by considerable indirect evidence [9,46,67,73-84]. Table 1 shows the clinical conditions in which stunned myocardium may be produced.

Stunned myocardium can be especially important in surgery and cardiac transplant and following acute myocardial infarction. During bypass and as well in transplantation, the heart is liable to overall ischaemia despite the protection provided by hypothermia and cardioplegia. Following a myocardial infarction with early reperfusion, whether spontaneous or therapeutically induced, it is possible to predict that all the myocardium saved will present as severely stunned over many hours or even some days. There is evidence as well that patients with severe ischaemia secondary to stress angina, unstable angina, Prinzmetal or repeated episodes of silent ischaemia can present with prolonged post-ischaemic contractile dysfunction [85]. In coronary angioplasty, the duration of the occlusion (generally less than 90 seconds) is too short to induce an appreciable depression of contractility. Yet, alterations in diastole have been observed.

The existence of myocardial stunning can have implications not only for therapy but also in diagnosis and prognosis. Various treatments have been demonstrated to have the capacity to attenuate stunning in different experimental models [49,53,86-92]. Among these the Ca^{2+} channel blockers [87,88] and the anti free radical agents standout [49, 53]. Studies in the isolated heart are concordant in showing the beneficial effect of the Ca^{2+} channel blockers. However, the results obtained *in vivo* are less consistent and, as yet, it has not been demonstrated that the administration of these compounds immediately before reperfusion has any beneficial effect. Angiotensin converting enzyme (ACE) inhibitors have been described as attenuating myocardial stunning when they are administered before reperfusion [86,93,94]. Once reperfusion has been restored, the myocardium dysfunction by stunning can be effectively corrected by inotropic stimulation and it has been tested that the recruitment of reperfused myocardium contractile reserve does not have negative effects on the myocites [15-21]. Hence, the natural history of spontaneous resolution and the inotropic response would indicate that myocardial dysfunction secondary to stunning is not an important clinical problem. This is the main reason explaining the lack of conclusive studies regarding the efficacy of treatment to prevent or reverse myocardial stunning.

Probably the most important clinical implication of stunned myocardium is the awareness of its existence as a possible cause of reversible contractile dysfunction [95]. Left ventricular function is the most important factor in many aspects of cardiovascular disease. In the context of coronary artery disease it is important to determine if the contractile function in a segment of the ventricular wall is due to the loss of contractile cells (necrosis and/or apoptosis) or if it is due to reversible dysfunction. This differentiation can have important prognostic implications. In an extreme example, severe ventricular dysfunction in the first few hours post-reperfusion treatment of an acute myocardial infarction can signify a very poor prognosis. The therapeutic option of cardiac transplantion has to be assessed in relation to whether this is due to myocardial necrosis or if it is caused, to a large extent, by stunning.

2. Hibernating myocardium

The term hibernation is used in zoology to describe the inactive state and profound hypothermia into which some animals, typically rodents and reptiles, enter at the start of winter and from which they recover rapidly and totally when the environmental temperature rises at the start of spring. This fascinating phenomenon, to-date, is not completely understood and consists of an adaptive decrease in energy expenditure in response to adverse conditions using a process that is active and reversible with the objective of preserving life until conditions improve. In an analogous manner, the term "myocardial hibernation" was coined originally to describe the chronic adaptive reduction of myocardial contractile function in response to decrease in myocardial flow that is observed in patients with ischaemic heart disease and, in whom, normalisation of the flow by surgical revascularisation normalises the contractile function. As we shall see later, recent studies have placed in doubt the concept that resting myocardial flow is diminished in patients with chronic ventricular dysfunction reversible with surgery. To-date, good animal models of chronic hibernation have not been available but, indeed, short-term (hours) myocardial hibernation has been achieved in certain models.

2.1.   FUNCTIONAL,   STRUCTURAL   AND   BIOCHEMICAL CHARACTERISATION OF HIBERNATING MYOCARDIUM

2.1.1. *Short-term hibernating myocardium in animal models*
The evidence of a strong correlation between perfusion and contraction in experiments with progressive decrease in myocardial flow has been rapidly accepted as the basis of the hibernating myocardium [96-100]. The myocardium was observed, subsequently, to be capable not only of remaining in a state of contractile hypofunction over a period of many hours in response to a reduction in flow that had been restored progressively, but also has the capacity to recover aerobic metabolism in this situation [12-14,101]. It has been demonstrated that it is possible to decrease coronary flow such as to induce severe myocardial dysfunction and to maintain the decrease over many hours without producing myocardial necrosis provided that the residual flow remains above a critical level (around 35-45% in the majority of conditions). Such a decrease in flow induces metabolic and biochemical changes characteristic of ischaemia, with activation of anaerobic glycolysis and acidosis and the fall in the concentrations of CK and ATP [102]. Nevertheless, the contractile failure occurs much earlier than significant reduction in the concentration of ATP, as a consequence of the increased concentration of inorganic phosphates and protons and which can be considered as a defensive response to preserve the cellular energy state by decreasing the energy expenditure associated with contraction. The fundamental biochemical characteristic of this model of the "short-term" hibernating myocardium is the progressive recovery of the concentrations of ATP and of the biochemical signs of ischaemia [103], such as acidosis, despite the continued reduction of myocardial flow and of contractile failure [104,105] (Figure 3). This biochemical normalisation appears to be the consequence of equilibrium between the synthesis and decreased utilisation of ATP [106] and constitutes the essential difference between ischaemic

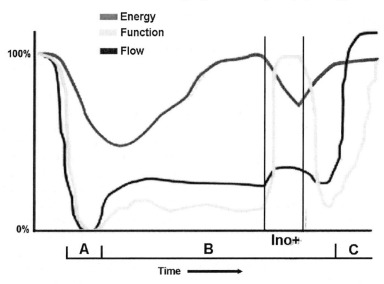

Figure 3. Pathophysiological scheme of short-term hibernating myocardium in which the induction phase (A), of equilibration perfusion/contraction (B) and normalisation of flow (C) are shown. It can be seen that the cellular energy status recovers during the equilibration phase. Inotropic stimulation (ino+) during this phase attempts to normalise contractile function (function) but at the expense of metabolic deterioration. Normalisation of flow is accompanied by functional recovery.

myocardial dysfunction and of short-term hibernation. The hibernating myocardium maintains a normal recruitable contractile reserve via inotropic stimulation [104,107]. In various models of short-term hibernation, the restoration of normal coronary flow is accompanied by functional recovery over a period of minutes or hours [16,98,102,108,109]. Possible structural changes in the short-term hibernating myocardium have not been clarified, as yet.

The physiopathological bases of hibernating myocardium contractile dysfunction is the decrease in the sensitivity of the contractile proteins to calcium [16]. Nevertheless, the molecular basis of this decrease is not known nor its causal mechanisms either. Being caused by a decrease in the sensitivity to Ca^{2+}, the contractile failure of the hibernating myocardium can be immediately overcome using methods that increase the contribution of Ca^{2+} to the myofibrils; actions such as adrenergic stimulation [104]. Nevertheless, in contrast to that which occurs in the stunned myocardium, inotropic stimulation ruptures the precarious balance between synthesis and degradation of ATP and is accompanied by biochemical changes characteristic of ischaemia (fall in the concentration in ATP, acidosis etc). If inotropic stimulation is sufficiently prolonged, the biochemical deterioration can progress to cell death [104]. The transitory functional recovery following deterioration triggered by inotropic stimulation has been termed "biphasic response" and has been used as a diagnosis of hibernating myocardium in patients [95].

Recent studies in the rabbit heart suggest that the objective of the energy equilibrium characteristic of the hibernating myocardium is favoured so that the natural progression towards necrosis is prevented when the sustained reduction by the coronary flow is preceded by an episode of severe ischaemia with zero flow [102]. It has been suggested that the rapid   restoration of the contractile failure during the severe ischaemic phase, within seconds, facilitates the subsequent energy recovery during the phase of moderate decrease in coronary flow [102,110,111]. At the other extreme, studies in the porcine model have demonstrated a better biochemical adaptation of the myocardium to the sustained decrease in coronary flow when this is progressively restored [112]. All these studies highlight that the progress and natural history of the hibernation process, as opposed to necrosis, depend on factors that are not very well understood.

2.1.2. Chronically hibernating myocardium in patients with coronary artery disease

In the context of chronic coronary artery disease, the hibernating myocardium can occur in territories dependent on narrowed coronary arteries and/or collateral circulation but in which the myocardial flow at rest is sufficient to avoid cell death. Similarly to the short-term hibernating myocardium, the chronically hibernating myocardium shows contractile failure with conserved inotropic reserve, and which reverts when the limitations of flow are eliminated. However, the two types of hibernation are capable of being differentiated on the basis of the chronically hibernating myocardium having considerable structural changes, the coronary flow at rest being very slightly decreased and the functional recovery induced by revascularisation can require days or even weeks.

Biopsy analysis of chronically hibernating human myocardium has demonstrated a reduction and disorganisation of the cytoskeletal proteins not only those of the intrasarcomeric (titina) but also extrasarcomeric (complex of fine filaments), such as morphologic abnormalities in the sarcoplasmic reticulum and mitochondria, increase of the cellular glycoprotein and of the proteins of the extracellular matrix. [85,113-115]. Biochemical studies have demonstrated changes in the protein isoforms of the hibernating myocardium with expression of proteins characteristic of smooth muscle, such as α-actin, not normally expressed by the myocardium [116]. These phenotypic changes have been interpreted as being the result of a process of de-differentiation and appear to be at least partially reversible with revascularisation.

Studies of myocardial flow with different imaging techniques, especially PET, in patients with hibernating myocardium have not been able, in general, to demonstrate reductions in the resting coronary flow of the magnitude necessary to produce short-term myocardial hibernation. Further, in recent studies, resting myocardial flow in the chronically hibernating myocardium was observed to be practically normal [117-123]. These findings have given rise to a controversy over the validity of the definition of the hibernating myocardium as being a dysfunction adaptation to the decrease in coronary flow and on the relevance of models of short-term hibernating myocardium [101, 124]. Indeed, the suggestion is that chronic hibernating myocardium does not really exist and that the chronic reversible dysfunction of the myocardium territory that is dependent on a narrowed coronary artery is the result of repeated cycles of ischaemia caused by augmenting the demand for oxygen; for example, during the exercise, followed by the corresponding period of stunning (chronic stunning) [124].

The resolution of this controversy will have to wait until it is possible to precisely monitor in a simultaneous and continuous manner the regional myocardial function and the local myocardial flow in patients with revascularisation-reversible contractile dysfunction. Long-term continuous monitoring of these variables has not been performed to-date in any species [124]. Nevertheless, there have been some observations that invite caution before discrediting the adaptive theory or negating the existence of chronic hibernation. Firstly, the determinations of myocardial flow with PET performed to-date have assigned measures of transmural coronary flow in which slight decreases of transmural flow are consistent with significant reductions of the sub-endocardiac flow and capable of inducing severe contractile dysfunction in short-term models [97,125]. This, together with the magnitude of error of measurement inherent currently in this technique, suggests that it may not be possible to categorically state that there exist significant sub-endocardiac decreases in flow in the majority of patients with hibernating myocardium included in studied series apart from patients in whom myocardial flow had been investigated. [101]. Secondly, the structural changes in the chronically hibernating myocardium need to be taken into account in that it is not possible to discount the magnitude of flow decrease necessary to maintain the hibernating myocardium to be less than that necessary to induce short-term hibernation.

The rate of recovery of contractile function induced by revascularisation of the chronically hibernating myocardium appears to be very variable but which, in any case, is much slower than observed in short-term stunning; reaching several weeks in some studies [126-131]. This duration is probably related to the severity of the structural changes described previously and would appear to be greater when myofibril loss is more marked. It has been suggested that the grade of conservation of inotropic response predicts the rate of post-revascularisation functional recovery probably because, as well, it is influenced by the severity of the structural changes in the myocytes [113,132]. It cannot be ruled out that, in certain cases, the de-differentiated and atrophied myocardium does not recover normal structure and function subsequent to effective revascularisation and the term "viable" is justified in describing the myocardium that is not only alive but also with a capacity to survive and recover contractile function.

2.1.3. Transition from short-term myocardial hibernation to chronic hibernation

For information on short-term myocardial hibernation studies to be applied in understanding the causal mechanisms of chronic hibernation in man and the way in which it occurs, it is necessary to show that short-term hibernation can progress to chronic hibernation and to determine the manner in which this transition is produced. The few animal studies that have been performed to clarify this question agree that it is possible to maintain, over a period of several days or weeks, myocardial dysfunction by the induction of coronary stenosis in the absence of necrosis [107,133-137] and including the absence of significant decrease in resting coronary flow but with a considerably reduced coronary reserve [107,136]. However, simultaneous and continuous monitoring of function and flow have not been performed for more than a few hours [98,107] and, in any case, the duration of these studies is much shorter than the natural history of the condition in patients with chronic hibernation [135].

3. Clinical implications

Taking into account that the causal mechanisms of the hibernating myocardium are unknown and that the recruitment of contractile reserve by sustained inotropic stimulation can have deleterious effects on cellular survival, the principal clinical implication of the hibernating myocardium is its detection as a cause of reversible ventricular dysfunction that is reversible with revascularisation [138].

Over the last few years, emphasis has been placed on the development of methods and diagnostic criteria capable of identifying the hibernating myocardium in patients with coronary artery disease and the present book reflects this emphasis. Studies on the detection of hibernating myocardium are beset with common limitations deriving from the retrospective nature of the unambiguous diagnosis that is established as a function of post-revascularisation contractile recovery [139]. Recovery cannot be produced if the revascularisation is incomplete or inadequate or, if during the revascularisation procedure, myocardial necrosis occurs.

Available information suggests that the hibernating myocardium is relatively infrequent as a significant cause of severe ventricular dysfunction [126,127]. Its frequency is estimated to be around 10% in patients who are candidates for cardiac transplant [102,128]. However, taking into account the scarcity of donor hearts, detection of such subgroups of such candidates who could benefit from surgical revascularisation would be of considerable cost-effectiveness interest [95,140]. Detection of the hibernating myocardium can, as well, have implications in the treatment of other subgroups of patients [95] and which is the subject of other chapters of this book.

4. Conclusions

In the majority of cases, coronary artery disease is the result of the asynchronic progression and complication of multiple atheromatous coronary lesions in different segments of the coronary tree. There is a dynamic component whose effects on the myocardium are modulated by systemic factors and, in particular, by haemodynamic changes. In this context it is to be hoped that stunning and hibernating can be produced simultaneously in different myocardial territories in the same patient and with variable long-term contribution to the contractile dysfunction of the territory. This can considerably complicate the interpretation of the diagnostic tests and of the therapeutic options. Inotropic stimulation can increase the function of a stunned myocardial segment and at the same time can put the survival of a hibernating segment at risk and can cause ischaemia in a third area dependent on a stenosed coronary artery.

Despite the complexity and incomplete knowledge, the mechanisms of reversible contractile failure in coronary disease need to be taken into account in the treatment of patients with coronary artery disease. The old model according to which ventricular dysfunction was the expression of loss of contractile elements has been replaced by another in which the dysfunction of the alive myocardium, the remodelled ventricle and the neuroendocrine adaptations contribute decisively to the ventricular failure and to the appearance of cardiac insufficiency.

Acknowledgements:

Funding was, in part, by the European Community (PL 95-0838) and the Fondo de Investigación de la Seguridad Social (FIS 95/0465).
The authors thank Sra. Beatriz Rodrigo for her excellent secretarial assistance.

References

1.   Tennant R, Wiggers CJ. The effect of coronary occlusion on myocardial contraction. Am J Physiol 1935; 112: 351-361.
2.   Théroux P, Franklin D, Ross J Jr, Kemper WS. Regional myocardial junction during acute coronary occlusion and its modification by pharmacologic agents in the dog. Cir Res 1974; 35: 896-908.
3.   García-Dorado D, Théroux P, Elízaga J et al. Myocardial reperfusion in the pig heart model: infarct size and duration of coronary occlusion. Cardiovasc Res 1987; 21: 537-544.
4.   Jennings RB, Sommers HM, SmythGa, Flack HH, Linn H. Myocardial necrosis induced by temporary occlusion of a coronary artery in the dog. Arch Pathol 1960; 70: 68-78.
5.   Sommers HM, Jennings RB. Experimental acute myocardial infarction. Histologic and histochemical studies of early myocardial infarcts induced by temporary or permanent occlusion of a coronary artery. Lab Invest 1964; 13: 1491-1503.
6.   Allen DG, Orchard CH. Myocardial contractile junction during ischemia and hypoxia. Cardiovasc Res 1987; 60: 153-168.
7.   Heyndrickx GR, Millard RW, McRitchie RJ, Maroko PR, Vatner SF. Regional myocardial functional and electrophysiological alterations after brief coronary artery occlusion in conscious dogs. J Clin Invest 1975; 56: 978-985.
8.   Siegmund B, Koop A, Klietz T, Schwartz P, Piper HM. Sarcolemmal integrity and metabolic competence of cardiomyocytes under anoxia-reoxygenation. Am J Physiol 1990; 258: H285-H291.
9.   Braunwald E, Kloner RA. The stunned myocardium: prolonged, postischemic ventricular dysfunction. Circulation 1982; 66: 1146-1149.
10. Rahimtoola SH. Coronary bypass surgery for chronic angina. Circulation 1982; 65: 225-241.
11. Rahimtoola SH. A perspective on the three large multicenter randomized clinical trials of coronary bypass surgery for chronic stable angina. Circulation 1985; 72 (Suppl. V): V-123-V-135.
12. Fedele FA, Gewirtz H, Capone RJ, Sharaf B, Most AS. Metabolic response to prolonged reduction of myocardial blood flow distal to a severe coronary artery stenosis. Circulation 1988; 78: 729-735.
13. Pantely GA, Malone SA, Rhen WS et al. Regeneration of myocardial phosphocreatine in pigs despite continued moderate ischemia. Circ Res 1990; 67: 1481-1493.
14. Schulz R, Guth BD, Pieper K, Martin C, Heusch G. Recruitment of an inotropic reserve in moderately ischemic myocardium at the expense of metabolic recovery: a model of short-term hibernation. Circ Res 1992; 70: 1282-1295.
15. Becker LC, Levine JH, Di Paula AF, Guarnieri T, Aversano T. Reversal of dysfunction in post-ischemic stunned myocardium by epinephrine and postextrasystolic potentiation. J Am Coll Cardiol 1986; 7: 580-589.
16. Heusch G, Rose J, Skyschally A, Post H, Schulz R. Calcium responsiveness in regional myocardial short-term hibernation and stunning in the in situ porcine heart-inotropic responses to postextrasystolic potentiation and intracoronary calcium. Circulation 1996; 93: 1556-1566.
17. Ito BR, Tate H, Kobayashi M, Schaper W. Reversibly injured, postischemic canine myocardium retains normal contractile reserve. Circ Res 1987; 61: 834-846.

18. Krams R, Duncker DJ, McFalls EO, Hogendoorn A, Verdouw PD. Dobutamine restores the reduced efficiency of energy transfer from total mechanical work to external mechanical work in stunned porcine myocardium. Cardiovasc Res 1993; 27: 740-747.

19. Krams R, Soei LK, McFalls EO et al. Endsystolic pressure length relations of stunned right and left ventricles after inotropic stimulation. Am J Physiol 1993; 265: H2099-H2109

20. García-Dorado D, Inserte J, Ruiz Meana M et al. Gap junction uncoupler heptanol prevents cell-to-cell progression of hypercontracture and limits necrosis during myocardial reperfusion. Circulation 1997; 96: 3579-3586.

21. Duncker DJ,Schulz R, Ferrari R et al. Myocardial stunning. Remaining questions. Cardiovasc Res 1998; 36: 3071-3082.

22. García-Dorado D, Oliveras J. Myocardial oedema: a preventable cause of reperfusion injury? Review article. Cardiovasc Res 1993; 27: 1555-1563.

23. García-Dorado D, González MA, Barrabés JA et al. Prevention of ischemic rigor contracture during coronary occlusion by inhibition of Na^+-H^+ exchange. Cardiovasc Res 1997; 35: 80-89.

24. García-Dorado D, Ruiz-Meana M. The (still) unknown mechanism of ischemic preconditioning: possible involving of reduced Na^+/H^+ exchange. Basic Res Cardiol 1997;92 (Suppl 2): 43-45.

25. Amende I, Bentivegna LA, Zeind AJ, Wenzlaff P, Grossman W, Morgan JP. Intracellular calcium and ventricular function. Effects of nisoldipine on global ischemia in the isovolumic, coronary-perfused heart. J Clin Invest 1992; 89: 2060-2065.

26. Steenbergen C, Murphy E, Levy L, London RE. Elevation in cytosolic free calcium concentration early in myocardial ischemia in perfused rat heart. Circ Res 1987; 60: 700-707.

27. Tani M, Neely JR. Role of intracellular Na^+ in Ca_2^+ overload and depressed coronary recovery of ventricular function of reperfused ischemic rat hearts. Circ Res 1989; 65: 1045-1056.

28. DeBoer LVW, Ingwall JS, Kloner RA, Braunwald E. Prolonged derangements of canine myocardial purine metabolism after a brief coronary artery occlusion not associated with anatomic evidence of necrosis. Proc Natl Acad Sci 1980; 77: 5471-5475.

29. Ellis SG, Henschke CI, Sandor T, Wynne J, Braunwald E, Kloner RA. Time course of functional and biochemical recovery of myocardium salvaged by reperfusion. J Am Coll Cardiol 1983; 1: 1047-1055.

30. Lange R, Ware J, Kloner RA. Absence of a cumulative deterioration of regional function during three repeated 5 or 15 minute coronary occlusions. Circulation 1984; 69: 400-478.

31. Laxson D, Homans D, Dai X, Sublett E, Bache R. Oxygen consumption and coronary reactivity in postischemic myocardium. Cir Res 1989; 64: 9-20.

32. Lerch R, Villiger B, Riedhammar H, Meier WE, Rutishauser W. Left ventricular function and creatine phosphate content during reperfusion. Circulation 1975:51/52 (Suppl II): II-208.

33. Lerch R. Myocardial stunning: the role of oxidative substrate metabolism. Basic Res Cardiol 1995: 90: 276-278.

34. Piper HM, Balser C, Ladilov YV et al. The role of Na^+/H^+ exchange in ischemia-reperfusion. Basic Res Cardiol 1996; 91: 191-202.

35. García-Dorado D, Ruiz Meana M, Barrabés J (1996) Does preconditioning reduce lethal mechanical reperfusion injury? Myocardial Preconditioning, in Wainwright OL and Parrat JR (eds.), Springer-Verlag, Heidelberg, pp. 19-34.

36. Piper HM, García-Dorado D, Ovize M. A fresh look on reperfusion injury. Cardiovascular Res 1998; 38: 291-300.

37. Marban E, Kitakaze M, Kusuoka H, Porterfield JK, Yue DT, Chacko VP. Intracellular free calcium concentration measured with 19F NMR spectroscopy in intact ferret hearts. Proc Natl Acad Sci USA 1987; 84: 6005-6009.

38. Marban E, Kitakaze M, Koretsune Y, Yue DT, Chacko VP, Pike MM. Quantification of $[Ca_2^+]i$ in perfused hearts: Critical evaluation of the 5F-BAPTA and nuclear magnetic resonance method as applied to the study of ischemia and reperfusion. Circ Res 1990; 66: 1255-1267.

39. Kusuoka H, Porterfield JK, Weisman HF, Weisfeldt ML, Marban E. Pathophysiology and pathogenesis of stunned myocardium: Depressed Ca_2^+ activation of contraction as a consequence of reperfusion-induced cellular calcium overload in ferret hearts. J Clin Invest 1987; 79: 950-961.

40. Kusuoka H, Koretsune Y, Chacko VP, Weisfeldt ML, Marban E. Excitation-contraction coupling in postischemic myocardium. Does failure of activator $Ca++$ transients underlie stunning? Circ Res 1990; 66: 1268-1276.

41. Gao WD, Atar D, Backx PH, Marban E. Relationship between intracellular calcium and contráctile force in stunned myocardium direct evidence for decreased myofilament Ca_2^+ responsiveness and altered diastolic function in intact ventricular muscle. Circ Res 1995; 76: 1036-1048.

42. Soei L, Sassen LMA, Fan DS, van Veen T, Krams R, Verdouw PD. Myofibrillar Ca_2^+ sensitization predominantly enhances function and mechanical efficiency of stunned myocardium. Circulation 1994; 90: 959-969.

43. Bezstarosti K, Soei LK, Krams R, Ten Cate FJ, Verdouw PD, Lamers JMJ. The effect of the thiadiazinone derivative [+]EMD 60263 on the responsiveness of Mg2+-ATPase to Ca_2^+ in myofibrils isolated from stunned and not-stunned porcine and human myocardium. Biochem Pharmacol 1996; 51: 1211-1220.

44. Hofman PA, Miller WP, Moss RL. Altered calcium sensitivity of isometric tension in myocyte-sized preparations of porcine postischemic stunned myocardium. Circ Res 1993; 72: 50-56.

45. McFalls EO, Duncker DJ, Krams R, Sassen LMA, Hoogendoorn A, Verdouw PD. Recruitment of myocardial work and metabolism in regionally stunned porcine myocardium. Am J Physiol 1992; 263: H1724-H1731.

46. Smart SC, Sawada S, Ryan T, et al. Low-dose dobutamine echocardiography detects reversible dysfunction after thrombolytic therapy of acute myocardial infarction. Circulation 1993; 88: 405-415.

47. Lamers JMJ, Duncker DJ, Bezstarosti K, McFalls EO, Sassen LMA, Verdouw PD. Increased activity of the sarcoplasmic reticular calcium pump in porcine stunned myocardium. Cardiovasc Res 1993; 27: 520-524.

48. Limbruno U, Zucchi R, Ronca-Testoni S, Galbani P, Ronca G, Mariani M. Sarcoplasmic reticulum function in the "stunned" myocardium. J Mol Cell Cardiol 1989; 21: 1063-1072.

49. Schattock MJ. Myocardial stunning: do we know the mechanism? Basic Res Cardiol 1997;92 (Suppl. 2): 18-22.

50. Bolli R, Zughaib M, Li XY et al. Recurrent ischemia in the canine heart causes recurrent bursts of free radical production that have a cumulative effect on contractile function. A pathophysiological basis for chronic myocardial "stunning". J Clin Invest 1995; 96: 1066-1084.

51. Bolli R. Mechanism of myocardial "stunning". Circulation 1990; 82: 723-738.

52. Bolli R, McCay PB. Use of spin traps in intact animals undergoing myocardial ischemia/reperfusion: A new approach to assessing the role of oxygen radicals in myocardial "stunning". Free Radic Res Commun 1990;9:169-180

53. Bolli R. Oxygen derived free radicals and myocardial reperfusion injury: an overview. Cardiovasc Drug Ther 1991; 5: 249-268.

54. De Jong JW, van der Meer P, Nieukoop AS, Huizer T, Stroeve RJ, Bos E, Xanthine oxidoreductase activity in perfused hearts of various species, including humans. Circ Res 1990; 67: 770-773.

55. Guarnieri C, Muscari C, Ferrari D, Giordano E, Caldarera CM. Does calcium-driven mitochondrial oxygen radical formation play a role in cardiac stunning? Basic Res Cardiol 1997; 92 (Suppl. 2): 23-25.

56. Henry TD, Archer SL, Neldon D, Weir EK, From AH. Postischemic oxygen radical production varies with duration of ischemia. Am J Physiol 1993; 264: H1478-H1484.

57. Bolli R, Jeroudi MO, Patel BS et al. Marked reduction of free radical generation and contractile dysfunction by antioxidant therapy begun at the time of reperfusion: evidence that myocardial "stunning" is a manifestation of reperfusion injury. Circ Res 1989; 65: 607-622.

58. Mekhfi H, Veksler V, Mateo P, Maupoil V, Rochette L, Ventura-Clapier R. Creatine kinase is the main target of reactive oxygen species in cardiac myofibrils. Circ Res 1996; 78: 1016-1027.

59. Bolli R. Role of neutrophils in myocardial stunning after brief ischaemia: the end of a six-year-old controversy. Cardiovasc Res 1993; 27: 728-730.

60. Bolli R. The early and late phases of preconditioning against myocardial stunning and the essential role of oxyradicals in the phase: an overview. Basic Res Cardiol 1996; 91: 57-63.

61. Yang ZK, Rix C, Shah A. Hypoxic superfusates from cultured endothelial cells inhibit myocardial connection. J Moll Cell Cardiol 1997; 29: A107.

62. Ertl G, Alexander RW, Braunwald E. Interaction between coronary occlusion and the renin-angiotensin system in the dog. Basic Res Cardiol 1983; 78: 518-533.

63. Ehring T, Baumgart D, Krajcar M, Hummelgen M, Kompa S, Heusch G. Attenuation of myocardial stunning by the ACE inhibitor ramiprilat through a signal cascade of bradykinin and prostaglandins but not nitric oxide. Circulation 1994; 90: 1368-1385.

64. Van der Giessen WJ, Schoutsen B, Tijssen JGP, Verdouw PD. Iloprost (ZK 36374) enhances recovery of regional myocardial function during reperfusion after coronary artery occlusion in the pig. Br J Pharmacol 1986; 87: 23-27.
65. Farber NE, Pieper GM, Thomas JP, Gross GJ. Beneficial effects of iloprost in the stunned canine myocardium. Circ Res 1988; 62: 204-215.
66. McFalls EO, Duncker DJ, Ward H, Fashingbauer P. Impaired endothelium-dependent vasodilation of coronary resistance vessels in severely stunned porcine myocardium. Basic Res Cardiol 1995; 90: 498-506.
67. Moore CA, Cannon J, Watson DD, Kaul S, Beller GA. Thallium-201 kinetics in stunned myocardium characterized by severe postischemic systolic dysfunction. Circulation 1990; 81: 1622-1632.
68. Nicklas JM, Becker LC, Bulkley BH. Effects of repeated brief coronary occlusion on regional left ventricular function and dimension in dogs. Am J Cardiol 1985; 56: 473-478.
69. Nicklas J, Gips J. Decreased coronary flow reserve after transient myocardial ischemia in dogs. J Am Coll Cardiol 1989; 13: 195-199.
70. Jeremy R, Stahl L, Gillinov M, Aversano T, Becker L. Preservation of coronary flow reserve in stunned myocardium. Am J Physiol 1989; 256: H1303-H1310.
71. Shen YT, Vatner SF. Differences in myocardial stunning following coronary artery occlusion in conscious dogs, pigs and baboons. Am J Physiol 1996; 270: H1312-1322.
72. Kloner RA, Przyklenk K (1993) Stunned myocardium. Properties, mechanisms, and clinical manifestations, Marcel Dekker Inc, New York.
73. Bolli R. Myocardial "stunning" in man. Circulation 1992; 86: 1671-1691.
74. Braunwald E (1993) Is myocardial stunning important from a clinical standpoint?, in R.A. Kloner and K Przyklenk (eds.), Stunned myocardium. Properties, mechanisms and clinical manifestations. New York, Marcel Dekker, Inc., pp: 441-452.
75. Dilsizian V, Bonow RO. Current diagnostic techniques of assessing myocardial viability in hibernating and stunned myocardium. Circulation 1993; 87: 1-20.
76. Sinusas AJ, Watson DD, Cannon JM, Beller GA. Effect of ischemia and postischemic dysfunction on myocardial uptake of technetium-99m-labeled methoxyisobutyl isonitrile and thallium-201. J Am Coll Cardiol 1989; 14: 1785-1793.
77. Fine DG, Clements IP, Callahan MJ. Myocardial stunning in hypertrophic cardiomyopathy: recovery predicted by single photon emission computed tomographic thallium-201 scintigraphy. J Am Coll Cardiol 1989; 13: 1415-1418.
78. Pierard LA, De Lansheere CM, Berthe C, Rigo P, Kulbertus HA. Identification of viable myocardium by echocardiography during dobutamine infusion in patients with myocardial infarction after thrombolytic therapy: comparison with positron emission tomography. J Am Coll Cardiol 1990; 15: 1021-1031.
79. Ferrari R, Alfieri O, Curello S, et al. Occurrence of oxidative stress during reperfusion of the human heart. Circulation 1990; 81: 201-211.
80. Ferrari R. The new ischemic syndromes. An old phenomenon disguised with a new glossary? Cardiovasc Res 1997; 36: 298-300.
81. Galli M, Giubbini R, Tavazzi L. Transient prolonged postischemic ventricular dilatation documented by 99mTcMIBI scan. Chest 1991; 99: 1536-1538.
82. Galli M, Marcassa C, Bolli R et al. Spontaneous delayed recovery of perfusion and contraction after the first 5 weeks after anterior infarction. Evidence for the presence of hibernating myocardium in the infarcted area. Circulation 1994; 90: 1386-1397.
83. Nienaber CA, Brunken RC, Sherman CT, et al. Metabolic and functional recovery in ischemic human myocardium following coronary angioplasty. J Am Coll Cardiol 1991; 18: 966-978.
84. Vatner SF, Heyndryckx GR. Ubiquity of myocardial stunning. Bas Res Cardiol 1995; 90: 253-256.
85. Ambrosio G, Betocchi S, Pace L et al. Prolonged impairment of regional contractile function after resolution of exercise-induced angina. Evidence of myocardial stunning in patients with coronary artery disease. Circulation 1996; 94: 2455-2464.
86. Duncker DJ, Soei LK, Werdouw PD (1997) Pharmacological modulation of myocardial stunning, in G.R. Heyndrickx, S. F. Vatner and W. Wijns. Stunning, hibernation and preconditioning: clinical pathophysiology of ischemia. Philadelphia, Lippincott Raven Publishers, pp. 229-252.
87. Heusch G. Myocardial stunning: a role for calcium antagonists during ischaemia? Cardiovasc Res 1992; 26: 14-19.
88. Opie LH. Myocardial stunning: a role for calcium antagonists during reperfusion? Cardiovasc Res 1992; 26: 20-24.

89. Kida M, Fujiwara H, Uegaito T et al. Dobutamine prevents both myocardial stunning and phosphocreatine overshoot without affecting ATP level. J Mol Cell Cardiol 1993; 25: 875-885.

90. Sun JZ, Tang XL, Knowton AA, Park SW, Qiu Y, Bolli R. Late preconditioning against myocardial stunning. An endogenous protective mechanism that confers resistance to postischemic dysfunction 24 h after brief ischemia in conscious pigs. J Clin Invest 1995; 95: 388-402.

91. Tang XL, Qiu Y, Park SW, Sun JZ, Kalya A, Bolli R. Time course of late preconditioning against myocardial stunning in conscious pigs. Circ Res 1996; 79: 424-434.

92. Urabe K, Miura T, Iwamoto T et al. Preconditioning enhances myocardial stunning via adenosine receptor activation. Cardiovasc Res 1993; 27: 657-662.

93. Przyklenk K (1993) Angiotensin converting enzyme inhibitors, in R.A. Kloner and K. Przyklenk K (eds.) Stunned myocardium. Properties, mechanisms, and clinical manifestations. New York, Marcel Dekker Inc. pp. 321-336.

94. Lefer AM, Ogletree ML, Smith JB et al. Prostacyclin: a potentially valuable agent for preserving myocardial tissue in acute myocardial ischemia. Science 1978; 200: 53-54.

95. Barrabés JA, García-Dorado D, Martín JA, Coma Canella I, Valle Tudela V. Papel de las exploraciones no invasivas en el manejo de la cardiopatía isquémica. Estimación de la viabilidad miocárdica. Rev Esp Cardiol 1997; 50: 75-82.

96. Gallagher KP, Matsuzaki M, Osakada G, Kemper WS, Ross Jr J. Effect of exercise on the relationship between myocardial blood flow and systolic wall thickening in dogs with acute coronary stenosis. Cir Res 1983; 52: 716-729.

97. Gallagher KP, Matsuzaki M, Koziol JA, Kemper WS, Ross Jr. J. Regional myocardial perfusion and wall thickening during ischemia in conscious dogs. Am J Physiol 1984; 247; H727-H738.

98. Matsuzaki M, Gallagher KP, Kemper WS, White F, Ross Jr. J. Sustained regional dysfunction produced by prolonged coronary stenosis: gradual recovery after reperfusion. Circulation 1983; 68: 170-182.

99. Ross Jr. J. Myocardial perfusion-contraction matching. Implications for coronary heart disease and hibernation. Circulation 1991; 83: 1076-1083.

100. Schulz R, Guth BD, Heusch G. No effect of coronary perfusion on regional myocardial function within the autoregulatory range in pigs: evidence against the Gregg phenomenon. Circulation 1991; 83: 1390-1403.

101. Rahimtoola SH. Hibernating myocardium is hypoperfused. Basic Res Cardiol 1997; 92 (Suppl. 2): 9-11.

102. Ferrari R, Cargnoni A, Bernocchi P et al. Metabolic adaptation during a sequence of no-flow and low-flow ischaemia: a possible trigger for hibernation. Circulation 1996; 94: 2587-2596.

103. Hearse DJ. Myocardial ischemia: can we agree on a definition for the 21st century? Cardiovasc Res 1994; 28: 1737-1744.

104. Schulz R, Rose J, Martin C, Brodde OE, Heusch G. Development of short-term myocardial hibernation: its limitation by the severity of ischemia and inotropic stimulation. Circulation 1993; 88: 684-695.

105. Schulz R, Rose J, Post H, Heusch G. Regional short-term hibernation in swine does not involve endogenous adenosine or KATP channels. Am J Physiol 1995; 268: H2294-H3201.

106. Hearse DJ. Hibernation: a form of endogenous protection? Six questions for investigation. Basic Res Cardiol 1997; 92 (Suppl. 2): 1-2.

107. Chen C, Li L, Chen LL et al. Incremental doses of dobutamine induce a biphasic response in dysfunctional left ventricular regions subtending coronary stenosis. Circulation 1995; 92: 756-766.

108. Ferrari R, La Canna G, Giubbini R (1994) Hibernating myocardium, in Pepper YM (ed.), Annual of cardiac surgery, pp. 28-32.

109. Ito BR. Gradual onset of myocardial ischemia results in reduced myocardial infarction. Association with reduced contractile function and metabolic downregulation. Circulation 1995; 91: 2058-2070.

110. Van Binsbergen XA, van Emous JG, Ferrari R, van Echteld CJA, Ruigrok TJC. Metabolic and functional consequences of successive no-flow and sustained low-flow ischaemia; a 31P MRS Study in rat hearts. J Mol Cell Cardiol 1996; 28:2373-2381.

111. Van Binsbergen XA, Van Echteld CJA, Ferrari R, Ruigrok TJC. Some triggering mechanism, in addition to perfusion-contraction matching, may be essential to initiate hibernation. Basic Res Cardiol 1997; 92 (Suppl. 2): 3-5.

112. Bolli R, Zhu XX, Myers ML, Hartley CJ, Roberts R. Beta-adrenergic stimulation reverses post-ischemic myocardial dysfunction without producing subsequent functional deterioration. Am J Cardiol 1985; 56: 964-968.

162 D. García-Dorado and J. Soler-Soler

113. Flameng W, Suy R, Schwarz F et al. Ultrastructural correlates of left ventricular contraction abnormalities in patients with chronic ischemic heart disease: Determinants of reversible segmental asynergy postrevasculatization surgery. Am Heart J 1981; 102: 846-857.
114. Elsässer A, Schaper J. Hibernating myocardium: adaptation or degeneration? Basic Res Cardiol 1995; 90: 47-48.
115. Elsässer A, Schlepper M, Klovekorn WP, Cai WJ, Zimmerman R, Muller KD. Hibernating myocardium: an incomplete adaptation to ischemia. Circulation 1997; 96: 2920-2931.
116. Borgers M, Ausma J. Structural aspects of the chronic hibernation myocardium in man. Basic Res Cardiol 1995; 90: 44-46.
117. Camici PG, Rimoldi O. Resting myocardial blood flow in patients with hibernating myocardium quantified by positron emission tomography. Basic Res Cardiol 1997; 92 (Suppl 2): 6-8.
118. Iskandrian AS, Hakki A-H, Kane SA, Goel IP, Mundth ED, Segal BL. Rest redistribution thallium-201 myocardial scintigraphy to predict improvement in left ventricular function after coronary arterial bypass grafting. Am J Cardiol 1983; 51: 1312-1316.
119. Camici PG, Wijns W, Borgers M et al. Pathophysiological mechanisms of chronic reversible left ventricular dysfunction due to coronary artery disease. Circulation 1997; 96: 3205-3214.
120. Tillisch J, Brunken R, Marshall R et al. Reversibility of cardiac wall-motion abnormalities predicted by positron emission tomography. N Engl J Med 1986; 314: 884-888.
121. Tamaki N, Yonekura Y, Yamashita K, et al. Positron emission tomography using fluorine-18 deoxyglucose in evaluation of coronary artery bypass grafting. Am J Cardiol 1989; 64: 860-865.
122. Van Overschelde JLJ, Wijns W, Depré C et al. Mechanisms of chronic regional postischemic dysfunction in humans. New insights from the study of noninfarcted collateral-dependent myocardium. Circulation 1993; 87: 1513-1523.
123. Marinho NVS, Keogh BE, Costa DC, Lammersma AA, Ell PJ, Camici PG. Pathophysiology of chronic left ventricular dysfunction. New insights from the measurement of absolute myocardial blood flow and glucose utilization. Circulation 1996; 93: 737-744.
124. Heusch G, Ferrari R, Hearse DJ, Ruigrok TJC, Schulz R. Myocardial hibernation: questions and controversies. Cardiovasc Res 1997; 36: 301-309.
125. Fallavollita JA, Canty JM. Differential 18F-2-deoxyglucose uptake in viable dysfunctional myocardium with normal resting perfusion evidence for chronic stunning in pigs. Circulation 1999; 40: 363-372.
126. La Canna G, Alfieri O, Giubbini R, Gargano M, Ferrari R, Visioli O. Echocardiography during infusion of dobutamine for identification of reversible dysfunction in patients with chronic coronary artery disease. J Am Coll Cardiol 1994; 23: 617-626.
127. Ando H, Jarraka J, Hisahara M, Omesue M, Shirota T. Effect of coronary by-pass grafting onto the site of old myocardial infarction and the recovery of cardiac function. Cardiovasc Surg 1998; 5: 511-519.
128. Vanoverchelde JJ, Depre C, Berber BL et al. Ti me course of functional recovery after coronary artery by-pass graft surgery in patients with chronic left ventricular ischemic dysfunction. Am J Cardiol 2000; 85: 1432-1439.
129. Rahimtoola SH. From coronary artery disease to heart failure: role of the hibernating myocardium. Am J Cardiol 1995; 75: 16E-22E.
130. Takeishi Y, Tono-oka I, Kubota I et al. Functional recovery of hibernating myocardium after coronary bypass surgery: does it coincide with improvement in perfusion? Am Heart J 1991; 122: 665-670.
131. Topol EJ, Weiss JL, Guzmán PA et al. Immediate improvement of dysfunctional myocardial segments after coronary revascularization: Detection by intraoperative transesophageal echocardiography. J Am Coll Cardiol 1984; 4: 1123-1134.
132. Bolli R, Zhu W-X, Thornby JI, O'Neill PG, Roberts R. Time course and determinants of recovery of function after reversible ischemia in conscious dogs. Am J Physiol 1988; 254: H102-H114.
133. Bolukoglu H, Liedtke AJ, Nellis SH, Eggleston AM, Subramanian R, Renstrom B. An animal model of chronic coronary stenosis resulting in hibernating myocardium. Am J Physiol 1992; 263: H20-H29.
134. Liedtke AJ, Renstrom B, Nellis SH, Subramanian R. Myocardial function and metabolism in pig hearts after relief from chronic partial coronary stenosis. Am J Physiol 1994; 267: H1312-H1319.
135. Mills I, Fallon JT, Wrenn D et al. Adaptive responses of coronary circulation and myocardium to chronic reduction in perfusion pressure and flow. Am J Physiol 1994; 266: H447-H457.
136. Liedtke AJ, Renstrom B, Nellis SH, Hall JL, Stanley WC. Mechanical and metabolic functions in pig hearts after 4 days of chronic coronary stenosis. J Am Coll Cardiol 1995; 26: 815-828.

137. Shen YT, Vatner SF. Mechanism of impaired myocardial function during progressive coronary stenosis in conscious pigs. Hibernation versus stunning. Circ Res 1995; 76: 479-488.
138. Rahimtoola SH. Importance of diagnosing hibernating myocardium: how and in whom? J Am Coll Cardiol 1997; 30: 1701-1706.
139. De Silva R, Yamamoto Y, Rhodes CG et al. Preoperative prediction of the outcome of coronary revascularization using positron emission tomography. Circulation 1992; 86: 1738-1742.
140. Kriett JM, Kaye MP. The registry of the international society for heart transplantation. J Heart Transplant 1990; 9: 323-330.

8. RADIONUCLIDE UPTAKE IN EXPERIMENTAL ISCHAEMIA AND NECROSIS

JOAN CINCA-CUSCULLOLA and AMPARO GARCIA-BURILLO

Over recent years, concepts of the pathophysiology of coronary artery disease have undergone considerable change. New and important concepts such as coronary microcirculation, ischaemic preconditioning, stunned myocardium, hibernating myocardium and myocardial viability have been introduced. Several experimental studies have explored these concepts towards developing an understanding of the phenomena that occur in ischaemic heart disease

Experimental nuclear cardiology has, as its principal goals, two objectives. One objective is to evaluate radiopharmaceuticals for use in studies of myocardial perfusion with respect to their pharmaco-kinetics and technical factors that can influence the quality of images obtained. The other objective is to mimic and study, in laboratory models, the different pathophysiological situations that arise in the human patient.

Thalium-201 and different technetium-labelled radiotracers such as sestamibi and tetrofosmin have demonstrated, in different experimental studies, their capacity to evaluate the alterations in the myocardial perfusion and play important roles in the study of ischaemia and necrosis.

1. Myocardial perfusion tracers

In the early nuclear medicine studies of myocardial perfusion in the 60s, labelled microspheres were injected into the left atrium or into a coronary artery and the coronary flow was determined with great precision. This technique continues to be the "gold standard" for the assessment of myocardial perfusion but is useful only in experimental models. Other tracers began to be assessed that could be taken-up by the myocardium in proportion to the local blood flow. Analogues of potassium such as ^{131}Cs, ^{81}Rb and ^{43}K were used but it was soon observed that the best tracer was ^{201}Tl [1]. It began to be used in clinical practice in 1975 and, until recently, has been the main diagnostic procedure in the study of myocardial perfusion. Over the years other experimental studies [2,3] with ^{201}Tl were initiated as well as other radiopharmaceuticals, such as pyrophosphates, to evaluate the damaged myocardium and which were subsequently used extensively in clinical practice for the diagnosis of myocardial infarction.

The radio-physical limitations of ^{201}Tl stimulated the discovery of a complexes labelled with ^{99m}Tc to serve as agents of cardiac perfusion assessment. It is a radionuclide that is suited to the existing gamma cameras. Hence, during the decade of the 80s, experimental studies were directed towards the identification and development of the ideal technetium-labelled tracers for the study of myocardial perfusion. Different studies such as that of

J. Candell-Riera et al. (eds.), Myocardium at Risk and Viable Myocardium, 165–182.
© 2001 *Kluwer Academic Publishers. Printed in the Netherlands.*

Deutsch et al. [4] using cationic complexes of ^{99m}Tc appeared promising and images of high quality in the canine experimental model were obtained. Subsequent studies, like those of Gerundini et al. [5], evaluated the role of three different perfusion agents labelled with ^{99m}Tc to investigate myocardial perfusion in a canine model as well as in humans. In 1984, Holman et al. [6] presented the first studies in humans using a new tracer: ^{99m}Tc-butyl-isonitrile. Leppo et al. [7] published their results in rabbits with a new derivative of the isonitriles with a better pharmaco-kinetic profile: 2-methoxy-isobutyl-isonitrile (MIBI); a complex that diffuses passively across the cellular membrane and locates in the cytosolic fraction. Subsequent experimental studies [8] demonstrated that the fundamental mechanism of uptake and subsequent retention of MIBI is the passive diffusion across the cellular and mitochrondrial membranes in response to the negative potential across the membrane. When a depolarisation of the membrane occurs (such as what happens in irreversible damage of the myocyte) the uptake and retention of the sestamibi is inhibited. It has been demonstrated experimentally [9,10] that sestamibi has a lower extraction and a slower washout than thallium and that extraction, washout and retention of both are influenced by variations in coronary flow.

Other new technetium-labelled tracers such as teboroxime, tetrofosmin and Q12 have since been discovered and evaluated in the early 90s and, of these, the most frequently used is tetrofosmin [11].

2. Experimental assessment of ischaemia

2.1. THALLIUM-201

Following the intravenous administration of ^{201}Tl, its initial uptake by the myocardium depends on the blood flow and on the extraction capacity of the myocardium.

One of the earliest studies that assessed its use as a marker of myocardial perfusion is that of Strauss et al. [12] which demonstrated that, in dogs with occlusion of the anterior descending coronary artery, the uptake of thallium is similar to that of [43]K. Subsequently, Weich et al. [13], established, as well in a canine model, that, under basal conditions, the fraction of thallium extracted by the myocardium, i.e. the myocardium's capacity of extraction from the blood in its first pass through the coronary circulation, was $88\pm2.1\%$. Studies such as that of Pohost et al. [14] demonstrated, in an animal model, the phenomenon of redistribution.

In various experimental studies in dogs the relationship between the initial uptake of thallium and the regional blood flow was determined using microspheres. Studies by Strauss et al. [12], Grunwald et al. [15] and Sinusas et al. [16] demonstrated, in canine models, that the uptake of thallium is proportional to the blood flow. Nielsen et al. [17], in a canine model, compared the myocardial distribution of thalium-201 with the regional cardiac blood flow during ischaemia and during exercise. In all the dogs, a clear correlation ($r \geq 0.98$) between the distribution of the tracer and the direct measurement of coronary flow was observed.

In 1984, Okada et al. [18] performed a kinetic study of thalium-201 in a canine model to evaluate the uptake in a reperfused myocardium following coronary artery occlusion. Following the reperfusion it was observed that, in the early phase, the washout of thallium was greater in the infarcted myocardium than in the salvaged myocardium and in the normal myocardium but with subsequent equilibration.

In summary, ^{201}Tl is a tracer whose uptake is in excellent proportion to coronary flow within almost the whole range of physiological variation of myocardial perfusion. Conversely, its incorporation into myocardial tissue has a clearance that is influenced in relation to the presence of regional myocardial ischaemia or necrosis.

2.2. TECHNETIUM-LABELED COMPOUNDS

Up to the middle of the 80s, the only tracer used for the assessment of myocardial perfusion was ^{201}Tl but this tracer is not ideal due to its known radio-physical characteristics. Hence, the search began for technetium-labelled compounds to be used as markers of myocardial perfusion. These would have better properties and be more easily and cheaply produced.

Early experimental studies such as that of Nishiyama et al. [19] were promising and used compounds that were technetium-labelled cations but it soon became clear that, in humans, there was no ideal between cardiac uptake contrast and background. From then on, the experimental studies were channelled into assessing two types of technetium labelled compounds: 1) Cation compounds of the isonitriles group such as ^{99m}Tc-Sestamibi, and 2) Neutral lipophilic compounds such as ^{99m}Tc-teboroxima and ^{99m}Tc-tetrofosmin.

2.2.1. Isonitriles

Among the initial experimental studies using isonitriles, those of Jones et al. [20] and of Holman et al. [6] stand out. The first isonitriles (TBI and CPI) did not have a great clinical usefulness due to high, and persistent, hepatic and pulmonary activity. The introduction of ^{99m}Tc-metoxy-iso-butyl-isonitrile (sestamibi) showed a good ratio of cardiac: background activity. Piwnica-Worms et al. [8] described the basic mechanisms of its uptake and its dependence on plasma and mitochondrial trans-membrane potential. Numerous experimental studies subsequently showed [16,21-26] that the intensity of the myocardial uptake of sestamibi is tightly correlated with the regional cardiac flow and cellular viability. Sinusas et al. [16], in 1989, intended correlating the myocardial uptake not only of sestamibi but also of thallium with the coronary blood flow using microspheres in a canine model. The conclusions were that both tracers were comparable under conditions of reduced coronary flow and during reperfusion following 15 minutes of coronary occlusion that provoked a post-ischaemic dysfunction and that both correlated well with the alterations in coronary flow. Beanlands et al. [26], in 1990, produced irreversible cellular damage in the myocytes of rats in which a constant flow was maintained and observed an intense reduction in the uptake of sestamibi due to the absence of intracellular retention of the tracer. Mousa et al. [24], in the same year, concluded, in a porcine model, that sestamibi was as sensitive as thallium in the detection and diagnosis of coronary artery disease.

The uptake of sestamibi in the myocardium is closely related to the coronary blood flow measured using microspheres, as already observed by Okada et al. [27], in 1988, in a canine model (r=0.92) but only when there are viable myocytes.

Beller et al. [23], in 1993, performed an interesting experimental study in a canine model to demonstrate that the myocardial uptake and retention of sestamibi following reperfusion in a model of myocardial infarction were indicative of viability. It was noted that the moment of injection of the tracer was fundamental. If the injection was too early and the quantification of the uptake of the tracer performed too soon, the amount of viable myocardium can be overestimated since, in the 3 subsequent hours there was a phase of sestamibi loss from the irreversible-damaged myocytes. This can have special relevance in the clinical studies when sestamibi is injected in the acute phase of a myocardial infarction. The detection would need to be delayed at least 3 hours so that the image obtained correctly defines the zones of the myocardium that are viable and those that are not cicatrised.

Many experimental studies have intended evaluating the role of sestamibi in the assessment of the area of myocardium threatened during a coronary occlusion or the quantity of myocardium salvaged following reperfusion [28-34]. Verani et al. [29], observed, in dogs subjected to 2 hours of coronary occlusion, that the size of the perfusion defect correlates with the size of the necrosis. Following a reperfusion of 48 hours, the size of the defect was notably reduced and correlated well with final size of the infarct.

Sinusas et al. [30] as well using a canine model of necrosis in which to evaluate the uptake and retention of sestamibi before and after reperfusion, concluded that the uptake was dependent as much on the myocardial viability as on the coronary flow. When the tracer was injected during the occlusion, and before the reperfusion, the uptake and retention was correlated with the jeopardised area as determined at post-mortem. If the injection was performed 90 minutes after the start of the reperfusion, a good correlation with the final area of necrosis would exist as well but no correlation with the coronary flow. Thus its uptake would appear to require the presence of viable myocytes and it would seem that under these conditions, more than being a marker of the grade of reperfusion, sestamibi can be a marker of myocardial viability. If the injection was performed immediately after the initiation of reperfusion, the quantity of salvaged myocardium is overestimated since the early uptake during hyperaemia reflects more the phenomenon of reperfusion that of viability.

Glover et al. [31], used a canine model to evaluate whether redistribution of sestamibi existed following reperfusion. It was demonstrated that redistribution did exist in the reperfused viable myocardium but that this was very slight and would not be appreciated on simple visual analysis. Conversely, no redistribution existed in the reperfused, non-viable myocardium or in that which is not reperfused.

2.2.2. Teboroxim

Among some studies using this tracer, Maublant et al. [35] investigated the effects of a metabolic inhibition of the uptake of teboroxime in cultured myocardial cells compared to the uptake of ^{201}Tl and of sestamibi. It was demonstrated that the uptake and retention of these two tracers were very influenced by the metabolic abnormalities while the uptake of teboroxime did not appear to be modified despite the presence of a marked metabolic derangement. In this sense, teboroxime would be a "pure" tracer of myocardial perfusion. Another experimental study is that of Leppo et al. [36] in which the myocardial uptake of teboroxime and ^{201}Tl were compared at different levels of coronary flow and, as well, their roles as tracers of flow were recorded. Di Rocco et al. [37] performed an experimental study in rats and dogs in which the coronary blood flow was measured using ^{201}Tl, sestamibi and teboroxime. A better approximation of the true flow was obtained using ^{201}Tl and teboroxime.

The scintigraphic assessment of myocardial hypoperfusion depends on the capacity of the tracers to distinguish disparities of regional blood flow. Weinstein et al. [38] performed a study with rabbits comparing thalium-201, MIBI and teboroxime as markers of myocardial hypoperfusion using a quantitative technique of high resolution (autoradiography) and concluded that the technetium-labelled compounds better distinguished the hypoperfused myocardium and was able to achieve better contrast to normal myocardium.

Beanlands et al. [39] performed a study in dogs to evaluate the temporal sequence of changes relating to the uptake of teboroxime and myocardial blood flow. The results demonstrated that both parameters correlated optimally at the moment of injection. Conversely, merely 5 minutes later, the retention of the tracer underestimated the flow. It is from these important data that rapid-acquisition protocols were developed for use with this type of tracer.

2.2.3. Tetrofosmin.
At the beginning of the 90s, studies were directed towards developing new technetium-labelled complexes that employ a diphosphate bond as a ligand. Outstanding among these compounds is 1,2-bis[bis(2-ethoxyethyl)phosphino] ethane (^{99m}Tc-tetrofosmin).

Tetrofosmin is a ligand that forms a lipophylic cation complex with technetium. One of the principal experimental explorations with this tracer was by Kelly et al. [11] who demonstrated its good cardiac uptake and retention and its rapid clearance, especially from the blood and liver. Another preliminary study was that of Dahlberg et al. [40] in which, in an experimental model with rabbits, its myocardial uptake was demonstrated as being linearly correlated with coronary blood flow.

One of the most important experimental studies validating this tracer as a marker of myocardial blood flow was that of Sinusas et al. [41]. In a canine model, it was demonstrated that the uptake of tetrofosmin was proportional to the coronary flow (as measured using microspheres) and that within only 10 minutes post-injection the tracer had already achieved a good heart/background definition.

Takashahi et al. [42] demonstrated in 1996, in an experimental model in rats, that the uptake and retention of tetrofosmin was influenced, equally as with ^{201}Tl and sestamibi, not only by the coronary flow but also by the cellular viability as well.

2.2.4. Q12
Of the latest technetium-labelled tracers used in the study of myocardial perfusion, ^{99m}Tc-Q12 is one of the most used. In 1994, Gerson et al. [43] studied its kinetic properties in a canine model and showed that its myocardial uptake was proportional to the coronary blood flow measured using microspheres.

3. Experimental evaluation of stunned and hibernating myocardium with single photon emission tracers

To differentiate between ischaemic, but viable, myocardium from the necrotic and non-viable myocardium has been, and continues to be, one of the principal objectives of isotopic studies over these last few years. Classically, the tracer most commonly used in the studies of viability has been ^{201}Tl but, as has been seen earlier, the technetium-labelled compounds began to play an important role in the evaluation of viability and, as such, has contributed to the clinical and experimental-animal studies.

At the start of the 80s the concept of the stunned myocardium was established experimentally and clinically as a post-ischaemic contractile dysfunction, sustained but reversible, in the reperfused myocardium [44]. In the canine model, clamping a coronary artery produces a contractile alteration in the myocardial wall of the territory of distribution of the occluded vessel. When after about 15 minutes, before cell death can occur, the artery is declamped contractile dysfunction persists despite reperfusion. On subsequent biopsy of this cardiac muscle, however, the tissues appear as normal myocardium. With follow-up in dogs, a gradual recovery in contractile function is observed until normality is reached over a period of hours or even days.

Various studies have demonstrated that after 15 minutes of coronary occlusion and subsequent reperfusion, a contractile dysfunction is produced that can last up to 12 hours before recovery [45,46].

Myocardial ischaemia provokes biochemical alterations and ultrastructural changes in the myocites [46,47] as well as alterations in the regional blood flow [45] that persist during reperfusion. Studies of myocardial perfusion, a sensitive method to evaluate metabolic alterations similar to that of evaluating alterations in flow, provide information on the myocardial viability in conditions of stunned post-ischaemic myocardium at which time there is evident ventricular contractile dysfunction. Sinusas et al. [16] demonstrated in an experimental study that, in these conditions of myocardial stunning, not only technetium-labelled compounds (sestamibi) but also thallium provide comparable information.

The concept of hibernation was introduced by Rahimtoola et al. [48,49] in 1985, although already in 1978 Diamond et al. [50] had intuited that the non-infarcted ischaemic myocardium could remain in a state of hibernation. This concept is characteristic of the myocardium that has an altered contractile function which is persistent at rest and which is associated with a severe reduction in the coronary flow; the contractile function being potentially recoverable if the flow improves.

Many experimental studies summarise how this state of hibernation can be produced and have explored the mechanisms of its recovery. The hibernating myocardium has been defined as acute, sub-acute or chronic depending on the rapidity of recovery of the contractile function following revascularisation and based on the morphologic changes observed. Matsuzaki et al. [51] observed that the ventricular function recovery, following 5 hours of reduction of myocardial perfusion, reduction of contractility and slight or no infarction, would be produced in a gradual manner over a period of one week.

Sinusas et al. [16] performed a study in a rabbit model in which an experimental hibernation of short duration (60 minutes) was produced using a partial, sustained occlusion of the anterior descending coronary artery. Having achieved the reduction in coronary flow, 5 mCi of ^{99m}Tc-MIBI and 0.5 mCi of thallium-201 were injected. It was demonstrated that the myocardial uptake of both tracers, under conditions of low coronary flow and during the period of post-ischaemic regional myocardial dysfunction, was similar. Kloner et al. [52] in 1994 conducted experimental studies in dogs, rats and rabbits. The coronary artery was occluded for 40 to 90 minutes but, prior to this, brief periods of ischaemia were induced in a subgroup of them. In the animals in which this pre-conditioning was performed, the size of the necrosis was smaller compared to the animals in which no prior ischaemic conditioning had been performed. These findings suggest that the myocardial ischaemia causes a metabolic adaptation in the specific cardiac musculature such that the new ischaemic episodes encounter a myocardial response that is more efficient and less ischaemia is provoked.

Fallavollita et al. [53] studied a porcine model of chronic hibernation in which the anterior descending coronary artery was partially occluded over a period of 3 months and which resulted in a moderate reduction in the myocardial perfusion but with a severe contractile dysfunction of the left ventricle. Although it was demonstrated that an adaptive mechanism existed in the myocardium, it was more evident in the sub-endothelial layers and varied in relation to the regional coronary reserve.

Although the clinical aspects of the hibernating myocardium are well established, the pathophysiological aspects remain under constant revision [54]. Myocardial blood flow reduction is one of the physiological bases of the hibernation but, nevertheless, there is not always a chronic and severe reduction in myocardial flow in basal conditions while, conversely, the phenomenon that is invariably encountered in the non-contractile viable myocardium is the absence of coronary reserve. These findings suggest the possibility that the restoration of the process of myocardial hibernation can contribute to the mechanism of reiteration of situations of ischaemia-reperfusion (stunning) when the myocardial demand for oxygen is increased or transitory phenomena of intra-coronary occlusion.

Moore et al. [55] obtained a canine model of stunned myocardium using repeated periods of occlusion and reperfusion. The uptake and washout of ^{201}Tl in the stunned myocardium did not differ from that observed in the normal myocardium with preserved wall motion but dependent on a stenosed vessel.

A few experimental models exist which reproduce fairly accurately the pathophysiological conditions of the phenomenon of hibernation in humans. In the study by Camici et al. [54] the causes that limit the majority of experimental studies of myocardial hibernation were analysed. One of the most important is that the induced coronary stenosis is not sufficiently prolonged. The majority of experimental studies performed [51,52,56-58] are not models of chronic hibernation. Kitakaze and Marban [56], for example, used an "in vitro" model in which the reduction in the flow is only for a matter of hours. In the canine models it is difficult to maintain a reduction of sustained coronary flow, not even for a few hours, because of the rapid appearance of collateral circulation [51]. Hence, many investigators use porcine models in which there is not such a rapid and extensive collateralisation. Schulz et al. [57] used a porcine model in which a constant hypoperfusion of flow was induced over 90 minutes. Chen et al. [58] employed a similar model but performed a coronary stenosis over 24 hours. As such, all these are models of acute flow reduction which do not necessarily reflect the situation of chronic arterial disease of humans.

The creation of a porcine model of chronic hibernation also has the drawback that, frequently, variable grades of necrosis are produced which make the interpretation of the results difficult [53,54]. Nevertheless, Shen et al. [59] used a porcine model of coronary occlusion and performed measurements of coronary flow and contractile function. It was documented that there was neither significant myocardial necrosis nor major collateralisation. Further, in the myocardium distal to the occluded artery there was a considerable functional dysfunction that could last up to 3 weeks.

In the porcine model of Fallavolita et al. [53] coronary flow and the uptake of ^{18}F-fluordeoxyglucose (FDG) was evaluated. It was observed that the reduction of coronary flow was inversely proportional to the increment of uptake of FDG in the akinetic zones although, as in the study of Shen et al. [59], the levels of flow were only moderately lower than those of the normoperfused myocardium. This causes certain investigators [54] to question the validity of these models as being representative of hibernation in the human heart. It must not be forgotten that, in clinical studies as well, the most recent estimations of regional myocardial flow show values normal or slightly diminished with respect to the healthy myocardium [60,61].

4. Uptake in acute ischaemia and in the experimental scar

We have performed studies in our laboratory with myocardial perfusion tracers [62,63] directed towards determining the grade of uptake in the regions of chronic infarction and in the acute arterial occlusion. In clinical practice, the differentiation between necrotic and ischaemic tissue is, on occasions, difficult since the low level of hypo-uptake occasioned by a much-reduced myocardium cannot be differentiated from the non-specific uptake by the scar. Hence, we were interested in performing a study, in a porcine model, directed towards determining, simultaneously, the grade of uptake of ^{99m}Tc-tetrofosmin and ^{201}Tl in infarct areas of scarred transmural myocardium and in areas

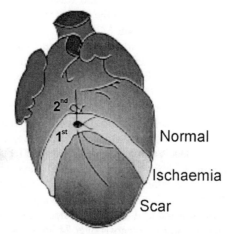

Figure 1. Representation of a porcine heart in which the first ligature of the anterior descending coronary artery as well as the second 20-30 mm above the first can be seen. These coronary occlusions delineate 3 areas of myocardial tissue: the scar, the acute ischaemic area without necrosis and the non-ischaemic tissue (normal).

contiguous with the acute ischaemia. The study was performed in 27 pigs surviving an infarct provoked by ligature of the anterior descending coronary artery. One month later the animals had a further intervention. A median sternotomy was performed to access the territory of the anterior descending artery 20 to 30 mm above the primary ligature which was dissected and re-occluded at this point (Figure 1). To ensure that the second ligature of the anterior descending coronary artery resulted in ischaemia we performed epicardiac electrograms in the pre-infarct zone [63].

One hour after re-occlusion of the coronary artery and, hence, of the induction of the acute ischaemia that included the zone of old infarct as well as a new wider area of peri-infarct ischaemia, we proceeded to inject (in sinusoidal rhythm) ^{99m}Tc-tetrofosmin into the left atrium (Group I, composed of 12 animals) or into the jugular vein (Group II, composed of 6 animals). To the 9 remaining animals (Group III) the radiopharmaceutical

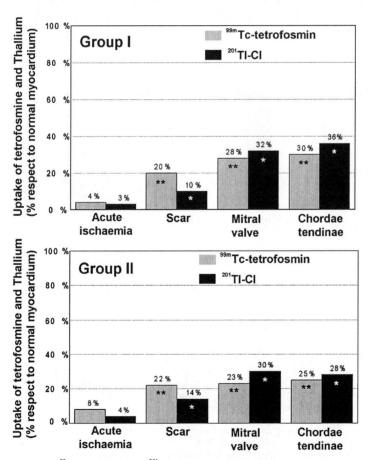

Figure 2. Uptake of ^{99m}Tc-tetrofosmin and ^{201}Tl chloride injected into the left atrium (Group I) or into the jugular vein (Group II) in pigs with an infarct of the anterior face of one month duration subjected to a re-occlusion of the proximal anterior descending coronary artery. The radionuclide uptake appears equal as regards the percentage of specific activity (cpm/g) with respect to the normal myocardium. The values are expressed as the mean. * (p<0.05) and ** (p<0.001) indicate significant differences with respect to the acute ischaemic area.

was injected in cardio-circulation stoppage so as to avoid the possible arrival of radiotracer across from the collateral coronary circulation.

Thallium-201 was simultaneously injected in 6 animals of Group I and all of Groups II and III and cylindrical transmural samples of tissue were obtained in the normal myocardium, in the zone of acute ischaemia and in the scar of the infarct and the specific activities of the radiotracers (cpm per gram) were determined.

At the conclusion of the biopsies, transversal sections were performed at a distance of 10 to 20 mm from the apex up to the atrio-ventricular ring. Sections were also obtained of the mitral valve leaflets and of the chordae tendinae to compare the activity in these fibrous tissues with that of the scar. Finally, scintigraphic measurements were performed on the slices and the selected cylindrical samples (Figure 2). The specific activity was measured and, to avoid the Compton effect of the ^{99m}Tc, the counting of the ^{201}Tl was performed at 24 hours. To define the borders of the peri-infarct zone of ischaemia, a 5 ml bolus dose of 20% fluoresceine was injected into the left atrium immediately before the administration of the radiotracers. Each of the tissue slices were examined under

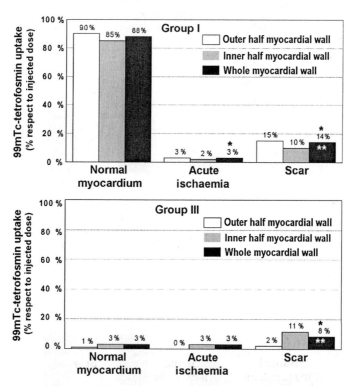

Figure 3. Uptake of ^{99m}Tc-tetrofosmin in transmural samples of the left ventricle of pig hearts with an earlier infarct of one month's duration, subjected to one hour of re-occlusion of the anterior descending artery in its proximal portion. The uptake of ^{99m}Tc-tetrofosmin is presented as percentage specific activity (cpm/g) with respect to the injected dose. The values are expressed as the mean.

* ($p<0.005$) and ** ($p<0.05$) indicate significant differences with respect to the normal myocardium uptake and the acute ischaemic area, respectively. Group I corresponds to the intra-atrial administration of the radionuclide under normal conditions while Group III corresponds to the intra-ventricular administration at cardiac arrest.

ultraviolet so that the non-fluorescent regions (acute ischaemic myocardium) were dissected and separated from the fluorescent regions (normal myocardium) and both parts were processed separately. To identify the margins of the first infarct, the preparation was incubated in triphenyl tretrazolium at 37°C. The white, non-stained zone (necrotic zone) was dissected and processed.

Histology studies were performed and it was observed that all the pigs had a transmural infarction scar that contained fibroblasts, extracellular matrix and some capillary vessels. The necrotic myocardial cells were heterogeneously distributed in the scar. Viable myocardial cells were observed only in the sub-endocardium in a band of about 0.25 mm in width.

These results demonstrated that the animals with acute ischaemic peri-infarct and injected with ^{99m}Tc-tetrofosmin, whether in the left atrium (Group I) or in the jugular vein

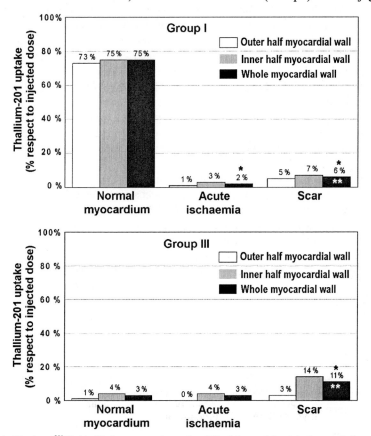

Figure 4. Uptake of ^{201}Tl chloride in transmural samples of the left ventricle of the hearts of pigs with anterior infarct subjected to one hour of re-occlusion of the anterior descending coronary artery in its proximal portion. The uptake of the isotope is presented as a percentage of the specific activity (cpm/g) with respect to the doses injected. The values are expressed as the means.
* (p<0.005) and ** (p<0.05) indicate significant differences with respect to the uptake in the normal myocardium and to the acute ischaemic area, respectively. Group I corresponds to the intra-atrial administration of the radionuclide under normal conditions while Group III corresponds to the intra-ventricular administration in cardiac arrest.

(Group II), had a greater activity in the necrotic zones than in the acute ischaemic zones. As seen in Figure 3, the mean of the radioisotope activity in the infarct zone was about 19% of that of the normal tissue in Group I and about 21% in Group II. Conversely, the activity in the acute ischaemia was very significantly less, visually zero on scintigraphy (2.9% in Group I and 5.8% in Group II; p<0.001). This difference in uptake of ^{99m}Tc-tetrofosmin between the normal myocardium, acute ischaemic and old scar is confirmed in the scintigraphy of the slices and myocardial biopsies (Plate 8.1). The activity of the tracer across the ventricular wall was more or less homogeneous (Figure 4) as indicated by the data obtained in the epicardiac and endocardiac sections of the ischaemic and infarcted zones. As illustrated in Figure 2, a considerable fraction of ^{99m}Tc-tetrofosmin is detected, as well, in samples of the chordae tendinae (25% in Group I and 21% in Group II) and in the mitral valve leaflets (29% and 23%, respectively).

The injection of ^{99m}Tc-tetrofosmin into the left ventricular cavity in hearts post-cardio-circulatory arrest and without coronary circulation (Group III) demonstrated, as well, higher uptake in the necrotic tissues than in the zones of acute myocardial ischaemia (5.8% vs. 2.1%; p<0.01) (Figure 3). These hearts had a greater radioisotope activity in the more internal sections than in the more external in the transmural samples taken in the normal (3.1% vs. 1.2%), acute ischaemic (3.1% vs. 0.3%) and necrotic (10.9% vs. 1.2%) myocardium zones.

In a parallel study with ^{99m}Tc-tetrofosmin, the same scheme was followed with a group of animals (n=10) in which the second occlusion was performed in the circumflex artery [65]. In all the cases, there was a greater activity in the necrotic zones (26%) than in the acute ischaemic zone (6.3%).

Similarly to that observed following the injection of ^{99m}Tc-tetrofosmin, the ^{201}Tl administered in sinus rhythm to hearts with peri-infarct acute ischaemia, whether via left atrium (Group I) or via the jugular vein (Group II), greater uptake of radiotracer is detected in the infarcted zone than in the acute ischaemic zone (Figure 4). The mean of the specific activity of ^{201}Tl in the necrotic tissues, relative to the normal, was 8.0% in group I and 13% in Group II. Conversely, the activity in the acute ischaemic myocardium was only 2.1% in Group I and 3.1% in Group II. The absorption of ^{201}Tl was homogeneous across the left ventricular wall. A significant fraction of the radiopharmaceutical was detected in the tendonous chords and in the mitral valve leaflets (Figure 2).

As can be seen in Figure 4, the intra-ventricular injection of ^{201}Tl in hearts in cardio-circulatory stoppage and coronary circulatory blockage (Group III) induced a greater activity in the scar of the infarct than in the acute ischaemic myocardium (9.8% and 3.9% of the standard doses, respectively). These hearts, as well, showed greater activity of ^{201}Tl in the internal slices than in the external. Scintigraphic images of the myocardium samples confirmed that the absorption of ^{201}Tl between the necrotic zones and the acute ischaemic zones (Plate 8.2) could be, on the other hand, completely superimposed on the images obtained with ^{99m}Tc-tetrofosmin (Plate 8.3).

Differences in uptake are observed between the zone of the scar and the area of healthy myocardium subjected to both an abrupt and total interruption of coronary flow. The absence of radioisotope activity in the acute ischaemic tissue is due to the elimination of the coronary perfusion and of the subsequent metabolic blockade. However, explanatory mechanisms as to how the tracer can arrive into a zone of a month-old myocardial infarction produced by ligature of the coronary artery are not readily available. In theory, the accumulation of radiotracers in the infarct zone would be possible only if collateral coronary circulation succeeded in reaching the infarct zone or if the radiotracers had the capacity to diffuse from the blood of the ventricular cavity.

Our data suggest that the collateral coronary circulation is not a significant source in the transport of the radiotracer to the necrotic zone. The pigs with cardio-circulatory arrest and coronary circulation blockade continued to show absorption of ^{99m}Tc-tetrofosmin and of ^{201}Tl greater in the necrotic zone than in the acute ischaemic zone and even than that occurring in the pigs in which the tracer was injected in sinus rhythm. Despite the hypothesis of the role of collateral coronary circulation influencing the absorption of the radiotracer in the zone of the infarct, other studies have demonstrated that collateral coronary circulation was slight [63-67] in healthy pigs as well as those with chronic infarction.

Early studies in sheeps [68] and in pigs demonstrated that the zones of chronic infarction possess a lower tissue electrical resistance, a property that implies a high ionic diffusibility [69]. This characteristic could explain the diffusion of the radiotracers from the ventricular cavity to the scar zone. Conversely, the healthy myocardium with a recent arterial occlusion maintains its tissue structure and has not, as yet, altered its electrical resistance that would impede the diffusion of the radiotracers from the vascular compartment.

Likewise, it needs to be pointed out that the external halves of the wall of the infarcted zone showed a greater uptake in the pigs that were injected during sinus rhythm than those injected during cardiac arrest. These differences may indicate that the external half of the infarcted wall of the beating heart receives a certain amount of radiotracer from small collateral epicardiac arteries or extra-coronary arteries. Alternatively, the gradient of uptake is inverted, with greater endocardial activity and less activity in the external half, in the hearts in haemodynamic arrest, suggesting a phenomenon of incomplete diffusion of the radiotracer from the ventricular cavity.

Another aspect relevant to our results is the verification that the zones of scarred myocardial infarction take-up ^{201}Tl and ^{99m}Tc-tetrofosmin. That the infarct zone contains fibroblasts, endothelial cells and an extra-cellular collagen matrix [68, 70, 71] is concordant with our histology findings. Fibroblasts and endothelial cells have the capacity to take-up ^{201}Tl and ^{99m}Tc-MIBI [72,73]. The possibility exists that these cationic compounds can be retained by the extra-cellular matrix since these structures contain proteoglycans (glucose-aminoglycans bound to proteins) that have negative electrical charge and, as such, are capable of attracting cations [70,71]. Our observation that the uptake in the tendinous structures (basically composed of connective tissue) is in the same range as that observed in the scar can help this hypothesis.

On the other hand, it appears of slight probability that the fine layer of viable sub-endothelial myocardial cells of the scar were responsible for the observed uptake. The zone of peri-infarction acute ischaemia was subjected to the same conditions of coronary occlusion and, as well, had sub-endothelial viable cells but, conversely, the uptake of ^{99m}Tc-tetrofosmin and of ^{201}Tl was practically zero.

Although it has been described [72,73] that, in "in vitro" cultures, several lines of cells have the capacity to retain ^{201}Tl or technetium-labelled tracers, we do not know the time of intra-cellular retention of these substances in live animals. It has been demonstrated that initial radiotracer activity in scar zones dependent on a patent artery is liable to a process of intense washout that is attributable to the absence of active mechanisms for retention by the myocytes. One possibility is that the activity, arriving at the scar via diffusion or via small collateral vessels, is cleared in a relatively short space of time (20-60 minutes). If so, we were unable to assess this due to the design of our study which required a second occlusion of the anterior descending artery and which precluded a prolonged maintenance of the haemodynamic conditions in the experimental animals.

5. Clinical implications

The observations in the porcine model can have a clinical application in humans in that, as in the pig, an occlusion of the coronary artery in man results in transmural infarction with a fine sub-endothelial layer of surviving cells [74]. This anatomical coincidence is due, presumably, to the fact that the hearts of both mammals have a poorly-developed collateral circulation and which appears slowly over a matter of weeks or months such that neovascularisation produces a significant coronary flow [66]. In contrast, the dog heart rapidly develops numerous collaterals such that, in these animals, non-transmural infarcts are observed following permanent occlusion of the coronary artery [75-78].

Although it is known that a quantitative value does not exist to define the myocardium that has the possibility of contractile recovery, our observations show that a grey area exists below which it not is possible to determine if the activity observed is due to the presence of viable tissue or to non-specific activity. It appears that this level is situated around 30% since below this value the probability of functional recovery is very low in patients [79, 80].

Conversely, we [81] and other authors [23,42] have demonstrated that the initial uptake in the zones of necrosis can overestimate the presence of myocytes due to the passive incorporation of the perfusion tracers into collagen and cellular structures of the scar. In any case, this uptake is below the accepted level in the evaluation of viability based on clinical observation [79,80,82-84] that generally have values of 40-50% of the maximum uptake indicative of the presence of viable tissue. It is advisable that, in clinical practice, scintigraphic detections of technetium tracers or of the ^{201}Tl injected at rest are performed following a waiting period of not less than 30 minutes so that the clearance of non-specific activity is retained in the necrotic zones.

References

1.   Lebowitz E, Greene MW, Fairchild R et al. Thallium-201 for medical use. J Nucl Med 1975;16: 151-155.
2.   Buja LM, Paekey RW, Stokely EM, Bonte FJ, Willerson JT. Pathophysiology of Technetium-99m Stannous pyrophosphate and thallium-201 scintigraphy of acute anterior myocardial infarcts in dogs. J Clin Inves 1976; 57: 1508-1522.
3.   Zweiman FG, Holman BL, O'Keefe A, Idoine J. Selective uptake of 99mTc complexes and 67Ga in acutely infarcted myocardium. J Nucl M 1975; 16: 975-979.
4.   Deutch E, Bushong W, Glavan KA et al. Heart imaging with cationic complexes of technetium. Science 1981; 214: 85-86.
5.   Gerundini P, Savi A, Gilardi MC et al. Evaluation in dogs and humans of three potential technetium-99m myocardial perfusion agents. J Nucl Med 1986; 27: 409-416.

6. Holman BL, Jones A, Lister-James J et al. A new 99mTc-labeled myocardial imaging agent, Hexakis (t-butyl-isonitrile)-[Technetium (I) 99mTc TBI: initial experience in the human. J Nucl Med 1984; 25: 1350-1355.

7. Leppo JA, Moeing AF. An evaluation of a Technetium-labelled isonitrile analogue as a myocardial imaging agent and comparison to thallium. Circulation 1986;74 (Suppl 2): 297 (Abstr.).

8. Piwnica-Worms D, Kronauge JF, Chiu ML. Uptake and retention of hexakis (2-methoxyisobutyl isonitrile) technetium (I) in cultured chich myocardial cells. Mitochondrial and plasma membrane potential dependence. Circulation 1990; 82: 1826-1838.

9. Marshall RC, Leidholdt EM Jr, Zhang D, Barnett CA. Technetium-99m hexakis 2-methoxy-2-isobutyl isonitrile and thallium-201 extraction, washout, and retention at varying coronary flow rates in rabbit heart. Circulation 1990; 82: 998-1007.

10. Melon PG, Beanlands RS, DeGrado TR, Nguyen N, Petry NA, Schwaiger M. Comparison of technetium-99m sestamibi and thallium-201 retention characteristics in canine myocardium. J Am Coll Cardiol 1992; 20: 1277-1283.

11. Kelly JD, Forster AM, Higley B et al. Technetium-99m-tetrofosmin as a new radiopharmaceutical for myocardial perfusion imaging. J Nucl Med 1993; 34: 222-227.

12. Strauss HW, Harrison K, Langan JK, Lebowitz E, Pitt B. Thallium-201 for myocardial imaging. Relation of thallium-201 to regional myocardial perfusion. Circulation 1975; 51: 641-645.

13. Weich HF, Strauss HW, Pitt B. The extraction of thallium-201 by the myocardium. Circulation 1977; 56: 188-191.

14. Pohost GM. Differentiation of transiently ischemic from infarcted myocardium by serial imaging after a single dose of thallium-201. Circulation 1977; 55: 294-302.

15. Grunwald AM, Watson DD, Holzgrefe HH Jr, Irving JF, Beller GA. Myocardial thallium-201 kinetics in normal and ischemic myocardium. Circulation 1981;4:10-618.

16. Sinusas AJ, Watson DD, Cannon JM Jr, Beller GA. Effect of ischemia and postischemic dysfunction on myocardial uptake of technetium-99m-labeled methoxyisobutyl isonitrile and thallium-201. J Am Coll Cardiol 1989; 14: 1785-1793.

17. Nielsen AP, Morris KG, Murdock R, Bruno FP, Cobb FR. Linear relationship between the distribution of thallium-201 and blood flow in ischemic and nonischemic myocardium during exercise. Circulation 1980; 61: 797-801.

18. Okada RD. Kinetics of thallium-201 in reperfused canine myocardium after coronary artery occlusion. J Am Coll Cardiol 1984; 3: 1245-1251.

19. Nishiyama H, Deutsch E, Adolph R et al. Basal kinetics studies of 99mTc DMPE as a myocardial imaging agent in the dog. J Nucl Med 1982; 23: 1093-1101.

20. Jones A, Abrams M, Davison A et al. Biological studies of a new class of technetium complexes: the hexakis alkylisonitrile technetium (I) cations. Int J Nucl Med Biol 1984; 11: 225-234.

21. Beller GA, Sinusas. AJ. Experimental studies of the physiologic properties of technetium-99m isonitriles. Am J Cardiol 1990: 66: 5E-8E.

22. Beller GA, Watson DD. Physiological basis of myocardial perfusion imaging with the technetium 99 m agents. Sem Nucl Med 1991; 21: 173-181.

23. Beller GA, Glover DK, Edwards NC, Ruiz M, Simanis JP, Watson DD. 99mTc-Sestamibi uptake and retention during myocardial ischemia and reperfusion. Circulation 1993; 87: 2033-2042.

24. Mousa SA, Cooney JM, Williams SJ. Relationship between regional myocardial blood flow and the distribution of 99mTc-sestamibi in the presence of total coronary artery occlusion. Am Heart J 1990; 119: 842-847.

25. Freeman I, Grunwald AM, Hoory S, Bodenheimer MM. Effect of coronary occlusion and myocardial viability on myocardial activity of technetium-99m-Sestamibi. J Nucl Med 1991; 32: 292-298.

26. Beanlands RSB, Dawood F, Wen WH et al. Are the kinetics of technetium-99m methoxyisobutyl isonitrile affected by cell metabolism and viability? Circulation 1990; 82: 1802-1814.

27. Okada RD, Glover D, Gaffney T et al. Myocardial kinetics of technetium-99m-hexakis-2-methoxy-2-methylpropyl-isonitrile. Circulation 1988; 77: 491-498.

28. Leon AR, Eisner RL, Martin SE et al. Comparison of Single-Photon emission computed tomographic (SPECT) myocardial perfusion imaging with thallium-201 and technetium-99m sestamibi in dogs. J Am Coll Cardiol 1992; 20: 1612-1625

29. Verani MS, Jeroudi MO, Mahmarian JJ et al. Quantification of myocardial infarction during coronary occlusion and myocardial salvage after reperfusion using cardiac imaging with technetium-99m hexakis 2-methoxyisobutyl isonitrile. J Am Coll Cardiol 1988; 12: 1573-1581.

30. Sinusas AJ, Trautman KA, Bergin JD et al. Quantification of area at risk during coronary occlusion and degree of myocardial salvage after reperfusion with technetium-99m Methoxyisobutyl Isonitrile. Circulation 1990; 82: 1424-1437.

31. Glover DK, Okada RD. Myocardial technetium 99m sestamibi kinetics after reperfusion in a canine model. Am Heart J 1993; 125: 657-666.

32. Li Q, Solot G, Frank TL, Wagner HN, Becker LC. Myocardial redistribution of technetium-99m-methoxyisobutyl isonitrile (SESTAMIBI). J Nucl Med 1990; 31: 1069-1076.

33. Merhi Y, Latour JG, Arsenault A, Rousseasu G. Effect of coronary reperfusion on technetium-99m methoxyisobutylisonitrile uptake by viable and necrotic myocardium in the dog. Eur J Nucl Med 1992; 19: 503-510.

34. De Coster PM, Wijns W, Cauwe F, Robert A, Beckers C, Melin JA. Area at risk determination by technetium-99m-hexakis-2-methoxyisobutyl isonitrile in experimental reperfused myocardial infarction. Circulation 1990; 82: 2152-2162.

35. Maublant J, Moins N, Gachon P. Uptake and release of two new 99mTc-labeled myocardial blood flow imaging agents in cultured cardiac cells. Eur J Nucl Med 1989; 15: 180-182.

36. Leppo J, Meerdink D. Comparative myocardial extraction of two technetium-labelled BATO derivates (SQ30217-SQ32014) and thallium. J Nucl Med 1990; 31: 67-74.

37. DiRocco RJ, Runsey WL, Kuczynski BL et al. Measurement of myocardial blood using co-injection technique for Technetium-99m-Teboroxime, Technetium-99m-Sestamibi and Thallium-201. J Nucl Med 1992; 33: 1152-1159.

38. Weinstein H, Reinhardt CP, Leppo JA. Teboroxime, sestamibi and thallium-201 as markers of myocardial hypoperfusion: Comparison by quantitative dual-isotope autoradiography in rabbits. J Nucl Med 1993; 34: 1510-1517.

39. Beanlands R, Muzik O, Nguyen N, Petry N, Schwaiger M. The relationship between myocardial retention of technetium-99m teboroxime and myocardial blood flow. J Am Coll Cardiol 1992; 20: 712-719.

40. Dahlberg S, Gilmore M, Leppo J. Effect of coronary flow on the "uptake" of tetrofosmin in the isolated rabbit heart J Nucl Med 1992; 33: 846 (Abstr.).

41. Sinusas AJ, Shi Q, Saltzberg MT et al. Technetium-99m-tetrofosmin to assess myocardial blood flow: experimental validation in an intact canine model of ischemia. J Nucl Med 1994; 35: 664-671.

42. Takahashi N, Reinhardt CP, Marcel R, Leppo JA. Myocardial uptake of 99mTc-tetrofosmin, sestamibi, and ^{201}Tl in a model of acute coronary reperfusion. Circulation 1996; 94: 2605-2613.

43. Gerson MC, Millard RW, Roszell NJ et al. Kinetic properties of 99mTc-Q12 in canine myocardium. Circulation 1994; 89: 1291-1300.

44. Braunwald E, Kloner RA. The stunned myocardium: Prolonged, post-ischemic ventricular dysfunction. Circulation 1982; 66: 1146-1149

45. Heyndricks GR, Millard RW, McRitchie RJ, Maroko PR, Vatner SF. Regional myocardial function and electrophysiological alterations after brief coronary artery occlusion in conscious dogs. J Clin Invest 1975; 56: 978-85.

46. Kloner RA, Ellis SG, Lange R, Braunwald E. Studies of experimental coronary artery reperfusion: effects of infarct size, myocardial function, biochemistry, ultrastructure and microvascular damage. Circulation 1983; 68(Suppl. I): 8-15.

47. DeBoer LWV, Ingwall JS, Kloner RA, Braunwald E. Prolonged derangements of canine myocardial purine metabolism after a brief coronary artery occlusion not associated with anatomic evidence of necrosis. Proc Natl Acad Sci USA 1980; 77: 54-71.

48. Rahimtoola SH. A perspective on three large multicentre randomized clinical trials of coronary bypass surgery for chronic stable angina. Circulation 1985; 72 (Suppl V): 123-135.

49. Rahimtoola SH. The hibernating myocardium. Am Heart J 1989; 117: 211-221.

50. Diamond GA, Forrester JS, de Luz PL, Wyatt HL, Swan HJC. Post-extrasystolic potentiation of ischemic myocardium by atrial stimulation. Am Heart J 1978; 95: 204-209.

51. Matsuzaki M, Gallagher KP, Kemper WS, White F, Ross J Jr. Sustained regional dysfunction produced by prolonged coronary stenosis: Gradual recovery after reperfusion. Circulation 1983, 68: 170-182.

52. Kloner RA, Yellon D. Does ischemic preconditioning occur in patients? J Am Coll Cardiol 1994; 24: 1133-1142.

53. Fallavolita JA, Perry BJ, Canty JM. 18-F-2-Deoxyglucose deposition and regional flow in pigs with chronically dysfunctional myocardium. Evidence for transmural variations in chronic hibernating myocardium. Circulation 1997; 95: 1900-1909.

54. Camici PG, Wijns W, Borgers M et al. Pathophysiological mechanisms of chronic reversible left ventricular dysfunction due to coronary artery disease (hibernating myocardium). Circulation 1997; 96: 3205-3214.

55. Moore CA, Cannon J, Watson DD, Kaul S, Beller GA. Thallium 201 kinetics in stunned myocardium characterized by severe post-ischemic systolic dysfunction. Circulation 1990; 81: 1622-1632.

56. Kitakaze M, Marban E. Cellular mechanism of the modulation of contractile function by coronary perfusion pressure in ferret hearts. J Physiol (Lond) 1989; 414: 455-472.

57. Schulz R, Heusch G. Acute adaptation to ischemia:short-term hibernating myocardium. Basic Res Cardiol 1995; 90: 29-31.

58. Chen C, Li L, Chen LL et al. Incremental doses of dobutamine induce a biphasic response in dysfunctional left ventricular regions subtending coronary stenoses. Circulation 1995; 92: 756-766.

59. Shen Y-T, Vatner SF. Mechanism of impaired myocardial function during progressive coronary stenosis in conscious pigs: hibernation versus stunning? Circ Res 1995; 76: 479-488.

60. Grandin C, Wijns W, Melin JA et al. Delineation of myocardial viability with PET. J Nucl Med 1995; 36: 1543-1552.

61. Maki M, Luotolahti M, Nuutila P et al. Glucose uptake in the chronically dysfunctional but viable myocardium. Circulation 1996; 93:1658-1666.

62. Cinca J, Blanch P, Carreño A, Mont L, García-Burillo A, Soler-Soler J. Acute Ischemic Ventricular arrhythmia in pigs with healed myocardial infarction. Comparative effects of ischemia at a distance and ischemia at the infarct zone. Circulation 1997; 96: 653-658.

63. Cinca J, Bardají A, Carreño A et al. ST segment elevation at the surface of a healed transmural myocardial infarction in pigs. Conditions for passive transmission from the ischemic peri-infarction zone. Circulation. 1995; 91: 1552-1559.

64. García-Burillo A, Cinca J, Castell J et al. Uptake of 99mTc-tetrofosmin in healed transmural myocardial infarction in pigs. Eur J Nucl Med 1996; 23: 1039 (Abstr.).

65. Schaper W (1971) The collateral circulation of the heart, in Scchaper W (ed.), Amsterdam, North Holland, pp. 5-18.

66. Patterson RE, Kirk ES. Analysis of coronary collateral structure, function, and ischemic border zones in pigs. Am J Physiol. 1983: 244: H23-H31.

67. White FC, Roth DM, Bloor CM. Coronary collateral reserve during exercise induced ischemia in the pig. Basic Res Cardiol. 1989; 84, 42-54.

68. Fallert MA, Mirotznik MS, Downing SW et al. Myocardial electrical impedance mapping of ischemic sheep hearts and healing aneurysms. Circulation 1993; 87: 199-207.

69. Plonsey R, Barr RC (1988) Introduction to membrane biophysics, in Plonsey R and Barr RC (eds.), Bioelectricity. A quantitative approach, Plenum Press, New York, pp, 33-64.

70. Jugdutt BI, Amy RWM. Healing after myocardial infarction in the dog: changes in infarct hydroxyproline and topography. J Am Coll Cardiol. 1986; 7: 91-102.

71. Ju H, Dixon IMC. Extracellular matrix and cardiovascular diseases. Can J Cardiol 1996; 12: 1259-1267.

72. Chiu ML, Kronauge JF, Piwnica-Worms D. Effect of mitochondrial and plasma membrane potentials on accumulation of hexakis (2-Methoxyisobutylisonitrile) technetium (I) in cultured mouse fibroblasts. J Nucl Med 1990; 31: 1646-1653

73. Caldwell JH, Mertens H, Linssen MCJG, van der Vusse GJ, Buell U, Kammermeier H. Uptake kinetics of technetium-99m-methoxyisobutylisonitrile and thallium-201 in adult rat heart endothelial and fibroblast-like cells in comparison to myocytes. J Nucl Med 1992; 33: 102-107.

74. Fishbein MC, Maclean D, Maroko PR. The histopathologic evolution of myocardial infarction. Chest 1978; 73: 843-849.

75. Becker LC, Schuster EH, Jugdutt BI, Hutchins GM, Bulkley BH. Relationship between myocardial infarct size and occluded bed size in the dog: difference between left anterior descending and circumflex coronary artery occlusions. Circulation. 1983; 67: 549-557.

76. Wilber DJ, Lynch JJ, Montgomery D, Lucchesi BR. Post-infarction sudden death: significance of inducible ventricular tachycardia and infarct size in a conscious canine model. Am Heart J 1985; 109: 8-18.

77. Garan H, McComb JM, Ruskin JN. Spontaneous and electrically induced ventricular arrhythmias during acute ischemia superimposed on 2-week-old canine myocardial infarction. J Am Coll Cardiol. 1988;11: 603-611.

78. Herre JM, Wetstein L, Lin Y, Mills AS, Dae M, Thames MD. Effect of transmural versus nontransmural myocardial infarction on inducibility of ventricular arrhythmias during sympathetic stimulation in dogs. J Am Coll Cardiol 1988; 11: 414-421.

79. Castell J, Candell-Riera J, Roselló-Urgell J et al. Valoración de la viabilidad miocárdica mediante tecnecio-99m isonitrilo y talio-201. Resultados del protocolo multicéntrico español. Rev Esp Cardiol 1997; 50: 320-330.

80. Candell-Riera J, Castell-Conesa J, González JM et al. Eficacia del SPET miocárdico esfuerzo-reposo con 99mTc-MIBI en la predicción de la recuperabilidad de la función contráctil posrevascularización. Resultados del protocolo multicéntrico español. Rev Esp Cardiol 2000; 53: 903-910.

81. Cinca J, García-Burillo A, Carreño A et al. Differential uptake of myocardial perfusion radiotracers in normal, infarcted, and acutely ischemic peri-infarction myocardium. Cardiovasc Res 1998; 38: 91-97.

82. Bonow RO, Dilsizian V, Cuocolo A, Bacharach SL. Identification of viable myocardium in patients with chronic coronary artery disease and left ventricular dysfunction. Comparison of Thallium scintigraphy with reinjection and PET imaging with 18F-Fluorodeoxyglucose. Circulation 1991; 83: 26-37.

83. Dakik HA, Howell JM, Lawrie GM et al. Assessment of myocardial viability with 99mTc-sestamibi tomography before coronary bypass graft surgery. Correlation with histopathology and postoperative improvement in cardiac function. Circulation 1997; 96: 2892-2898.

84. Maes AF, Borgers M, Flameng W et al. Assessment of myocardial viability in chronic coronary artery disease using technetium-99m sestamibi SPECT. Correlation with histologic and positron emission tomographic studies and functional follow-up. J Am Coll Cardiol 1997; 29: 62-68.

9. ISOTOPIC DIAGNOSIS OF VIABLE MYOCARDIUM

JOAN CASTELL-CONESA and JOSE M. GONZALEZ-GONZALEZ

Several clinical and experimental observations have indicated that viable non-contractile myocardium can exist and it has become necessary to differentiate with precision those areas of the left ventricle that have suffered irreversible necrosis from those that are potentially recoverable with respect to function [1-4].

The images that nuclear medicine provides possess a fundamental character that distinguishes them from other types of diagnostic techniques: the origin of the signal that one analyses is not an anatomical structure but a specific metabolic function or chemical reaction. In fact, the conventional studies of myocardial "perfusion" reflect the sum of two separate variables: tissue flow and the existence of metabolically active cells. Multiple studies have verified the proportionality between regional myocardial flow and the grade of incorporation of various tracers [5-11]. Experimental observations, as well, have demonstrated that myocardial uptake of these radiopharmaceuticals is due, essentially, to their retention in the cardiac myocytes via mechanisms that require the production and consumption of energy [12-20].

To-date, the available radiotracers for cardiac SPET studies only provide information on the existence of viable myocardial cells and their uptake that is directly related to the regional cardiac flow. However, it is known that these data are not sufficient in predicting whether revascularisation of a particular coronary artery territory will produce a significant improvement in the overall systolic function of the left ventricle; the primary objective directly related to the survival and the decrease in morbidity of patients with coronary artery disease [21,22].

Hence, currently available are radiopharmaceuticals (thallium-201, MIBI, tetrofosmin) with "cellular" specificity but which do not reflect the metabolic status of these cells: hypoxia, β-oxidation of fatty acids, consumption of oxygen and glucose etc. Possibly, the development of the SPET techniques over the next few years and the introduction of specific metabolic radiotracers will provide images of the biochemistry of the "in vivo" myocardium [23-25]

This chapter provides a view of the methods that nuclear cardiology currently offers for the detection of the presence of viable myocardium together with a review of the most relevant aspects of positron emission studies (PET: positron emission tomography). PET radiotracers possess specificity for the study of normal metabolism and the abnormalities that can occur and, as such, constitute the bases for the understanding of the mechanisms of the biochemical abnormalities in the myocardial cells. As explained earlier, real possibilities currently exist of extending this type of exploration into the field of conventional SPET. Further, the fundamental bases and results of the tomographic methodology with single photon emission radiotracers

J. Candell-Riera et al. (eds.), Myocardium at Risk and Viable Myocardium, 183–211.
© 2001 *Kluwer Academic Publishers. Printed in the Netherlands.*

(SPET: single photon emission tomography) are explored and which, to-date, represent the essential core information from nuclear cardiology. A special mention is made of the new perspectives in metabolic radiopharmaceuticals labelled with technetium-99m and iodine-123. Finally, the applications of isotopic ventriculography in the study of the viable myocardium are analysed.

1. Positron emitters

The reference method for the study of flow and myocardial metabolism is positron emission tomography (PET) [26-29] (Table 1). In the decade of the 80s, it had been demonstrated that regions which appear very hypoperfused in the images obtained with tracers such as ^{13}N-ammonium or ^{82}Rubidium can take-up ^{18}-fluor-deoxyglucose (^{18}F-FDG) [30-36]. This pattern of "mismatch" flow-metabolism is indicative of viable myocardium that is capable of obtaining energy, even in conditions of minimum flow, via the glycolysis route [37-39] (Plate9.1). According to the review by Bax et al. [40] based on 12 series totalling 148 patients studied with ^{18}F-FDG and evaluated pre- and post-revascularisation using different methods of analysis of contractility, images from ^{18}F-FDG define, with high sensitivity, the dysfunctional regions that recover following revascularisation (Figure 1) [34,41-51].

TABLE 1. PET radiotracers

FLOW TRACERS	
	^{13}N-ammonium
	^{15}O-water
	^{82}Rb
METABOLIC TRACERS	
Fatty acids:	^{11}C-palmitic acid
Oxidative metabolism:	^{11}C-acetate
Glycolysis:	^{18}F-fluordeoxyglucose

In all the publications, however, it can be seen that a proportion of about 10-30% of segments that, although capable of taking-up ^{18}F-FDG, do not recover contractility. Several explanations of this finding have been proposed and which include inadequate revascularisation of these regions as well as the existence of areas of the ventricular wall with viable myocardium but incapable of recovery of contractile function [21,22,52-54] i.e. due to the presence of partially necrotic areas that would affect, above all, the endocardial zone on which contractility essentially depends. Images of ^{18}F-FDG show the presence of viable myocardium (predominantly epicardial) that, once revascularised, does not significantly modify the contractility of this region. From the early comparative studies with ^{11}C-acetate [44], it was shown that glycolysis could be the mechanism of cellular energy acquisition and which does not discriminate between aerobic and anaerobic metabolism [55]. Cells with anaerobic glycolysis, possibly sustained over a protracted period, may not have the capacity of metabolic recovery following revascularisation and, indeed, a strong correlation between functional recovery and the grade of uptake of ^{18}F-FDG has been

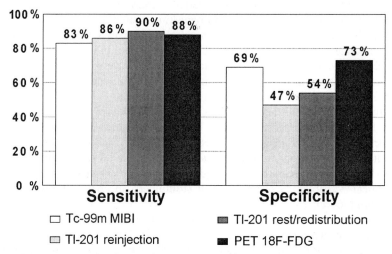

Figure 1. Diagnostic accuracy of myocardial viability (regions that show contractility following revascularisation). Comparison of the most frequently used nuclear cardiology techniques: MIBI, ^{201}Tl rest-redistribution, ^{201}Tl reinjection, and PET studies with ^{18}F-FDG. The data are from the series of patients studied by Bax et al. [40].

demonstrated [56-57]. With respect to longevity that the hibernating myocardium can have, Elsässer et al. [58], in a histopathology study, demonstrated that in the hibernating cells there are important changes of cellular structure, essentially that of the disarrangement of the cytoskeleton and loss of myofilaments, that result in sarcomere_instability_and the decrease in contractile capacity. These authors detected a close correlation between the grade of cellular lesion and the recoverability following revascularisation and would appear to confirm previous clinical evidence [59,60] of hibernation being more a mechanism of degeneration than of adaptation and that, if the restoration of flow is delayed, an irreversible cell breakdown is produced.

The more recent studies of PET precisely quantify myocardial flow per gram of tissue (^{13}N-ammonium or ^{15}O-water). This has made it possible to detect that, surprisingly, in the akinetic regions a persistent and severe reduction in the flow does not exist [61-63]. In basal conditions, viable tissues show normal flow or moderate reductions that do not explain the disappearance of contractile function. The qualitative image of hypoperfusion that is observed in PET studies could be due to the effect that can be produced by the scar mixed in with viable myocardium zones and which results in a reduced overall uptake in those segments with a lower mass of viable myocardium [52]. On the other hand, these regions show an almost complete absence of reserve flow [53] and this has lead some authors to hypothesise that small, repeated increments in the myocardial demand for oxygen is almost invariably conducive to the appearance of the phenomenon of stunning that would occasion a sustained akinesis (hibernation) [52].

Investigations in the field of PET continue and, currently, other experimental lines are being explored. For example, [82]Rb is a flow tracer which is taken-up by the myocardium when normal myocytes are present while, in the absence of viable tissue, suffers a rapid "washout" and disappearance from the ventricular wall. This difference in behaviour facilitates distinguishing viable from non-viable zones. Studies by Goldstein et al. [64] and Gould et al. [65] show satisfactory results with this radionuclide that has a very favourable economic and time-course profile in the study perfusion and viability. The advantage of perfusion-viability studies with [82]Rb resides in that this product is obtained from a transportable generator and, as such, can be used in a PET installation that does not have a cyclotron.

It has been demonstrated that fatty acids maintain the uptake in viable myocardium [66,67]. Palmitic acid labelled with ^{11}C has been used as a metabolic substrate to demonstrate the aerobic route for energy acquisition and its detection in the myocardium with positron cameras indicates the presence of viable myocardial cells [68,69]. However, its non-uniform uptake and being very dependent on several physiological variables have reduced its usefulness in the detection of viable myocardium [70,71].

[11]C-acetate is converted to acetyl-CoA and is incorporated into the tricarboxylic cycle such that its uptake by the myocardium is unequivocally indicative of mitochondrial oxidative metabolic capacity [72-77]. Several studies have shown that the prediction of recovery post-revascularisation is more precise using viability evaluation with acetate than with ^{18}F-FDG [44,78]. It would appear that the specificity of the acetate is superior to that of the ^{18}F-FDG such that this tracer presents false positives that could be due to the incorporation into cells without contractile function recovery capacity while, conversely, ^{11}C-acetate uptake identifies only those cells with in which the oxidative cycle is preserved.

PET is an expensive technique because the tracers employed are, in the main, produced in the cyclotron. This considerably reduces its utilisation in non-specialised clinical institutions. In those countries in which it is routinely available, reasons for its high economic cost and the reduced proportion of patients in which it is applied would need to be explored. The possibility of transporting ^{18}F-FDG to centres situated within a radius of some hours of travel opens up the possibility that these well-equipped institutions can fulfil the additional function of providing this tracer to institutions that may have only a positron camera or the new type gamma cameras that incorporate systems of mechanical or electronic collimation of photons at 511 KeV.

2. Metabolic studies with SPET

Until quite recently it was possible to study myocardial perfusion only with thallium-201 or cation complexes labelled with technetium-99m. Progress in the labelling of fatty acids have made possible, currently, that investigations can be performed to evaluate the myocardial consumption of these metabolic substrates. Advances in the construction of new systems of detection facilitate the construction of scintillation cameras capable of acquiring images from the single photon emitters (such as thallium-201 and technetium-99m) and of emitters of positrons such as ^{18}F-FDG. It can be stated, then, that a great part of the basic aspects of cardiac physiology can be assessable, currently, using SPET (Table 2).

TABLE 2. SPET radiotracers

PERFUSION TRACERS	
	^{201}Tl
	^{99m}Tc-MIBI
	^{99m}Tetrofosmin
METABOLIC TRACERS	
Fatty acids:	^{123}I-IHA, ^{123}I-IHDA, ^{123}I-IPPA
Glycolysis:	^{18}F-Fluordeoxyglucose
Hypoxia:	^{99m}Tc-Nitroimidazol

2.1. ^{18}F-FLUORDEOXYGLUCOSE

Image acquisition from ^{18}F-FDG using gamma cameras has been made possible by the innovation of systems of physical (or electronic) collimator that allows for detections of high energies in conventional gamma cameras. The apparatus consists of two opposed detectors that spatially locate an appropriate proportion of photons of 511 KeV generated by the annihilation of positrons. The relatively large disintegration loss by ^{18}Fluor ($t_{1/2} = 110$ minutes) allows for it to be transportable to centres dispersed from the cyclotron-unit producer so that studies with ^{18}F-FDG may be performed in conventional centres of nuclear cardiology [79,80].

Early clinical studies demonstrated that the reliability of ^{18}F-FDG detection using these gamma cameras is very similar to that obtained with PET cameras [81,82]. Protocols have been designed for diagnostic purposes that include stress test with MIBI followed by infusion of ^{18}F-FDG in repose. A single, simultaneous detection of the double isotope (^{99m}Tc-^{18}F) is immediately performed and images of identical characteristics corresponding to perfusion under stress and viability at rest, are obtained [83].

Already there are developmental studies assessing the predictability functional recovery following revascularisation in regions defined as hibernating i.e. akinetic or dyskinetic segments with non-reversible perfusion defects that have increased uptake of ^{18}F-FDG [84]. Although the spatial resolution and efficiency of the counts of the ^{18}F-FDG-SPET assessments are lower that with PET cameras, the diagnostic effectiveness as well as the predictive value of these studies is completely coincident with that of detection with PET.

2.2. FATTY ACIDS

The possibility of labelling long chain fatty acids, such as palmitic acid, with ^{123}I has facilitated, using SPET, myocardial distributions of the metabolic substrates of beta-oxidation. Although the detection using SPET is difficult because of the rapid myocardial clearance, several clinical studies have been performed with heptadodecanoic acid (IHA), hexadodecanoic acid (IHDA) and phenylpentadecanoic acid (IPPA) [71]. IHDA [85] and IPPA [86,87] appear to have the best biokinetic conditions for the measurement of beta-oxidation but this capacity has been used, principally, to study myocardial ischaemia in repose. Certain fatty acids have a beta-methyl group in its chemical structure that slows its myocardial clearance and facilitates a better detection using SPET scintillation cameras. Although experience is limited in its use in the evaluation of myocardial viability, preliminary studies appear promising in comparison to the protocol of rest-reinjection with thallium-201 [88,89].

2.3. TRACERS FOR HYPOXIA

For several years investigation have been under way into markers of tissue hypoxia that, in a similar manner ^{18}F-FDG, can directly identify viable myocardium in situations of metabolic deficit. Recently, several complexes of the nitroimidazole group, labelled with ^{99m}Tc, have demonstrated the capacity to be incorporated specifically into hypoxic cells in experimental models and in some "in vivo" trials [90,91].

These tracers, developed from antibiotics designed for the treatment of infections by anaerobic organisms, enter the cells by passive diffusion and are not retained in the cytosol if a deficit of oxygen does not exist [92,93]. When the molecule enters the cell it is reduced by enzyme action but intracellular oxygen is capable of reversing the process and allows the molecule to escape. In the absence of normal concentrations of oxygen, reoxidation is not produced and the nitroimidazole remains trapped in the cytosol. This characteristic confers on this family of tracers a metabolic specificity that identifies those zones that remain viable in conditions of oxygen deficiency [94-96].

Currently, these tracers are in the experimental phase and the intent is optimise the contrast between the zones of interest and the background and to develop the optimum protocol as a function the time that is needed to pass between the injection of the pharmaceutical agent and its subsequent detection.

3. Studies with Thallium-201

The most widely used radionuclide has been thallium-201. Its pharmacokinetic characteristics make it ideal for the study of the viability of the tissues under conditions of low flow [97]. Following intravenous injection, its distribution responds to the regional myocardial flow [9,12,98]. There is an evident difference between the regions with normal arteries and those dependent on severely stenosed vessels when the ^{201}Tl is injected under stress induction (exercise or pharmaceutical). It has a peculiar characteristic in that it is not retained in the cytosol and, in the course of its stay in the organ, maintains an equilibrium between cellular and blood concentrations. This results in continuous presence of ^{201}Tl in the plasma in the hours following its administration. The zones of the normoperfused myocardium that initially incorporate more tracer are subject to a process termed "washout" which involves a loss of content of ^{201}Tl in absolute terms and progressively arriving to a concentration of radiotracer corresponding to the situation in repose [99-102]. Conversely, the areas of low flow that initially have a low uptake of ^{201}Tl, particularly in comparison with those territories that have the capacity several times the baseline perfusion level, receive a limited but constant exposure to the radionuclide. This results, after a more or less long period (up to 24 hours) [103,104], for a level of tissue concentration to be arrived-at which can be detected using scintigraphic images and with which the presence of viable myocardium may be assessed (phenomenon of redistribution).

It had been observed that, using the conventional study protocol, a high proportion of the regions with severe perfusion defects (levels according to some authors of 50% of the segments) did not show redistribution at 2-3 hours, but did so at 18-24 hours [104,105] or showed ^{18}F-FDG uptake in PET [31] studies, or improved uptake or function following revascularistation [106]. This considerable underestimation of viable myocardium requires that detections be performed much later for them to be correct and which represents an inconvenience with respect to the quality of image obtained at 24 hours, especially if the SPET technology is employed. However, starting with the studies of Dilsizian et al. [107] and Rocco et al. [108] in which the reinjection of thallium was introduced, a method became available which provided an effectiveness closer to PET in terms of detection of viable myocardium [109,110]. Once past the conventional time of redistribution (3-4 hours) a supplementary dose of tracer (1 mCi) is administered and which increases the supply at rest and, from a practical point of view, "accelerates" the process of late/delayed redistribution that finally facilitates visualising severely hypoperfused myocardium (Plate9.2). When this procedure was quantitatively analysed, there appeared that, in fact, a decrease in the difference of activity between the normal and hypoperfused zones (reversibility) is not produced, but also that the increment of overall counts visually improves the uptake in the regions with severe reduction of coronary flow [24]. In the patient series published to-date, in those that assessed the prediction of functional recovery following revascularisation with the protocol of exercise-redistribution-reinjection, the adjusted levels of positive and negative predictive values were 69% and 89% respectively (Figure 1) [107,111-114].

Subsequently, various studies demonstrated a moderate increase in efficacy in the detection of viable myocardial segments using detections at 3-4 hours after reinjection [115] or of a reinjection at rest (protocol of rest-redistribution) when only the assessment of the presence of viable myocardium was of interest [118]. The various patient series with rest-redistribution protocol provide results that are very similar with respect to the prediction of recovery post-revascularisation. The protocols that included images of stress had mean levels of positive predictive values of 69% and of negative predictive values of 92% (Figure 1) [116-124]. In two comparative studies, a concordance of at least 80% was obtained with respect to whether the segments were considered viable or not between this protocol and that of exercise-redistribution reinjection [125,126]. Iskandrian et al. [127], Ragosta et al. [119] and Mori et al. [116] observed a predictive of around 75-80% with respect to the improvement of overall systolic function.

Because of the cellular viability representation in the delayed images of thallium-201 [104,115], some authors currently propose a "compressed" protocol of exercise-reinjection immediate-redistribution at 4 hours that would combine the information on the ischaemic territories with the maximum sensitivity with respect to the detection of viable myocardium within the same period of time as the conventional protocol (stress-redistribution) and that provides identical results to those described in the options presented earlier [128].

An important aspect that needs to be emphasised in the interpretation of the results of perfusion with ^{201}Tl is that of the intensity of post-stress defects and its behaviour at rest. Slight or moderate hypoperfusions that do not show redistribution or that are accentuated in the images obtained at 3 hours (paradoxical pattern) need to be interpreted as indicative of viable myocardium [110]. Earlier studies, at the reinjection stage, had already indicated that salvaged viable myocardium in a territory that had suffered an infarct can present with a paradoxical pattern [129]. The relationship between defect intensity and reversibility and uptake of 18F-FDG [110,130] have been specifically investigated. Mild and moderate defects show low percentages of reversibility but, virtually always, visible. Conversely, severe defects (uptake <50% of maximum) without redistribution require the reinjection to demonstrate whether viability is real or not. In this group, 51% of the segments incorporated the tracer following the reinjection and concordance with the ^{18}F-FDG image was 76%. In the study on the paradoxical pattern in an infarct zone [131], regions with moderate defects had more intense an image of redistribution; systematically (82%) behaving as viable in the images of reinjection and PET. An explanation for this type of phenomenon is complex but, essentially, it is interpreted as being that the myocardium which survives after an acute myocardial infarction and that does not remain in a state of severe ischaemia (because of the patency of the responsible vessel or by the collateral flow) is capable of increasing its uptake of thallium-201 during the stress and of presenting washout in the subsequent hours such that the contrast between the defect (coexistence of myocardium and necrosed tissue) and the rest of the territories is greater in the image of redistribution than in the post-stress image. A similar mechanism would explain the presence of paradoxical patterns in early post-reinjection with respect to redistribution that may be observed on certain occasions and that, in this case, would reflect the difference of flow in repose between the normal zones and the severely ischaemic.

It can be said that thallium-201 is an ideal tracer of myocardial viability but has limitations proceeding from its radiophysical characteristics. In a study performed in patients with chronic coronary artery disease and territories with severe decrease in contractility, Alterhoefer et al. [132] obtained a high coincidence between the uptake of ^{201}Tl and ^{18}F-FDG with respect to the presence or not of viable myocardium in the antero-septal territory (90%). Conversely, in the inferior and posterior region there was a discordance of 44% when the ^{201}Tl defects were severe (uptake <50% of maximum) and of 46% when the hypo-uptake was moderate (51%-75% of maximum). The difference resided, in great part, in the underestimation of the myocardial mass by ^{201}Tl and is interpreted, by the authors, as being due to the greater attenuation of the radiation proceeding from the inferior and posterior regions. Nevertheless, in this study as in the series of Tamaki et al. [51] and Bonow et al. [110], the overall coincidence by segments between the images of [201]Tl (injected at rest or following reinjection) and those of ^{18}F-FDG are excellent, with discordances around 15% in the severe defects and around 10% when it has been documented that the patients have or have not viable myocardium in the regions with severe reduction in contractility.

4. Studies of perfusion tracers labelled with technetium-99m

By the end of the decade of the 80s, the first complexes of myocardial perfusion labelled with technetium-99m, termed the isonitriles [133-136], were being produced and, in the early 90s, tetrofosmin was introduced [137-139]. These products, and probably others that will become available in the next few years, have the property of being taken-up by the myocardial cells as a function of their viability and of coronary flow. They can be labelled with technetium-99m, a radionuclide that has the best radiophysical characteristics for detection with scintillation cameras [140]. Methoxy-isobutyl-isonitrile (MIBI) [141-144] and tetrofosmin [145,146] are the most frequently used because of high myocardial extraction and appropriate pharmaceutical profile. The principal advantage compared to thallium-201 is that the photon flow of these radiopharmaceuticals is much higher so that tomographic images of better quality are obtained. Due to ^{99m}Tc having a short half-life (6 hours), doses 10-25 mCi can be administered to patients and, with an energy of 140 KeV, is more penetrating than ^{201}Tl and, as such, with less problems of tissue attenuation. Another characteristic different from ^{201}Tl is that there is practically no redistribution [137,147]. Technetium labelled complexes are cations that passively diffuse across the cellular and mitochondrial membranes and are retained, in greater part, in the mitochondria as long as the membrane potentials are maintained [19,20,148]. Situations of ischaemia that give rise to cellular metabolic effects that depolarise the membrane cause a reduction in the cellular retention of MIBI and tetrofosmin that can become almost zero when no viable cells exist [149,150]. Conversely, as has been demonstrated experimentally not only in models of occlusion-reperfusion ("stunned" myocardium) but also in situations of chronic reduction and intensity of coronary flow (hibernating" myocardium), the uptake of MIBI is maintained proportional to the coronary flow in a manner similar to that of thallium whether or not profound systolic dysfunction exists [17,151,152].

There are other technetium labelled complexes for the study of myocardial perfusion but they are still in the clinical trial phase and, as such, there are not much data on their usefulness in studies of viability. Of these, teboroxime is the tracer on which the most studies of validation have been performed [153,154]. Others such as the boronic acid family bonded to technetium dioxime (BATO) are neutral and lipophilic and have, as a special peculiarity, rapid myocardial clearance (5-10 minutes) and excellent proportionality with variations in coronary flow [155]. Preliminary studies on predominantly flow tracers, appear unfavourable for their employment   as indicators of viability.

4.1. MIBI STUDIES

Since its introduction into clinical practice, MIBI has demonstrated its efficacy in the diagnosis and evaluation of the extent of disease of the coronary arteries. Its use has been widened because of the excellent conditions, from the clinical and technical points of view, that are provided by SPET. The high quality of the tomographic images provides a high diagnostic precision in delineating ischaemic territories that, in several studies, appear superior to ^{210}Tl-SPET [141,156,157]. The absence of redistribution [147] allows for the investigation of patients who have been subjected to thrombolytic treatment i.e. the detection can be performed once the patient has received the treatment and is in a more stable clinical condition and the images obtained at this point in time define the jeopardised area and which can be compared with studies performed a few days later such that differences between the two assessments would provide information on the salvaged myocardium and on the final extent of necrosis [158].

Hence, perfusion studies with technetium tracers provide excellent results [159-164] for the investigation of stunned myocardium (post-ischaemic myocardium with permeable vessel). Another special situation is that of the hibernating myocardium. In experimental studies, such as those of Sinusas et al. [151] in a canine model, the uptake of MIBI in severely hypoperfused and akinetic tissues is very similar to that with ^{201}Tl but, in a majority of trials in which this tracer had been compared with thallium reinjection or ^{18}F-FDG uptake, there had been an under-estimation of viability [165-172]. As such, the non-redistribution of MIBI in plasma is a disadvantage because, following its initial biodistribution, the severely hypoperfused tissues have not the opportunity to incorporate this tracer, in contrast with the redistribution phenomenon of ^{201}Tl [169,170,173].

Remarkable differences of opinion exist in the literature with respect to the effectiveness of MIBI in the evaluation of the myocardial viability as, in general, with all the technetium tracers without redistribution. Comparative series with ^{18}F-FDG or ^{201}Tl reinjection or rest-redistribution are short and, in general, reflect an underestimation of the viable segments on the part of MIBI. The properties of MIBI are different compared to ^{201}Tl and, as such, need to be evaluated within their own specific criteria. On detailed analysis of the studies of Rocco et al. [172] and Altehoefer et al. [174,175], it appears that the question resides in what level of uptake is taken as the frontier between viable and non-viable. In the series of patients studied by Altehoefer, it can be observed that no segment that incorporated ^{18}F-FDG had a level <30% of the SPET-MIBI image and that the discrepancies were in the grade of uptake of both tracers, which is not surprising if their completely different biokinetic characterises are taken into account. In several studies comparing MIBI with ^{201}Tl-reinjection, it can be seen that the poorer results of the isonitriles were obtained when the study was performed with planar methodology [166-168]. With SPET, the MIBI did not show significant differences from the immediate thallium reinjection image although a significantly increased uptake was detected in the image obtained at 3 hours of reinjection [169]. Conversely, Udelson et al. [118], in a quantitative study performed by SPET compared the rest-MIBI and ^{201}Tl rest-redistribution uptake and showed a correlation of 86%. The concordance viable/non-viable segments was of 87% (Kappa 0.76) in the 18 revascularised patients and there were no significant differences between the uptakes of MIBI and of ^{201}Tl in any of the 4 levels into which the segments had been sub-grouped. In the meta-analysis of Bax et al. [40] (Figure 1), no differences were observed in sensitivity and specificity of different protocols and tracers (thallium, MIBI and FDG) in the prediction of contractile recovery of the dysfunctional segments.

Arrighi et al. [176] in a study with MIBI and ^{18}F-FDG analysed the influence that the grade of ventricular dysfunction can have on the capacity of MIBI to detect viable myocardium. These authors investigated 20 patients divided in two groups according to whether the ejection fraction (EF) was greater or lower than 25%. The subgroup with mean EF of 36% had an elevated concordance with ^{18}F-FDG (89%) and, with MIBI, 88% of the viable segments were detected by PET. The 11 with mean EF of 17%, concordance was observed in 78% of the segments and only 42% of the segments shown by PET as being viable (mismatch pattern), were detected.

With the objective of evaluating the effectiveness of tomographic perfusion studies in the prediction of functional recovery post-revascularisation, we conducted a multicentre study [177] in which 116 patients with stable coronary artery disease were included and who were revascularised. Gated blood-pool radionuclide ventriculography studies were performed pre-revascularisation and 3-6 months post-revascularisation (Plate 9.3). Following the usual procedures in each of the 11 participating hospitals, tomographic studies of myocardium perfusion with MIBI or ^{201}Tl were performed. Above 30% uptake, no significant differences in the percentages of functional recovery were observed. The grade of improvement of ventricular function was modest but similar to that observed by other authors [83,178]. The EF improved more than 5 points in 3-6 months in 28% of the patients while in 50% of the cases there was no objective change and in 22% of the patients a decrease in the EF was observed (Figure 2). From the point of view of diagnosis of myocardial viability, a higher sensitivity was obtained adopting 30% of the maximum uptake as the lower limit of viability, not only for ^{201}Tl but also for MIBI, and the specificity was lower for all the grades analysed. This last aspect is related, probably, to the low overall probability of improvement of regional contractility of the dyskinetic segments in this series of patients irrespective of the level of uptake observed in the pre-revascularisation study.

Some studies directly evaluated the "extent of viable myocardium", factor that plays an important role in the prediction of post-revascularisation contractile recovery [21].

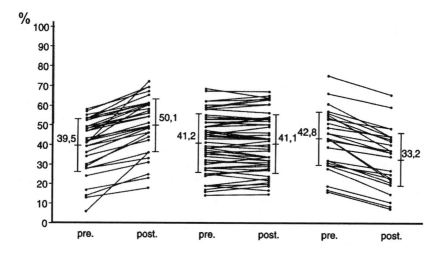

Figure 2. Ejection fraction pre- and post-revascularisation of patients in the Spanish multicentre study of myocardial viability. On the right are patients that shoed increased systolic function >5% EF, in the centre those showed had no change and on the left are those that showed a reduction of >5% EF.

Studies with ^{18}F-FDG and ^{201}Tl have demonstrated a strong correlation between the number of dysfunctional segments and the post-revascularisation EF improvement. In the Spanish multicentre study quoted earlier, an inverse relationship was observed between the improvement of systolic function and the number of segments with an uptake <30%. The results showed that there was no clear division in the uptake threshold between viable and non-viable myocardium, neither with ^{201}Tl nor MIBI. For levels of uptake <30%, there was improvement of 18% (^{201}Tl) and 20% (MIBI) of segments following revascularisation. This probability of improvement was significantly less than that of the segments with uptake >30%.

In a sub-group of 40 patients studied in our hospital as part of the multicentre trial, we introduced a quantitative factor using an estimation of the viable territory in the polar maps. Four vascular regions were considered per patient: the antero-septal region (dependent on the left anterior descending coronary artery); the inferior (dependent on the right coronary artery); the lateral (dependent on the left circumflex coronary artery); and the apical which, because of its variable vascularisation, had not been assigned to any specific artery (see Chapter 2). Different levels of uptake (30%, 40% and 50%) were compared and >50% was adopted as the criterion of viability and the extent of each of the vascular regions defined with respect to being above this re-defined cut-off level. Of a total of 166 regions, 82 had severe decrease in contractility and, of these, 73 were revascularised. The same sensitivity (98%) was observed for the levels of uptake of 30% and 40%. However, for the level of 50%, the sensitivity was lower (79%) (p=0.004). The specificity was low for all the levels, although significantly better for the level of 50% with respect to that of 30% (36 Vs 20; p=0.045). No statistically significant differences were observed with respect to specificity for the level of uptake of 50% relative to that of 40% (36% vs 24%) [179]. However, in other patient series, the observed best uptake cut-off levels for viability prediction were different. Cuocolo et al. [180] observed the same predictive power to detect functional recovery in akinetic or dyskinetic segments for thallium and MIBI, but with minimal differences in the uptake levels for each tracer: >58% for thallium and >55% for MIBI. In this and in other series [181] a relationship between the best predictor cut-off level and the left ventricular regions was found. Schneider et al. [181] observed that the average MIBI uptake in the central infarct region of patients with improvement of function and inferior infarct was significantly lower (43%) than in patients with anterior infarcts (68%, p<0.003). Using an infarct location adjusted optimal threshold of 50% for anterior infarcts and 35% for inferior infarcts, they obtained a positive predictive value of 90% and negative predictive value of 91% for improvement of left ventricular function.

Other studies [182,183] have highlighted a close correlation between the presence of viable myocardium evaluated using histology and the uptake of MIBI. The observations were made in a series of hearts removed from patients undergoing heart transplant and who, a few hours earlier, had received a dose of MIBI [182]. The results appeared to be very much in agreement with the Spanish multicentre viability study in that there was practically an absence of myocardium when the uptake was <30% and a coexistence of zones of scar and myocardial tissue in parallel proportion to the grade of MIBI uptake between 30% and 85%. When >85%, the myocardial tissue was normal in all segments. Dakik et al. [183] and Maes et al. [184] confirmed the concordance between the grade of histological lesion (determined by myocardial biopsy obtained during revascularisation surgery), the uptake of MIBI, the regional uptake of ^{18}F-FDG and the subsequent functional recovery. Even while confirming that a specific level of uptake does not exist that would identify the viable myocardium, the minimum optimum threshold is situated around 55% of the maximum in the series of Dakik et al. and around 50% in the series of Maes et al. The positive and negative predictive values were situated around 79% to 82% and 72% to 99%, respectively.

4.2. STUDIES WITH TETROFOSMIN

Tetrofosmin is a cationic complex that has very similar properties to MIBI, although its hepatic and blood clearance is faster and allows for very early image acquisition following its intravenous administration [11,137-139,145,146]. Its retention in the myocardial cells requires that mitochondrial metabolism is conserved and, for this reason, is an indicator of viability [19, 20]. We confirmed, in a porcine model, that this tracer presents uptakes of <30% in areas of necrosis relative to the normally-perfused myocardium [185] (see chapter 8) and other authors have demonstrated its correlation with the zones that are histologically viable in models of occlusion-reperfusion[186] or of sustained low flow [187].

We studied a series of 20 patients with myocardial infarction in whom, using polar map images, the reversibility and the extention of rest defects between stress-rest tetrofosmin and the ^{201}Tl stress-reinjection were compared. There were no differences with respect to reversibility and a slight but significant difference was observed between both tracers when the cut-off adopted for both as the criterion for viability was 50% of the peak uptake; a greater extent of defects being observed with tetrofosmin. However, taking 45% as the threshold for this tracer and compared with the level of the 50% for [201]Tl (Figure 3), the differences disappeared with respect to the extent of non-viable areas and a concordance of 88% was obtained in assigning the segments as viable or non-viable [188]. These results agree with those of Heo et al. [189] although other authors have described underestimation of the viable segments when compared with protocols of rest-reinjection with [201]Tl [190]. In the series of patients studied by Matsunarie et al. [191] the evaluation of viability, based on the visual assessment of defect reversibility, showed an under-estimation in the tetrofosmin images relative to those of ^{201}Tl re-injection while, with respect to quantification, the grade of uptake in repose did not appear different between the two tracers. Hence, a parallelism exists between tetrofosmin and MIBI in the evaluation of viability; discordances with the ^{201}Tl with respect to the visual assessment of reversibility and concordance when the uptake at rest is quantified.

5. Attenuation correction, gated-SPET and administration of nitrates

A series of methodological options exist that can increase the efficiency of myocardial perfusion studies in the evaluation of the viable myocardium. On the one hand, advances in image acquisition facilitate the correction for attenuation caused by anatomical structures and which can result in an underestimation in the myocardial uptake while, on the other hand, using acquisition synchronised with the ECG one can perform ventricular contractility analyses. Also, protocols have been designed using pharmacological intervention that could further improve the detection of viable myocardium.

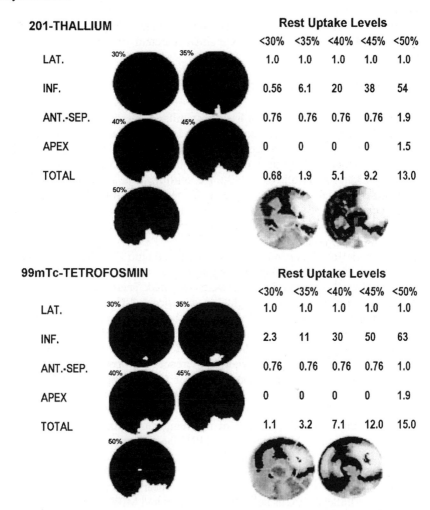

201-THALLIUM

Rest Uptake Levels

	<30%	<35%	<40%	<45%	<50%
LAT.	1.0	1.0	1.0	1.0	1.0
INF.	0.56	6.1	20	38	54
ANT.-SEP.	0.76	0.76	0.76	0.76	1.9
APEX	0	0	0	0	1.5
TOTAL	0.68	1.9	5.1	9.2	13.0

99mTc-TETROFOSMIN

Rest Uptake Levels

	<30%	<35%	<40%	<45%	<50%
LAT.	1.0	1.0	1.0	1.0	1.0
INF.	2.3	11	30	50	63
ANT.-SEP.	0.76	0.76	0.76	0.76	1.0
APEX	0	0	0	0	1.9
TOTAL	1.1	3.2	7.1	12.0	15.0

Figure 3. Rest polar maps with masks of different uptake levels (30% to 50% of maximum uptake) in a patient with an inferior infarct. In the upper panel is the study with ^{201}Tl and in the lower that of tetrofosmin. It can be seen that the distribution is practically the same in the zones above and below each level with both tracers.

5.1. ATTENUATION CORRECTION AND GATED-SPET

A recent technical advance in SPET in myocardial perfusion studies is the correction for attenuation using transmission images. The improvement contributed by the system in the evaluation of viability is via the correction for artefactual hypo-uptakes produced by the diaphragm or breast tissues which can contribute to myocardial under-estimation in the inferior and/or anterior regions [192-194] (Figure 4) but, as yet, there is little or no experience with this methodology to assess its impact on the evaluation of viability.

SPET myocardial perfusion synchronised with the ECG facilitates the acquisition of images representative of the movement and thickening of the ventricular wall during the cardiac cycle. The methodology has special importance in the evaluation of viability since not only the grade of uptake in a ventricular region can be analysed but also its movement should an increase in systole be produced. The increase in terms of unit area is due to systolic thickening of the myocardial wall and, as such, its existence is an indicator of viability (Plate 9.4).

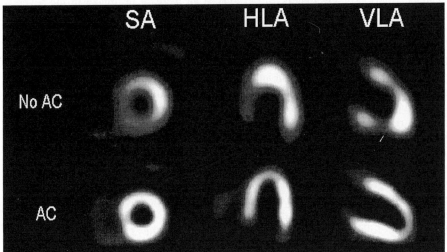

Figure 4. Attenuation correction effect in tomographic slice in a female patient. It can be seen that the uptake is diminished in the septal region (short axis and long horizontal axis), in the anterior and inferior regions (short axis and long vertical axis) in the images without attenuation correction (No AC). In the lower panel is the normalisation of the defects observed on the application of attenuation correction (AC) [194].

The possibility of acquiring parameters of overall systolic function together with images of perfusion substantially increase the information that can be obtained from a myocardial SPET, especially in patients with coronary artery disease. Further, there already exist observations that highlight the benefits that can be gained in the evaluation of motion and systolic thickening in the evaluation of regional viability [195-197] and an excellent correlation has been observed between the images of re-injection with ^{201}Tl and the intensity of regional systolic thickening [198]. However, Gonzalez et al. [199] did not encounter any added benefit of gated-SPET over the conventional tomographic images in the prediction of functional recovery while the polar map quantification of extent, severity and reversibility of the defects described better definitions of regions with recoverable myocardium. These data are not surprising since it is possible that viable but akinetic zones without thickeningcan exist in basal conditions if these areas are in the state of hibernation [200].

The acquisition of gated-SPET images with simultaneous attenuation correction will signify, probably, an improvement of isotopic analysis of myocardial viability. In the short space of time since its clinical application there have been sufficient studies that confirm its forecasted effectiveness in this field.

5.2. NITRATES

For some years it had been proposed that administering nitrates would improve the detection of viable myocardium using contrast ventriculography [201] and, recently, this methodology has been applied to the studies of myocardial perfusion. These substances increase regional coronary flow basically because of their effects of vasodilation and reduction of after-load [202,203]. Administered before rest injection of myocardial perfusion tracers, nitrates cause an increase in uptake in the severely hypoperfused, but viable, regions.

In 1993 the first article [204] was published based on the experience in 20 patients with coronary artery disease, 11 of whom with myocardial infarction and with thrombolytic treatment two weeks previously. Two protocols with ^{201}Tl were performed: Exercise/Re-injection and Exercise/Nitrates/Re-injection. Fifteen patients showed reversible defects with the re-injection protocol and 18 with nitrates/re-injection protocol. Of the 54 fixed segments following the re-injection only, 14 (26%) showed reversibility with the protocol of nitrates/re-injection. The extent of the redistribution was significantly greater in the patients that had been treated with nitroglycerine. Subsequently, in another study with more patients (96) in whom a protocol of stress/redistribution/re-injection with ^{201}Tl was performed, two randomised groups received placebo or 0.8 mg of sublingual nitroglycerine. The results demonstrated that of the 66 patients with persistent defects in the redistribution images, 58% of the group that had received nitrates showed improvement of the reversibility following the re-injection compared to the 33% of those who had received placebo (p<0.05) [205]. In 100 patients with recent myocardial infarction, followed-up between 8 and 32 months, Basu et al. [206] evaluated the presence of jeopardized myocardium and its relationship with severe complications. Reversibility of stress-redistribution images and stress-nitrates-reinjection at rest images were compared. With the first protocol, only 29 patients with ischaemia were detected while 68 patients showed reversibility with nitrate administration; a definite net superiority of the latter protocol in the identification of patients at risk of severe complications.

Studies evaluating the effect of nitrates when administered together with the doses of the technetium-labelled tracers at rest have been performed [207,208]. Several studies [209, 210] demonstrated that an increment in the number of segments defined as viable is systematically produced in the studies performed with nitrates. The MIBI rest uptake resembles more the ^{201}Tl rest-redistribution [209] and has a better positive and negative predictive value with respect to improvement in post-revascularisation contractility [207, 210]. In a recent Spanish study, the uptake of tetrofosmin with and without nitrates was compared with the images of ^{201}Tl in rest-redistribution [211]. As in the studies performed with MIBI, a moderate improvement in the myocardial uptake was observed when nitrates were administered, albeit without being able to detect all the segments that were defined as viable in the delayed images of ^{201}Tl (Figure 5).

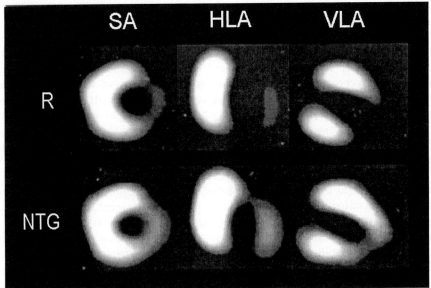

Figure 5. Tomographic images along the short axis (SA), long vertical axis (LVA) and long horizontal axis (LHA) in a study with tetrofosmin: (R) rest injection and (NTG) following the administration of sublingual nitroglycerine. A severe lateral and apical defect is observed that improves moderately with the vasodilator [211].

A cut-off level of 50% respect to the maximum uptake was used to define viability in most of these series. A lowered cut-off of 35-40% was tried in some studies and the concordance with the studies of ^{201}Tl rest-redistribution was observed to be practically total [207, 211]. This would appear to confirm the hypothesis that the 50% level seems to be excessively high to be used systematically in all subgroups of patients, and especially in the inferior wall.

6. Radionuclide ventriculography

In the field of myocardial viability, radionuclide ventriculography is a technique employed, essentially, in the evaluation of systolic function and of regional contractility pre- and post-revascularisation [40, 212]. The high reproducibility of this method, and limitations in its use being practically absent, makes it the ideal method to identify changes in ventricular function.

As with any other method, ventriculography can be used to analyse contractile response to pharmacological stress. Contrast ventriculography with nitrates has been employed to assess if increment in coronary flow produces an improvement in ventricular contractility in ischaemic patients [201]. However, the slight experience with radionuclide ventriculography [213], to-date, does not permit an efficacy assessment with respect to the prediction of functional recovery.

It has been known for some time that contraction in akinetic regions or with severe hypokinesia can be stimulated by the phenomenon of post-extrasystolic potentiation

[214], by pharmaceutical agents such as epinephrine [215] or by physical exercise [216]. Using echocardiography, it has been shown that the appearance of contractility in akinetic regions or increment in severely hypokinetic regions when dobutamine is administered at low doses, is an excellent predictor of post-revascularisation functional recovery [40]. Hence, radionuclide ventriculography can be used as an alternative method to echocardiography for the study of contractile reserve of the myocardium [217]. Its use is much reduced for various reasons such as the greater availability of echocardiography, the lower spatial resolution of ventriculography in regional contractility analysis and its incapacity to directly analyse movement and thickening of the ventricular wall. Nevertheless, it needs to be emphasised that ventriculography possesses considerable efficiency in the evaluation of wall motion (Plate 9.5) and, added to which, is its excellent reproducibility not only in the quantification of the overall ejection fraction but also in the acquisition of parametric images of amplitude and phase [218-220]. We have used radionuclide ventriculography to evaluate the response of EF and of regional contractility to the administration of low doses of dobutamine in patients with recent anterior myocardial infarction and overall involvement or segmentation of contractility. We observed a high correlation between the regions that have conserved contractile reserve and the normalisation of motility in ventriculogaphy performed at 6 months [221].

It has been demonstrated, however, that dobutamine, even at low doses, can induce myocardial ischaemia when the coronary lesions are severe, as we had observed in the patients in our series (Plate 9.6). It can produce an underestimation of viable myocardium since the absence of contractile increment is not due scarred tissue but only to the ischaemia provoked by the haemodynamic effects of the pharmaceutical agent [20, 222].

Amrinone is a catecholamine that is similar to dobutamine in that it has a positive inotropic effect but differs in that it does not increase myocardial consumption of oxygen [223, 224]. This represents an advantage over dobutamine in that it does not induce ischaemia when administered to patients with severely reduced coronary flow. Perez-Baliño et al. [225] studied, using radionuclide ventriculography with amrinone, 44 patients with coronary artery disease and ventricular dysfunction (basal EF 28±7%). Following the administration of the drug, the mean EF increased to35±5% (p<0.0001) and, at 21 days post-revascularisation, a mean EF value of 33±6% was observed. The 13 patients that had increased EF of 10% with amrinone had an increment of >8% following surgical intervention. Conversely, only two of the 31 patients without significant changes in EF with amrinone had improved systolic function following revascularisation.

In summary, it can be stated that radionuclide ventriculography can be used to evaluate contractile reserve of regions with severe motion abnormalities and, more importantly, is an ideal method for follow-up of ventricular function in patients with coronary artery disease.

References

1.   Braunwald E, Kloner RA. The stunned myocardium: prolonged, postischemic ventricular dysfunction. Circulation 1982; 66: 1146-1149.

2.   Braunwald E, Rutheford JD. Reversible ischemic left ventricular dysfunction: Evidence for the "hibernating myocardium". J Am Coll Cardiol 1986; 8: 1467-1470.

3.   Rahimtoola SH. The hibernating myocardium. Am Heart J 1989; 117: 211-221.

4.   Bolli R. Myocardial "stunning" in man. Circulation 1992; 86: 1671-1691.

5.   Grunwald AM, Watson DD, Holtzgrefe HH Jr, Irving JF, Beller GA. Myocardial thallium-201 kinetics in normal and ischemic myocardium. Circulation 1981; 64: 610-618.

6.   Nielsen AP, Morris KG, Murdok R, Bruno FP, Cobb FR. Linear relationship between the distribution of thallium-201 and blood flow in ischemic and non ischemic myocardium during exercise. Circulation 1983; 68: 310-320.

7.   Nichols AB, Weiss MB, Sciacca RR, Cannon PJ, Blood DK. Relationship between segmental thallium-201 uptake ang regional myocardial blood flow in patients with coronary artery disease. Circulation 1983; 68: 310-320.

8.   Mays AE Jr, Cobb FR. Relationship between regional myocardial blood flow and thalium-201 redistribution in the presence of coronary artery stenosis and dipyridamole-induced vasodilation. J Clin Invest 1984; 73: 1359-1366.

9.   DiRocco RJ, Runsey WL, Kuczynski BL et al. Measurement of myocardial blood using co-injection technique for Technetium-99m-Teboroxime, Technetium-99m-Sestamibi and Thallium-201. J Nucl Med 1992; 33: 1152-1159.

10. Glober DK, Okada RD. Myocardial kinetics of Tc-MIBI in canine myocardium after dipyridamole. Circulation 1990; 81: 628-637.

11. Sinusas AJ, Shi QX, Saltzberg et al. Technetium-99m-tetrofosmin to assess myocardial blood flow: Experimental validation in an intact canine model of ischemia. J Nucl Med 1994; 35: 664-671.

12. Melin JA, Becker LC. Quantitative relationship between global left ventricular thallium uptake and blood flow: Effects of propanolol, ouabain, dipyridamole, and coronary artery oclusion. J Nucl Med 1986; 27: 641-652.

13. Krivokapich J, Shine KI. Effects of hiperkalemia and glycoside on thallium exchange in rabbit ventricle. Am J Physiol 1981; 240:H612-H619.

14. Goldhaber SZ, Newell JB, Alpert NM, Andrews E, Pohost GM, Ingwall JS. Effects of ischemic-like insult on myocardial thallium-201 accumulation. Circulation 1983; 67: 778-786.

15. Piwnica-Worms D, Krounage JF, Chiu ML. Uptake and retention of hexakis (2-methoxyisobutyl isonitrile) technetium (I) in cultured chick myocardial cells. Mitochondrial and plasma membrane potential dependance. Circulation 1990; 82:1626-1836.

16. Carvalho PA, Chiu ML, Kronauge JF et al. Subcellular distribution and analysis of technetium-99m-MIBI isolated perfused rat hearts. J Nucl Med 1992; 33: 1516-1521.

17. Beanlands RS, Dawood F, Wen WH et al. Are the kinetics of technetium-99m methoxyisobutil isonitrile affected by cell metabolism and viability? Circulation 1990; 82: 1802-1814.

18. Beller GA, Glover DK, Edwards NC, Ruiz M, Simanis JP, Watson DD. Technetium-99m sestamibi uptake and retention during myocardial ischemia and reperfusion. Circulation 1993; 87: 2033-2042.

19. Platts EA, North TL, Pickett RD, Kelly JD. Mechanism of uptake of technetium-tetrofosmin. I: Uptake into isolated adult rat ventricular myocites and subcellular localization. J Nucl Cardiol 1995; 2: 317-326.

20. Younès A, Songadele JA, Maublant J, Platts EA, Pickett RD, Veyre A. Mechanism of uptake of technetium-tetrofosmin. II: Uptake into isolated adult rat heart mitochondria. J Nucl Cardiol 1995; 2: 327-333.

21. Bonow RO. Identification of viable myocardium. Circulation 1996; 94: 2674-2680.

22. Iskandrian AS. Myocardial viability: Unresolved issues. J Nucl Med 1996; 37: 794-797.

23. Wagner HN Jr. The future. Semin Nucl Med 1996; 26: 194-200.

24. Beller GA (1996) Assessment of myocardial viability, in Beller GA (ed.), Clinical Nuclear Cardiology. WB Saunders Company, Philadelphia, pp. 293-336.

25. Bergmann SR (1994) Delineation of viable myocardium with metabolic imaging, in Iskandrian AS and Van der Wall EE (eds.), Myocardial viability. Detection and clinical relevance. Kluwer Academic Publishers, Dordrecht, pp. 71-102.

26. Schelbert HR. Merits and limitations of radionuclide aproches to viability and future develpements. J Nucl Cardiol 1994; 1: S86-S96.

27. Tamaki N. Current status of viability assessment with positron tomography. J Nucl Cardiol 1994; 1: 40-47.

28. Bergmann SR. Use and limitations of metabolic tracers labeled with positron-emitting radionuclides in the identification of viable myocardium. J Nucl Med 1994; 35(Suppl): 15S-22S.

29. Schwaiger M, Hicks R. The clinical role of metabolic imaging of the heart by positron emission tomography. J Nucl Med 1991; 32: 565-578.

30. Marshall RC, Tillisch JH, Phelps ME et al. Identification and differentiation of resting myocardial ischemia in man with positron computed tomography, 18F-labeled fluorodeoxyglucose and 13N-ammonia. Circulation 1983; 67: 766-778.

31. Brunken R, Schwaiger M, Grover-McKay M, Phelps ME, Tillisch J, Schelbert HR. Positron emission tomography detects tissue metabolic activity in myocardial segments with persistent thallium perfusion defects. J Am Coll Cardiol 1987; 10: 557-567.

32. Brunken R, Tillisch J, Schwaiger M et al. Regional perfusion, glucose metabolism, and wall motion in patients with chronic electrocardiographic Q wave infarctions: evidence for persistence of viable tissue in some infarct regions by positron emission tomography. Circulation 1986; 73: 951-963.

33. Tamaki N, Yonekura Y, Yamashita K et al. Relation of left ventricular perfusion and wall motion with metabolic activity in persisten defects on thallium-201 tomography in healed myocardial infarction. Am J Cardiol 1988; 62: 202-208.

34. Tillisch J, Brunken R, Marshall R et al. Reversibility of cardiac wall-motion abnormalities predicted by positron tomography. N Engl J Med 1986; 314: 884-888.

35. Liedtke AJ: Alterations of carbohydrate and lipid metabolism in the acutely ischemic heart. Prog Cardiovasc Dis 1981; 23: 321-336.

36. Kalff V, Schwaiger M, Ngoc N, Mcclanahan TB, Gallagher KP. The relationship between myocardial blood flow and glucose uptake in ischemic canine myocardium determined with fluorine-18-deoxyglucose. J Nucl Med 1992; 33: 1346-1353.

37. Schwaiger M, Hutchins GD. Evaluation of coronary artery disease with positron emission tomography. Semin Nucl Med 1992; 22:210-223.

38. Marwick TH, MacIntyre WJ, Lafont A, Nemec JJ, Salcedo EE. Metabolic responses of hibernating and infarcted myocardium to revascularization. Circulation 1922; 85: 1347- 1353.

39. Maes A, Flameng W, Nuyts J et al. Histological alterations in chronically hypoperfused myocardium: correlation with PET findings. Circulation 1994; 90: 735-745.

40. Bax JJ, Wijns W, Cornel JH, Visser FC, Boersma E, Fioretti PM. Accuracy of currently available techniques for prediction of functional recovery after revascularization in patients with left ventricular dysfunction due to chronic coronary artery disease: comparison of pooled date. J Am Coll Cardiol 1997; 30: 1451-1460.

41. Marwick TH, MacIntyre WJ, Lafont A, Nemec JJ, Salcedo EE. Metabolic responses of hibernating and infarcted myocardium to revascularization. Circulation 1992; 85: 1347-1353.

42. Gerber BL, Vanoverschelde J-LJ, Bol A et al. Myocardial blood flow, glucose uptake and recruitment of inotropic reserve in chronic left ventricular ischemic dysfunction: implications for the pathophysiology of chronic hibernation. Circulation 1996; 94: 651-659.

43. Tamaki N, Yonekura Y, Yamashita K et al. Positron Emission Tomography using Fluorine-18 Deoxyglucose in evaluation of coronary artery bypass grafting. Am J Cardiol 1989; 64: 890-865.

44. Gropler RJ, Geltman EM, Sampathkumaran K et al. Comparison of carbon-11-acetate with fluorine-18-fluorodeoxyglucose for delineating viable myocardium by positron emission tomography. J Am Coll Cardiol 1993; 22: 1587-1597.

45. Maes AF, Borgers M, Flameng W et al. Assessment of myocardial viability in chronic coronary artery disease using technetium-99m sestamibi SPECT: correlation with histologic and positron emission tomographic studies and functional follow-up. J Am Coll Cardiol 1997; 29: 62-68.

46. Tamaki N, Kawamoto M, Tadamura E et al. Prediction of reversible ischemia after revascularization: perfusion and metabolic studies with positron emission tomography. Circulation 1995; 91: 1697-1705.

47. Knuuti MJ, Saraste M, Nuutila P et al. Myocardial viability: Fluorine-18-deoxyglucose positron emission tomography in prediction of wall motion recovery after revascularization. Am Heart J 1994; 127: 785-796.

48. Baer FM, Voth E, Deutsch HJ et al. Predictive value of low dose dobutamine transesophageal and fluorine-18 fluorodeoxyglucose positron emission tomography for recovery of regional left ventricular function after successful revascularization. J Am Coll Cardiol 1996; 28: 60-69.

49. Lucignani G, Paolini G, Landoni C et al. Presurgical identification of hibernating myocardium by combined use of technetium-99m hexakis 2-metoxyisobutylisonitrile SPECT and fluorine-18 fluoro-2-deoxy-D-glucose positron emission tomography in patients with coronary artery disease. Eur J Nucl Med 1992; 19: 874-881.

50. Carrel T, Jenni R, Haubold-Reuter S, Von Schultess G, Pasic M, Turina M. Improvement of severely reduced left ventricular function after surgical revascularization in patients with preoperative myocardial infarction. Eur J Cardiothorac Surg 1992; 6: 479-484.

51. Tamaki N, Ohtani H, Yamashita K et al. Metabolic activity in the areas of new fill-in after thallium-201 reinjection: comparison with positron emission tomography using fluorine-18-deoxyglucose. J Nucl Med 1991; 32: 673-678.

52. Camici PG, Wijs W, Borgers M et al. Pathophysiological mechanisms for chronic reversible left ventricular dysfunction due to coronary artery disease (hibernating myocardium) Circulation 1997; 96: 3205-3214.

53. Fallavollita JA, Perry BJ, Cantry JM. 18F-2-2deoxyglucose deposition and regional flow in pigs with chronucally dysfunction myocardium. Evidence of transmural variations in chronic hibernating myocardium. Circulation 1997; 95:1900-1909.

54. Vanoverschelde JLJ, Wijns W, Depre C et al. Mechanisms of chronic regional postischemic dysfunction in humans: new insights from the study of noninfarcted collateral-dependent myocardium. Circulation 1993; 87: 1513-1523.

55. Schwaiger M, Neese RA, Araujo L et al. Sustained nonoxidative glucose utilization and depletion of glycogen in reperfused canine myocardium. J Am Coll Cardiol 1989; 13: 745-754.

56. Knuuti MJ, Nuutila P, Ruotsalainen U et al. The value of quantitative analysis of glucose utilization in detection of myocardial viability by PET. J Nucl Med 1993; 34:2068-2075.

57. Di Carli M, Asgarzadie F, Schelbert HR et al. Quantitative relation between myocardial viability and improvement in heart failure symptoms after revascularization in patients with ischemic cardiomyopathy. Circulation 1995; 92: 3436-3444.

58. Elsässer A, Schlepper M, Klövekorn WP et al. Hibernating myocardium. An incomplete adaptation to ischemia. Circulation 1997; 96: 2920-2931.

59. Eitzman D, Al-Aquar Z, Kanter HL et al. Clinical outcome of patients with advanced coronary artery disease after viability studies with positron emission tomography. J Am Coll Cardiol 1992; 20: 559-565.

60. Lee KS, Marwick TH, Cook SA et al. Prognosis of patients with left ventricular dysfunction, with and without viable myocardium after myocardial infarction. Relative efficacy of mediacal therapy and revascularization. Circulation 1994; 90: 2687-2694.

61. Grandin C, Wijns W, Melin JA et al. Delineation of myocardial viability with PET. J Nucl Med 1995; 36: 1543-1552.

62. De Silva R, Yamamoto Y, Rhodes CG et al. Preoperative prediction of the outcome of coronary revascularization using positron emission tomography. Circulation 1992; 86: 1738-1742.

63. Maki M, Luotolahti M, Nuutila P et al. Glucose uptake in the chronically dysfunctional but viable myocardium. Circulation 1996; 93: 1658-1666.

64. Golstein R. Kinetics of rubidium-82 after coronary occlusion and reperfusion. Assessment of patency and viability in open-chested dogs. J Clin Invest 1985; 75: 1131-1137.

65. Gould KL, Yoshida K, Hess MJ et al. Myocardial metabolism of fluorodeoxyglucose compared to cell membrane integrity for the potasium analogue rubidum-82 for assessing infarct size in man by PET. J Nucl Med 1991; 32: 1-9.

66. Weiss ES, Ahmed SA, Welch MJ, Williamson JR, Ter-Pogosian MM, Sobel BE. Quantification of infarction in cross sections of canine myocardium in vivo with positron emission transaxial tomography and ^{11}C-palmitate. Circulation 1977; 55: 66-73.

67. Lerch RA, Ambos HD, Bergmann SR, Welch MJ, Ter-Pogosian MM, Sobel BE. Localization of viable, ischemic myocardium by positron eission tomography with 11C-palmitate. Circulation 1981; 64: 689-699.

68. Schön HR, Schelbert HR, Robinson G et al. C-11 labeled palmitic acid for the noninvasive evaluation of regional myocardial fatty acid metabolism with positron-computed tomography. I. Kinetics of 11-C palmitic acid in normal myocardium A Heart J 1981; 103: 532-547.

69. Schelbert HR, Henze E, Schon HR et al. C-11 palmitate for the noninvasive evaluation of regional myocardial fatty acid metabolism with positron computed tomography. III. In vivo demonstration of the effects of substrate availability on myocardial metabolism. Am Heart J 1983; 105: 492-504.

70. Fox KA, Abendschein DB, Ambos HD, Sobel BE, Bermann SR. Efflux of metabolized an nonmetabolized fatty acid from canine myocardium. Implications for quantifying myocardial metabolism tomographically. Cir Res 1985; 57: 232-243.

71. Bergmann SR (1994) Delineation of viable myocardium with metabolic imaging, in Iskandrian AS and Van Der Wall EE (eds.), Myocardial viability. Detection and clinical relevance. Kluwer Academic Publishers, Dordrecht, pp. 53-70.

72. Brown MA, Marshall D, Sobel BF, Bergmann S. Delineation of myocardial oxygen utilazation with C-11-labeled acetate. Circulation 1987; 76: 687-696.

73. Walsh MN, Geltman EM, Brown MA et al. Noninvasive estimation of regional myocardial oxygen consumption by positron emission tomography with carbon-11 acetate in patients with myocardial infarction. J Nucl Med 1989; 30: 1798-1808.

74. Gropler RG, Siegel BA, Sampathkumaran K et al. Dependence of recovery of contractile function on maintenance of oxidative metabolism after myocardial infarction. J Am Coll Cardiol 1992; 19: 989-997.

75. Gropler RG, Geltman EM, Sampathkumaran K et al. Functional recovery after coronary revascularization for chronic coronary artery disease is dependent on maintenance of oxidative metabolism. J Am Coll Cardiol 1992; 20: 569-577.

76. Brown MA, Myears DW, Bergmannn SR. Validity of estimates of oxidative metabolism with carbon-11 acetate and positron emission tomography despite altered patterns of substrate utilization. J Nucl Med 1989; 30: 187-193.

77. Henes CG, Bergmann S, Walsh MN, Sobel BF, Geltman EM. Assessment of myocardial oxidative metabolic reserve with positron emission tomography and carbon-11 acetate. J Nucl Med 1989; 30:1489-1499.

78. Gropler RG, Geltman EM, Sampathkumaran K et al. Comparison of carbon-11-acetate with fluorine-18-fluorodeoxyglucose for delineating viable myocardium by positron emission tomography. J Am Coll Cardiol 1993; 22: 1587-1597.

79. Bax JJ, Visser FC, van LingenA et al. Relation between myocardial uptake of thallium-201 chloride and F18-fluorodexyglucose imaged with SPECT in normal individuals. Eur J Nucl Med 1995; 22: 56-60.

80. Delbeke D, Videlefsky S, Patton JA et al. Rest myocardial perfusion/metabolism imaging using simultaneous dual-isotope acquisition SPECT with technetium-99m-MIBI/fluorine-18-FDG. J Nucl Med 1995; 36: 2110-2119.

81. Martin WH, Delbeke D, Patton JA et al. FDG-SPET: correlation with FDG-PET. J Nucl Med 1995; 36: 988-995.

82. Burt RW, Perkins OW, Oppenheim BE et al. Direct comparison of fluorine-18-FDG SPECT, fluorine-18-PET and rest thallium-201 SPECT for the detection of myocardial viability. J Nucl Med 1995; 36: 176-179.

83. Sandler MP, Videlefsky S, Delbeke D et al. Evaluation of myocardial ischemia using a rest metabolism/stress perfusion protocol with fluorine-18 deoxyglucose/technetium-99m MIBI and dual isotope simultaneous adquisition single-photon emission computed tomography. J Am Coll Cardiol 1995; 26: 870-888.

84. Bax JJ, Cornel JH, Visser FC et al. Prediction of recovery of miocardial dysfunction following revascularization; Comparison of F18-fluorodeoxyglucose/thallium-201 single photon emission computed tomography, thallium-201 stress-reinjection single photon emission computed tomography and dobutamine echocardiography. J Am Coll Cardiol 1996; 28: 558-565.

85. Van der Wall EE, Heidendal GAK, den Hollander W, Westera G, Roos JP. Metabolic myocardial imaging with 123I-heptadecanoic acid in patients with angina pectoris. Eur J Nucl Med 1981; 6: 391-396.

86. Henrich MM, Vester E, von der Lohe et al. The comparison of of 2-^{18}F-2-deoxyglucose and 15-(orto-^{123}I-phenyl)-pentadecanoic acid uptake in persisting defects on thallium-201 tomography in miocardial infarction. J Nucl Med 1991; 32: 1353-1357.

87. Hansen CL, Corbett JR, Pippin JJ et al. Iodone-123 phenylpentadecanoic acid and single photon emission computed tomography in identifying left ventricular regional metabolic abnormalities in patients with coronary artery disease. J Am Coll Cardiol 1988; 12: 78-87.

88. Marie PY, Karcher G, Danchin N et al. comparison between thallium-201 rest-reinjection and (^{123}I)-16-iodo-3-methylhexadecanoic acid imaging in patients with myocardial infarction: analysis of defect reversibility. J Nucl Med 1995; 36:1561-1568.

89. Marie PY, Angioï M, Danchin N et al. Assessment of myocardial viability in patients with previous myocardial infarction by using single-photon emission computed tomography with a new metabolic tracer: (^{123}I)-16-iodo-3-methylhexadecanoic acid (MIHA). Comparison with the rest-reinjection thallium-201 technique. J Am Coll Cardiol 1997; 30: 1241-1248.

90. Strauss HW, Nunn A, Linder K. Nitroimidazoles for imaging hypoxic myocardium. J Nucl Med 1995; 2:437-445.

91. Nunn A, Linder K, Strauss HW. Nitroimidazoles and imaging hypoxia: a review. Eur J Nucl Med 1995; 22: 265-280.

92. Martin GV, Biskupiak JE, Caldwrl JH, Rasey JS, Krohn KA. Characterization of iodovinylmisonidazole as a marker for myocardial hypoxia. J Nucl Med 1993; 34: 918-923.

93. Shelton ME, Dence CS, Hwang DR, Welch MJ, Bergman SR. Myocardial kinetics of fluorine-18-misonidazole: a marker of hypoxic myocardium. J Nucl med 1989; 30: 351-358.

94. Rumsey WL, Patel B, Lindel KE. The effect of graded hypoxia on the retention of a novel 99mTc-nitroheterocycle in the perfused rat heart. J Nucl Med 1995; 36: 632-636.

95. Rumsey WL, Kuczynski B, Patel B et al. SPECT imaging of ischemic myocardium using a Technetium-99m-Nitroimidazole ligand. J Nucl Med 1995; 36: 1445-1450.

96. Shi C, Sinusas AJ, Dione DP et al. Technetium-99m nitroimidazole (BMS181321): a positive imaging agent for detecting myocardial ischemia. J Nucl Med 1995; 36: 1078-1086.

97. Bonow RO, Dilsizian V. Tallium-201 for assessment of myocardial viability. Semin Nucl Med 1991; 21: 230-241.

98. Nielsen AP, Morris KG, Murdock R, Bruno FP, Cobb FR. Linear relationship between the distribution of thallium-201 and blood flow in ischemic and nonischemic myocardium during exercise. Circulation 1980; 61: 797-801.

99. Verani MS, Jhingram S, Attar M, Rizk A, Quinones MA, Miller RR. Poststress redistribution of thallium-201 in patients with coronary artery disease with and without prior myocardial infarction. Am J Cardiol 1979; 43: 1114-1122.

100. Beller GA, Watson DD, Ackell P, Pohost GM. Time course of thallium-201 redistribution after transient myocardial ischemia. Circulation 1980; 61:791-797.

101. Gutman J, Berman DS, Freeman M et al. Time to complete redistribution of thallium-201 in exercise thallium-201 scintigraphy: relationship to the degree of coronary artery stenosis. Am Heart J 1983; 108: 989-995.

102. Pohost GM, Zir LM, Moore RH, McKusick KA, Guiney TE, Beller GA. Differenciation of transiently ischemic from infarcted myocardium by serial imaging after a single dose of thallium-201. Circulation 1977; 55: 294-302.

103. Gutman J, Berman DS, Freeman M et al. Time to complete redistribution of thallium-201 in exercise myocardial scintigraphy: relationship to the degree of coronary stenosis. Am Heart J 1983; 106: 989-995.

104. Kiat H, Berman DS, Maddahi J et al. Late reversibility of tomographic myocardial thallium-201 defects: an accurate predictor of myocardial viability. J Am Coll Cardiol 1988; 12: 1456-1463.

105. Yang LD, Berman DS, Kiat H et al. The frequency of late reversibility in SPECT thallium-201 stress-redistribution studies. J Am Coll Cardiol 1990; 15: 334-340.

106. Gibson RS, Watson DD, Taylor GJ et al. Prospective assessment of regional myocardial perfusion before and after coronary revascularization surgery by quantitative thallium-201 scintigraphy. J Am Coll Cardiol 1983; 1: 804-815.

107. Dilsizian V, Rocco TP, Freedman NMT, Leon MB, Bonow RO. Enhanced detection of ischemic but viable myocardium by the reinjection of thallium after stress-redistribution imaging. N Engl J Med 1990; 323: 141-146.

108. Rocco TP, Dilsizian V, McKusick KA, Fishman AJ, Boucher CA, Strauss HW. Comparison of thallium redistribution with rest "reinjection" imaging for the detection of viable myocardium. Am J Cardiol 1990; 66: 158-163.

109. Ohtani H, Tamaki N, Yonekura Y et al. Value of thallium-201 reinjection after delayed SPECT imaging for predicting reversible ischemia after coronary artery bypass grafting. Am J Cardiol 1990; 66: 394-399.

110. Bonow RO, Dilsizian V, Cuocolo A, Bacharach SL. Identification of viable myocardium in patients with chronic coronary artery disease and left ventricular dysfunction. Comparison of Thallium scintigraphy with reinjection and PET imaging with 18F-Fluorodeoxyglucose. Circulation 1991; 83: 26-37.

111. Vanoverschelde L-LJ, D'Hondt A-M, Marwick T et al. Head-to-head comparison of exercise-redistribution-reinjection thallium single-photon emission tomography and low dose dobutamine echocardiography for prediction of reversibility of chronic left ventricular ischemic dysfunctiun. J Am Coll Cardiol 1996; 28: 432-442.

112. Arnese M, Cornel JH, Salustri A et al. Prediction of improvement of regional left ventricular function after surgical revascularization: a comparison of low-dose dobutamine echocardiography with 201-Tl SPECT. Circulation 1995; 91: 2748-2752.

113. Tamaki N, Ohtani H, Yonekura Y et al. Significance of fill-in after thallium-201 reinjection following delayed imaging: comparison with regional wall motion and angiographic findings. J Nucl Med 1990; 31:1617-1623.

114. Haque T, Furukawa T, Takahashi M, Kinoshita M. Identificaion of hibernating myocardium by dobutamine stress echocardiography: comparison with thallium-201 reinjection imaging. Am Heart J 1995; 130: 553-563.

115. Kiat H, Friedman JD, Wang FP et al. Frecuency of late reversibility in stress-redistribution thallium-201 SPECT using an early reinjection protocol. Am Heart J 1991; 122: 613-619.

116. Mori T, Minamiji K, Kurogane H, Ogawa K, Yoshida Y. Rest-injected thallium-201 imaging for assessing viability of severe asynergic regions. J Nucl Med 1991; 32: 1718-1724.

117. Inglese E, Bambrilla M, Dondi M et al. Assessment of myocardial viability after Thallium-201 reinjection or rest-resdistribution imaging: a multicenter study. J Nucl Med 1995; 36: 555-563.

118. Udelson JE, Coleman PS, Metherall J et al. Predicting recovery of severe regional ventricular dysfunction. Comparison of resting scintigraphy with 201Tl and 99mTc-Sestamibi. Circulation 1994; 89: 2552-2561

119. Ragosta M, Beller GA, Watson DD, Kaul S, Gimple LW. Quantitative rest-redistribution 201Tl imaging in detection of myocardial viability and prediction of improvement in left ventricular function after coronary bypass surgery in patients with severely depressed left ventricular function. Circulation 1993; 87: 1630-1641.

120. Perrone-Filard P, Pace L, Prastaro M et al. Assessment of myocardial viability in patients with chronic coronary artery disease: rest-4-hour-24-hour ^{201}Tl tomography versus dobutamine echocardiography. Circulation 1996; 94: 2712-2719.

121. Marzullo P, Parodi O, Eisenhofer B et al. Value of rest thallium-201/technetium-99m sestamibi and dobutamine echocardiography for detecting myocardial viability. Am J Cardiol 1993; 71: 166-172.

122. Qureshi U, Nagueh SF, Afridi I et al. Dobutamine echocardiography and quantitative rest-redistribution ^{201}Tl tomography in myocardial hibernation: relation of contractile reserve to 201Tl uptake and comparative prediction of recovery of function. Circulation 1997; 95: 626-635.

123. Alfieri O, La Canna G, Giubinni R, Pardini A, Zogno M, Fuci C. Recovery of myocardial function. Eur J Cardiothorac Surg 1993; 7: 325-330.

124. Charney R, Schwinger ME, Chun J et al. Dobutamine echocardiography end resting-redistributon thallium-201 scintigraphy predicts recovery of hibernating myocardium after coronary revascularization. Am Heart J 1994; 128: 864-869.

125. Dilsizian V, Perrone-Filardi P, Arrighi JA et al. Concordance and discordance between stress-redistribution-reinjection and rest-redistribution thallium imaging for assessing viable myocardium. Comparison with metabolic activity by positron emission tomography. Circulation 1993; 88: 941-952.

126. Galassi AR, Centamore G, Fiscella A et al. Comparison of rest-redistribution thallium-201 imaging and reinjection after stress-redistribution for the assessment of myocardial viability in patients with left ventricular dysfunction secondary to coronary artery disease. Am J Cardiol 1995; 75: 436-442.

127. Iskandrian AS, Hakki A, Kane SA et al. Rest and redistribution thallium-201 myocardial scintigraphy to predict improvement in left ventricular function after coronary arterial bypass grafting. Am J Cardiol 1983; 51: 1312-1316.

128. Van Eck-Smit BLF, Van der Wall EE, Kuijper AFM, Zwinderman AH, Pauwels EKJ. Immediate thallium-201 reinjection following imaging: a time-saving approach for detection of myocardial viability. J Nucl Med 1993; 34: 737-743.

129. Weiss AT, Maddahi J, Lew AS et al. Reverse redistribution of thallium-201: a sign of nontransmural myocardial infarction with patency of the infarct-related coronary artery. J Am Coll Cardiol 1986; 7: 61-67.

130. Dilsizian V, Freedman NMT, Bacharach SL, Perrone-Filardi P, Bonow RO. Regional thallium uptake in irreversible defects. Magnitude of change in thallium activity after reinjection distinguishes viable from nonviable myocardium. Circulation 1992; 85: 627-634.

131. Marin-Neto JA, Dilsizian V, Arrighi JA et al. Thallium reinjection demostrates viable myocardium in regions with reverse redistribution. Circulation 1993; 88 (part 1): 1736-1745.

132. Altehoefer C, von Dahl J, Buell U, Uebis R, Kleinhans E, Hanrath P. Comparison of thallim-201 single-photon emission tomography after rest injection and fluorodeoxyglucose positron emission tomography for assessment of myocardial viability in patients with chronic coronary artery disease. Eur J Nucl Med 1994; 21: 37-45.

133. Jones AG, Abrams MJ, Davison A. Biological studies of a new class of technetium complexes: the hexakis (alkylisonitrile) technetium (I) cations. J Nucl Med Biol 1984; 11: 225-234.

134. Okada RD, Glover MD, Gaffney T, Williams S. Myocardial kinetics of technetium-99m hexakis-2-methoxy-2-methylpropyl-isonitrile. Circulation 1988; 77: 491-498.

135. Beller GA, Watson DD. Physiological basis of myocardial perfusion imaging with the technetium 99m agents. Semin Nucl Med 1991; 21: 173-181.

136. Wackers FJ, Berman DS, Maddahi J et al. Techetium-99m hexakis 2 methoxy-isobutyl isonitrile, a new radiopharmaceutical for myocardial perfusion imaging: human biodistribution, dosimetry, safety and preliminary comparison to thallium-201 for myocardial perfusion imaging (phase I and II studies). J Nucl Med 1989; 30: 301-311.

137. Higley B, Smith FW, Smith T et al. Technetium-99m-1,2-bis[bis(2-ethoxyethyl)phosphino]ethane: Human biodistribution, dosimetry and safety of a new myocardial perfusion imaging agent. J Nucl Med 1993; 34: 30-38.

138. Tamaky N, Takahashi N, Kawamoto M et al. Myocardial tomography using Technetium-99m-Tetrofosmin to evaluate coronary artery disease. J Nucl Med 1994; 35:594-600.

139. Rigo P, Leclercq B, Itti R, Lahiri A, Braat S. Technetium-99m-Tetrofosmin myocardial imagin: a comparison with Thallium-201 and angiography. J Nucl Med 1994; 35:587-593.

140. Berman DS, Kiat H, Van Train KF, Friedman J, García EV, Maddahi J. Comparison of SPECT using technetium-99m agents and thallium-201 and PET for the assessment of myocardial perfusion and viability. Am J Cardiol 1990; 66: 72E-79E.

141. Kiat H, Maddahi J, Roy LT et al. Comparison of technetium 99m methoxy isobutyl isonitrile and thallium 201 for evaluation of coronary artery disease by planar and tomographic methods. Am Heart J 1989; 117: 1-11.

142. Berman DS, Kiat H, VanTrain KF et al. Technetium-99m-sestamibi in the assessment of chronic coronary artery disease. Semin Nucl Med 1991; 21: 190-212.

143. Santana C, Candell J, Castell J et al. Diagnóstico de la enfermedad coronaria mediante la tomografía de esfuerzo con isonitrilos-tecnecio-99. Med Clin (Barc) 1995; 105 :201-204.

144. Castell J, Santana C, Candell C et al. La tomogammagrafía miocárdica de esfuerzo en el diagnóstico de la enfermedad coronaria multivaso. Rev Esp Cardiol 1997; 50:635-642.

145. Sridhara B, Sochor H, Rigo P et al. Myocardial single-photon emission computed tomographic imaging with technetium 99m tetrofosmin: Stess-rest imaging with same-day and separate-day rest imaging. J Nucl Cardiol 1994; 1: 138-143.

146. Montz R, Perez-Castejón MJ, Jurado JA et al. Technetium-99m tetrofosmin rest/stress myocardial SPET with a same-day 2-hour protocol: comparison with coronary angiography. A Spanish-Portugues multicentre clinical trial. Eur J Nucl Med 1996; 23: 639-647.

147. Li Q, Solot G, Frank TL, Wagner HN, Becker LC. Myocardial redistribution of technetium-99m-methoxyisobutyl isonitrile (SESTAMIBI). J Nucl Med 1990; 31:1069-1076.

148. Carvalho PA, Chiu ML, Kronauge JF et al. Subcellular distribution and analysis of technetium-99m-MIBI in isolated perfused rat hearts. J Nucl Med 1992; 33: 1516-1521.

149. Piwnica-Worms D, Kronauge JF, Delmon L, Holman L, Marsh JD, Jones AG. Effect of metabolic inhibition on technetium-99m-MIBI kinetics in cultured chick myocardial cells. J Nucl Med 1990; 31: 464-472.

150. Freeman I, Grunwald AM, Hoory S, Bodenheimer M. Effect of coronary occlusion and myocardial viability on myocardial activity of technetium-99m-sestamibi. J Nucl Med 1991; 32: 292-298.

151. Sinusas AJ, Watson DD, Canon JM, Beller GA. Effect of ischemia and postischemic dysfunction on myocardial uptake of technetium-99m-labeled methoxyisobutyl isonitrile and thallium-201. J Am Coll Cardiol 1989; 14: 1785-1793.

152. Rigo P, Benoit T, Braat S (1994) The role of technetium-99m Sestamibi in the evaluation of myocardial viability, in Iskandrian AS and Van der Wall EE (eds.), Myocardial viability. Detection and clinical relevance. Kluwer Academic Publishers, Dordrecht, pp. 39-52.

153. Johnson LL. Clinical experience with Technetium 99m Teboroxime. Semin Nucl Med 1991; 21: 182-189.

154. Labonté Ch, Taillefer R, Lambert R et al. Comparison between Technetium-99m-Teboroxime and Thallium-201 Dipyridamole planar myocardial perfusion imaging in detection of coronary artery disease. Am J Cardiol 1992; 69: 90-96.

155. Narra RK, Nunn AD, Kuczynski BL, Feld T, Wedeking P, Eckelman WC. A neutral technetium-99m complex for myocardial imaging. J Nucl Med 1989; 30: 1830-1837.

156. Iskandrian AS, Heo J, Kong B, Lyons E, Marsch S. Use of technetium-99m isonitrile (RP-30A) in assessing left ventricular perfusion and function at rest and during exercise in coronary artery disease, and comparison with coronary arteriography and exercise thallium-201 SPECT imaging. Am J Cardiol 1989; 64: 270-275.

157. Khan JK, McGhie I, Akers MS et al. Quantitative rotational tomography with ^{201}Tl and [99m]Tc 2-Methoxy-Isobutyl-Isonitrile. A direct comparison in normals individuals and patients with coronary artery disease. Circulation 1989; 79: 1282-1293.

158. Wackers FJTh, Gibbons RJ, Verani M et al. Serial quantitative planar technetium-99m isonitrile imaging in acute myocardial infarction: efficacy for noninvasive assessment of thrombolytic therapy. J Am Coll Cardiol 1989; 14: 861-873.

159. Freeman I, Grunwald AM, Hoory S, Bodenheimer M. Effect of coronary occlusion and myocardial viability on myocardial activity of technetium-99m-sestamibi. J Nucl Med 1991; 32: 292-298.

160. Sinusas AJ, Trautman KA, Bergin JD et al. Quantification of "area at risk" during coronary occlusion and degree of myocardial salvage after reperfusion using cardiac imaging with technetium-99m-methoxy isobutyl isonitrile. Circulation 1990; 82: 1424-1437.

161. Kayden DS, Mattera JA, Zaret BL, Wackers FJT. Demonstration of reperfusion after thrombolysis with technetium-99m isonitrile myocardial imaging. J Nucl Med 1988; 29: 1865-1867.

162. Santoro GM, Bisi G, Sciagrà R et al. Single photon emission computed tomography with technetium-99m hexakis 2-methoxyisobutyl isonitrile in acute myocardial infarction before and after thrombolytic treatment: assessment of salvaged myocardium and prediction of late functional recovery. J Am Coll Cardiol 1990; 15: 301-314.

163. Wackers FJ. Thrombolytic therapy for myocardial perfusion imaging with technetium-99m sestamibi. Am J Cardiol 1990; 66: 36E-41E.

164. Behrenbeck T, Pellikka PA, Huber KC, Bresnahan JF, Gersh BY, Gibbons RJ. Primary angioplasty in myocardial infarction: assessment of improved myocardial perfusion with technetium-99m isonitrile. J Am Coll Cardiol 1991; 17: 365-372.

165. Cuocolo A, Pace L, Ricciardelli B, Chiariello M, Trimarco B, Salvatore M. Identification of viable myocardium in patients with chronic coronary artery disease: comparison of thallium-201 scintigraphy with reinjection and technetium-99m-methoxyisobutylisonitrile. J Nucl Med 1992; 33: 505-511.

166. Dilsizian V, Arrighi JA, Diodati JG et al. Myocardial viability in patients with chronic coronary artery disease: comparison of 99mTc-sestamibi with thallium-201 reinjection and (18F)fluorodeoxyglucose. Circulation 1994; 89: 578-587.

167. Marzullo P, Sambuceti G, Parodi O. The role of sestamibi scintigraphy in the radioisotopic assessment of myocardial viability. J Nucl Med 1992; 33: 1925-1930.

168. Marzullo P, Sanbuceti G, Parodi O et al. Regional concordance and discordance between rest thallium 201 and sestamibi imaging for assessing tissue viability: Comparison with postrevascularization function recovery. J Nucl Cardiol 1995; 2: 309-316.

169. Dondi M, Tartagni F, Fallani F et al. A comparison of rest sestamibi and rest-redistribution thallium single photon emission tomography: possible implications for myocardial viability detection in infarcted patients. Eur J Nucl Med 1993; 20: 26-31.

170. Maurea S, Cuocolo A, Pace L et al. Rest-injected thallium-201 redistribution and resting technetium-99m methoxyisobutylisonitrile uptake in coronary artery disease: Relation to the severy of coronary artery stenosis. Eur J Nucl Med 1993; 20: 502-510.

171. Dilsizian V, Rocco TP, Strauss HW, Boucher CA. Technetium-99m isonitrile myocardial uptake at rest. I. Relation to severity of coronary artery stenosis. J Am Coll Cardiol 1989; 14: 1678-1684.

172. Rocco TP, Dilsizian V, Strauss HW, Boucher CA. Technetium-99m isonitrile myocardial uptake at rest. II. Relation to clinical markers of potential viability. J Am Coll Cardiol 1989; 14: 1678-1684.

173. Bonow RO, Dilsizian V. Thallium-201 and technetium-99m-Sestamibi for assessing viable myocardium. J Nucl Med 1992; 33: 815-817.

174. Altehoefer C, Kaiser HJ, Doerr R et al. Fluorine-18 deoxyglucose PET for assessment of viable myocardium in perfusion defects in 99mTc-MIBI SPET: a comparative study in patients with coronary artery disease. Eur J Nucl Med 1992; 19: 334-342.

175. Altehoefer C, von Dahl J, Biedermann M et al. Significance of defect severity in technetium-99m-MIBI SPECT at rest to assess myocardial viability: comparison with fluorine-18-FDG PET. J Nucl Med 1994; 35: 569-574.

176. Arrighi JA, NG CK, Dey HM, Wackers FJT, Soufer R. Effect of left ventricular function on the assessment of myocardial viability by technetium-99m sestamibi and correlation with positron emission tomography in patients with healed myocardial infarcts or stable angina pectoris, or both. Am J Cardiol 1997; 80: 1007-1013.

177. Castell J, Candell J, Roselló J et al. Valoración de la viabilidad miocárdica mediante tecnecio-99m isonitrilo y talio-201. Resultados del protocolo multicéntrico español. Rev Esp Cardiol 1997; 50: 320-330.

178. Cuocolo A, Nicolai E, Petretta M et al. One-Year effect of myocardial revascularization on resting left ventricular function and regional thallium uptake in chronic CAD. J Nucl Med 1997; 38:1684-1692.

179. Castell J, González JM, Fraile M et al. SESTAMIBI uptake quantification predicting recovery of severe regional ventricular dysfunction. J Nucl Cardiol 1995; 2: 21 (Abstr.).

180. Cuocolo A, Acampa W, Nicolai E et al. Quantitative thallim-201 and technetium 99m sestamibi tomography at rest in detection of myocardial viability in patients with chronic ischemic left ventricular dysfunction. J Nucl Cardiol 2000; 7: 8-15.

181. Schneider CA, Voth E, Gawlich S et al. Significance of rest technetium-99m sestamibi imaging for the prediction of improvement of left ventricular dysfunction after Q wave myocardial infarction: importance of infarct location adjusted thresholds. J Am Coll Cardiol 1998; 32: 648-654.

182. Medrano R, Lowry RW, Young JB et al. Assessment of myocardial viability with 99mTc-Sestamibi in patients undergoing cardiac transplantation. A scintigraphic/pathological study. Circulation 1996; 94: 1010-1017.

183. Dakik HA, Howell JM, Lawrie GM et al. Assessment of myocardial viability with 99mTc-sestamibi tomography before coronary bypass graft surgery. Correlation with histopathology and postoperative improvement in cardiac function. Circulation 1997; 96: 2892-2898.

184. Maes AF, Borgers M, Flameng W et al. Assessment of myocardial viability in chronic coronary artery disease using technetium-99m sestamibi SPECT. Correlation with histologic and positron emission tomographic studies and functional follow-up. J Am Coll Cardiol 1997; 29: 62-68.

185. Cinca J, García-Burillo A, Carreño A et al. Differential Uptake of Myocardial Perfusion Radiotracers in Normal, Infarcted, and Acutely Ischemic Peri-infarction Myocardium Cardiovasc Res 1998; 38:91-97.

186. Takahashi N, Reinhardt CP, Marcel R, Leppo JA. Myocardial uptake of ^{99m}Tc-Tetrofosmin, sestamibi, and ^{201}Tl in a model of acute coronary reperfusion. Circulation 1996; 94: 2605-2613.

187. Koplan BA, Beller GA, Ruiz M, Yang JY, Watson DD, Glover DK. Comparison between Thallium-201 and Technetium-99m-Tetrofosmin uptake with sustained low flow and profound systolic dysfunction. J Nucl Med 1996; 37: 1398-1402.

188. Moragas G, González JM, Buxeda M et al. Stress and rest myocardial SPECT quantification with Thallium-201 and Technetium-99m-Tetrofosmin: A comparative study. Nucl Med Comun 1998; 19: 633-640.

189. Heo J, Care V, Wasserleben V, Iskandrian AS. Planar and tomographic imaging with technetium 99m-labelled tetrofosmin: correlation with tallium 201 and coronary angiography. J Nucl Cardiol 1994; 1: 317-324.

190. Nakajima K, Taki J, Shuke N, Bunko H, Takata S, Hisada K. Myocardial perfusion imaging and dynamic analysis with technetium-99m tetrofosmin. J Nucl Med 1993; 34: 1478-1484.

191. Matsunari I, Fijino S, Taki J et al. Myocardial viability assessment with technetium-99m-tetrofosmin and thallium-201 reinjection in coronary artery disease. J Nucl Med 1995; 36: 1961-1967.

192. Ficaro EP, Fessler JA, Shreve PD, Kritzman JN, Rose PA, Corbett JR. Simultaneous transmission/emission myocardial perfusion tomography. Diagnostic accuracy of attenuation-corrected 99mTc-sestamibi single-photon emission computed tomography. Circulation 1996; 93: 463-473.

193. Kluge R, Sattler B, Seese A, Knapp WH. Attenuation correction by simultaneous emission-transmission myocardial single-photon emission computed tomography: impact on diagnostic accuracy. Eur J Nucl Med 1997; 24: 1107-1114.

194. Jiménez-Hoyuela JM, McClellan JR, Alavi A, Araujo LI. Impacto de la corrección de atenuación en la imagen de perfusión miocárdica con SPECT. Rev Esp Cardiol 1998; 51 (Suppl. 1): 26-32.

195. Chin BB, Kim HJ, Zukerberg B, Alavi A. Gated resting Tl-201 SPECT in the evaluation of myocardial viability. Clin Nucl Med 1996; 21: 275-279.

196. Hambye AS, Van Den Branden F, Vandevivere J. Diagnostic value of Tc-99m sestamibi gated SPECT to assess viability in a patient after acute myocardial infarction. Clin Nucl Med 1996; 21: 19-23.

197. Shehata AR, Mitchell J, Heller GV. Use of gated SPECT imaging in the prediction of myocardial viability. J Nucl Cardiol 1997; 4: 99-100.

198. Nicolai E, Cuocolo A, Pace L et al. Assessment of systolic wall thickening using technetium-99m methoxyisobutylisonitrile in patients with coronary artery disease: relation to thallium-201 scintigraphy with re-injection. Eur J Nucl Med 1995; 22: 1017-1022.

199. González P, Massardo T, Muñoz A et al. Is the addition of ECG gating to technetium-99m sestamibi SPET of value in the assessment of myocardial viability? An evaluation based on two-dimensional echocardiography following revascularization. Eur J Nucl Med 1996; 23: 1315-1322.

200. Perrone-Filardi P, Bacharach, Dilsizian V et al. Metabolic evidence of viable myocardium in regions with reduced wall thickness and absent wall thickening in patients with chronic ischemic left ventricular dysfunction. J Am Coll Cardiol 1992; 20: 161-168.

201. Helfant RH, Pine R, Meister SG, Feldman MS, Trout RG, Banka VS. Nitroglycerin to unmask reversible asynergy: correlation with postcoronary bypass ventriculography. Circulation 1974; 50: 108-113.

202. Parker JD, West RO, Digiogi S. The effect of nitroglycerin on coronary blood flow and the hemodynamic response to exercise in coronary artery disease. Am J Cardiol 1971; 27: 59-65.

203. Mathes P, Rival J. Effect of nitroglycerin on total and regional coronary blood flow in the normal and ischemic canine myocardium. Cardiovasc Res 1971; 5: 54-61.

204. He ZX, Darcourt J, Guignier A et al. Nitrates improve detection of isquemic but viable myocardium by thallium-201 reinjection SPECT. J Nucl Med 1993; 34: 1472-1477.

205. He ZX, Medrano R, Hays JT, Mahmarian JJ, Verani MS. Nitroglycerin-augmented Tl-201 reinjection enhances detection of reversible myocardial hypoperfusion. A randomized, double-blind, parallel, placebo-controlled trial. Circulation 1997, 95: 1799-1805.

206. Basu S, Senior R, Raval U, Lahiri A. Superiority of nitrate-enhanced 201Tl over conventional redistribution 201Tl imaging for prognostic evaluation after myocardial infarction and thrombolysis. Circulation 1997; 96: 2932-2937.

207. Bisi G, Sciagrà R, Santoro GM, Rossi V, Fazzini PF. Technetium 99m-sestamibi imaging with nitrate infusion to detect viable hibernating myocardium and predict postrevascularization recovery. J Nucl M 1995; 36: 1994-2000.

208. Sciagrà R, Bisi G, Santoro GM, Agnolucci M, Zoccarato O, Fazzini PF. Influence of the assessment of defect severity and intravenous nitrate administration during tracer injection on the detection of

viable hibernating myocardium with data-based quantitative technetium 99m-labeled sestamibi single-photon emission computed tomography. J Nucl Cardiol 1996; 3: 221-230.

209. Maurea S, Cuocolo A, Soricelli A et al. Enhanced detection of viable myocardium by technetium-99m-MIBI imaging after nitrate administration in chronic coronary artery disease. J Nucl Med 1995; 36: 1945-1952.

210. Bisi G, Sciagrà R, Santoro GM, Fazzini PF. Rest technetium-99m-sestamibi tomography in combination with short-term administration of nitrates: feasibility and reliability for prediction of postrevascularization outcome of asynergic territories. J Am Coll Cardiol 1994; 24: 1282-1289.

211. Flotats A, Carrió I, Estorch M et al. Nitrate administration to enhace the detection of myocardial viability by technetium-99m tetrofosmin single-photon emission tomography. Eur J Nucl Med 1997; 24: 767-773.

212. Dilsizian V, Bonow RO, Cannon RO et al. The effect of coronary bypass grafting on left ventricular systolic function at rest: evidence for preoperative subclinical myocardial ischemia. Am J Cardiol 1988; 61:1248-1254.

213. Breisblatt WM, Vita NA, Armuchastegui M, Cohen LS, Zaret BL. Usefulness of serial radionuclide monitoring during graded nitroglycerin infusion for unstable angina pectoris for determining left ventricular function and individualized therapeutic dose. Am J Cardiol 1988; 61: 685-690.

214. Popio KA, Gorlin R, Bechtel D, Levine JA. Postextrasystolic potentiation as a predictor of potential myocardial viability: preoperative analyses compared with studies after coronary bypass surgery. Am J Cardiol 1977; 39: 944-953.

215. Nesto RW, Cohn LH, Collins JJ, Wynne J, Holman L, Cohn PF. Inotropic contractile reserve: a useful predictor of increased 5 year survival and improved postoperative left ventricular function in patients with coronary artery disease and reduced ejection fraction. Am J Cardiol 1982; 50: 39-44.

216. Rozanski A, Berman D, Gray R et al. Preoperative prediction of reversible myocardial asynergy by postexercise radionuclide ventriculography. N Enl J Med 1982; 307: 212-216.

217. Coma-Canella I, del Val Gómez M, Terol I, Rodrigo F, Castro JM. Radionuclide studies in patients with stress-induced ST-segment elevation after acute myocardial infarction. J Am Coll Cardiol 1994; 128: 459-465.

218. Wakers FJ, Berger HJ, Johnstone DE et al. Multiple gated cardiac blood pool imaging for left ventricular ejection fraction: validation of the technique and assessment of variability. Am J Cardiol 1979; 43: 1159-1166.

219. Rocco TP, Dilsizian V, Fischman AJ, Strauss HW. Evaluation of ventricular function in patients with coronary artery disease. J Nucl Med 1989; 30:1149-1165.

220. Bonaduce D, Morgano G, Petretta M et al. Phase analysis of radionuclide angiography in acute myocardial infarction. Eur J Nucl Med 1990; 16: 161-165.

221. Cortadellas J, Figueras J, Domingo E et al. Ondas T negativas precoces y profundas en un primer infarto de miocardio anterior. Relación con la contractilidad regional en la fase aguda y en el seguimiento a medio plazo. Rev Esp Cardiol 1997; 50: 93 (Abstr.).

222. Kaul S (1994) Echocardiographic assessment of myocardial viability, in Iskandrian AS and Van der Wall EE (eds.), Myocardial viability. Detection and clinical relevance. Kluwer Academic Publishers, Dordrecht, pp. 71-102

223. Benotti JR, Grossman W, Brawnwald E et al. Hemodynamic assessment of amrinone: a new inotropic agent. N Engl J Med 1978; 299: 1373-1377.

224. Benotti JR, Grossman W, Braunwald E, Carabello BA. Effects of amrinone on myocardial energy metabolism and hemodynamics in patients with severe congestive heart failure to coronary artery disease. Circulation 1980; 62: 28-34.

225. Perez-Baliño NA, Masoli OH, Meretta AH et al. Amrinone stimulation test: ability to predict improvement in left ventricular ejection fraction after coronary bypass surgery in patients with poor baseline left ventricular function. J Am Coll Cardiol 1996; 28: 1488-1492.

10.   CLINICAL VALUE OF VIABLE MYOCARDIUM DETECTION

JORDI SOLER-SOLER and JAUME CANDELL-RIERA

1.   Clinical relevance of viable myocardium

Myocardial viability is highly topical as evidenced by numerous editorials that have been published in the high-impact cardiology journals [1-9]. The most relevant aspects of viable myocardium from the point of view of clinical practice are:

1.   In which patients are these diagnoses of myocardial viability to be conducted
2.   Which methods need to be employed for the diagnoses
3.   Do these diagnoses have prognostic implications for the patient's therapeutic management

These are the three points to be addressed in this chapter. The diagnosis of myocardial viability needs to be considered in those patients in whom there is severely impaired contractility in a myocardial region: akinesia or dyskinesia. Many authors include those regions that are severely hypokinetic such that a myocardial region with these characteristics could contribute, especially if it is extensive, to a deterioration of the overall left ventricular function. If this left ventricular function is caused by myocardial stunning or hibernation, i.e. viable myocardium, this can be reversed on revascularisation.

It is very rare that a severe impairment of contractility can occur in patients that have not suffered a prior myocardial infarction but in some cases severe sustained hypoperfusion can be a cause. Lewis et al. [10], using echocardiography, detected impairment in regional wall motion of about 31% in a series of 252 patients without a history of previous myocardial infarction. However, the defects of contractility were severe only in 36% of these regions i.e. <10% of patients without prior infarct had severe segmental alterations of systolic ventricular function. Conversely, it is rare that segmental contractility defects contribute to a significant overall decrease in left ventricular function in patients without previous infarction. In a series of consecutive patients without infarction studied in our nuclear cardiology unit, only a 3% had an ejection fraction <50% [11].

Lemlek et al. [12] in a retrospective study on 532 patients with coronary artery disease in chronic phase and of whom 17% had Q wave necrosis on ECG, found that the diagnosis of viability, based on ^{201}Tl-SPET-stress images, was about 21% of cases when there were scintigraphic criteria of necrosis (irreversible severe defects) or, predominantly, of more residual ischaemic necrosis (partially reversible severe defects). When ventriculography demonstrated further abnormalities in the segmental contractility in these regions, the percentage decreased to 12%.

J. Candell-Riera et al. (eds.), Myocardium at Risk and Viable Myocardium, 213–224.
© 2001 *Kluwer Academic Publishers. Printed in the Netherlands.*

In a series of 100 patients with uncomplicated myocardial infarction studied in our hospital [13,14] using stress ^{201}Tl and radionuclide ventriculography, we observed that the percentage of patients with severe contractility defects and patterns of severe and non-reversible perfusion defects was 20% in patients with anterior infarcts and 8% in those with inferior infarcts.

In clinical practice, the diagnoses of myocardial viability are considered in two types of well-differentiated situations. The first, and more frequent, is in patients that have suffered a myocardial infarction and have a severe impairment in contractility in a region that may be more or less extensive. The second, and much less frequent, occurs in patients with coronary artery disease i.e. with a severe and diffuse impairment of the overall contractility of the left ventricle causing a very low left ventricular ejection fraction and in whom clinical heart failure is predominant. It is evident that the greater the extent of viable myocardium the higher the dyskinetic region that can benefit from revascularisation.

However, the diagnosis of viable myocardium is not synonymous with the necessity for revascularisation. In the majority of patients with severe segmental contractility defects due to a previous infarction, the indication for revascularisation is based, essentially, on the clinical condition of the patient and/or on the extent of the jeopardised myocardium and what needs to kept in mind is the jeopardised myocardium is myocardium that is also alive. Hence, when criteria of reversibility in perfusion scintigraphy already exist, further studies of diagnosing myocardial viability (which are often complex and expensive) are not necessary.

The more extensive the territory with viable myocardium the greater the tendency is towards the decision to revascularise. As we will see, the extent of necrotic or non-viable myocardium increases progressively from non-Q wave infarcts (in which the diagnosis of viable myocardium is, practically, never undertaken) up to the extensive anterior infarcts. The extreme case is that of the ischaemic myocardium in which the therapeutic decision between transplant and revascularisation is, sometimes, very difficult.

In our hospital we evaluated the extent of necrotic or non-viable territory in patients with previous infarction using myocardial SPET with resting- ^{99m}Tc-MIBI in a series of 209 patients (89 anterior, 76 inferior and 44 non-Q) [15,16]. The percentage of territory with uptake <40% was quantified, in the resting polar maps, for each of the 5 regions (anterior, septal, inferior, lateral and apical) into which the left ventricle was divided. We considered as non-viable those regions with >50% of territory having an uptake <40% relative to the maximum. In the anterior infarcts, 46% of the apical region, 21% in the anterior region and only 8% in the septal region and a 15% in the overall left ventricle did not satisfy the criteria of viability with resting-^{99m}Tc-MIBI-SPET. In the inferior infarcts, 23% of the inferior region and 9% of the entire left ventricle was non-viable while, in the non-Q infarcts, this percentage was only 3%. Among the last 200 patients with previous myocardial infarction studied with gated SPET tetrofosmin we observed that <30% had an ejection fraction < 40%, and only 6% had an ejection fraction < 20%.

2. Clinical methods for the diagnosis of viable myocardium

The usefulness of scintigraphic techniques that evaluated perfusion, cellular integrity and myocardium metabolism in the diagnoses of myocardial viability have been described in the previous chapter. Although the attempt had been to give stress electrocardiogram [17,18] a role in the diagnosis of myocardial viability, we believe that the specificity of such technique for this purpose is insufficient [19] and that, in clinical practice, we need to use other explorations. Among the methods directed towards evaluating ventricular contractile reserve are echocardiography [20-44], radionuclide ventriculography [45-49], contrast ventriculography [50,51] and nuclear magnetic resonance [52-55].

ST segment elevation in leads with the Q wave necrosis in the course of a stress test has been associated with the presence of a higher extent of infarction [56-58], of dyskinesia, of ventricular aneurysm [59], and more severe coronary stenosis [60]. Other studies with dobutamine appear to support the hypothesis that the elevation in ST segment in the infarction region is related more with asynergy than with ischaemia induced by exercise [61,62]. There have been reports, nevertheless, that in patients with an elevated ST segment during the stress test, there were reversible defects frequently observed with ^{201}Tl and that this could be a specific and acceptably sensitive sign for the detection of viable myocardium in the same zone of the infarct [17,18]. However, in none of these publications was the extent of necrosis and of ischaemia quantified in these patients.

In intending to clarify this controversy and to study the significance of ST segment elevation with exercise in the region of the necrosis, we studied [19] 62 patients with anterior infarct using stress-^{99m}Tc-MIBI-SPET to quantify the extent of necrosis (uptake <40% relative to the maximum at rest) and of ischaemia (difference in repose-stress of >310%) in the same zone of the infarct and at distance according to whether or not there was ST segment elevation in the precordial shunts during the stress. Twenty-two patients showed elevation of ST > 1mm during the stress test and 40 did not show this response. Further, ventricular aneurysm in catheterisation (p=0.001), extent of necrosis in the antero-septal region (p=0.001) as well as apical (p=0.002), extent of ischaemia in the lateral region (p=0.003) in the polar maps were greater in patients with elevated ST. In a multivariate analysis in which the interval between the infarct and the performing of the stress test, the peak heart rate achieved and the presence of basal elevated ST were introduced as confounding factors, the results did not change. Although it is certain that some patients of the group that had elevated ST segment during the stress test presented with residual ischaemia in the same region as the infarct (a sign of viability), the electrocardiographic response essentially indicated a greater extent of necrotic myocardium and greater extent of ischaemia at distance. These results agree with those obtained experimentally in our hospital [63] in which we observed that the ischaemia adjacent to a chronic infarct induces elevation of the ST segment on the same surface of the necrosis in the absence of viable tissue in this zone. Hence, we believe that the stress ECG is not useful for the diagnosis of viable myocardium and that more complex investigation need to be used.

Echocardiography with perfusion of low dose dobutamine (5-10 µg/kg/min over 3 to 5 minutes) is one of the techniques most commonly used to evaluate improvement in contractility in territories with severe hypokinesia, akinesia or dyskinesia in basal conditions. Dobutamine is a selective beta-1 stimulating agent that produces an increase in the myocardial inotropism. This is a study of considerable use for the cardiologist especially in those centres without nuclear medicine facilities because it has a good correlation with the PET studies and with very acceptable levels of sensitivity and specificity in the prediction of contractile recovery post-revascularisation. (Table 1) [20-27]. Currently, administration of dobutamine up to a maximum dose of 40 µg/kg/min is recommended; doses that provoke ischaemia and also a more specific response (described as "biphasic response") from the hibernating myocardium i.e. when improvement in contractility to low doses is observed and its worsens at high doses.

TABLE 1. Viable myocardium. Diagnostic accuracy of echo-dobutamine.

	N	Sensitivity (%)	Specificity (%)	PPV (%)	NPV (%)
Stunning					
Piérard et al.[20]	17	100	73	63	100
Barilla et al.[21]	21	100	-	100	-
Hibernation					
Cigarroa et al.[22]	25	82	86	82	86
La Canna et al.[23]	33	87	82	90	77
Afridi et al.[24]	20	80	90	89	82
Perrone-Filardi et al.[25]	18	88	87	91	82
Arnese et al.[26]	38	74	96	85	93
DeFilippi et al.[27]	23	97	73	85	94

NPV: negative predictive value, PPV: positive predictive value.

However, the response to dobutamine administration can be difficult to interpret since various factors are involved such as the extent of viable myocardium, the severity of the coronary stenose responsible for hibernation, collateral circulation and treatment with beta blockers [3,8]. The first two of these are fundamental and, in some patients with critical coronary stenosis, the dobutamine even at low doses, can produce ischaemia that would not produce improvement of contractility despite existing myocardial viability. Another fundamental factor is the acquisition of a satisfactory echocardiographic recording since subjectivity of interpretation of the images is considerable [30]. Transoesphageal echocardiography have been used with the objective of improving the quality of the studies but we feel that the inconvenience that this technique represents for the patient makes it inappropriate for routine use. The studies that have compared the diagnostic efficacy of ^{201}Tl reinjection with echo-dobutamine have highlighted that the sensitivity of the former is greater while the latter is more specific. Panza et al. [31] who had employed both techniques in the same patients demonstrated that the proportion of segments with positive response to dobutamine was significantly lower than those that show uptake suggestive of viability with ^{201}Tl suggesting that the cellular mechanisms responsible for the positive inotropic response to the adrenergic stimulation require a higher grade of functional integrity of the myocites than that required for the radionuclide uptake.

Recently, contrast echocardiography has been used for the diagnosis of viable myocardium. It is a technique that facilitates the assessment of the spatial distribution of the microvascular circulation and, as such, resembles the myocardial scintigraphy of perfusion/viability [27,32,33]. The integrity of the coronary microcirculation is related to myocardial viability.

Improvements of ventricular function after post-extrasystolic pause [35], post-exercise [45], with nitroglycerine [46,47], with the infusion of isoproterenol [48] or amrinone [49] have been associated with well with the performance of a contrast or radionuclide ventriculography. However, the spatial resolution of this exploration is not as good as the echocardiogram which, if it is of good quality, permits an evaluation of myocardial wall thickening as well.

3. Systolic function behaviour following revascularisation

Left ventricular ejection fraction is the single most important prognostic factor in patients with coronary artery disease. If the objectives were to increase survival of patients with hibernating myocardium using revascularisation, it would be fundamental to demonstrate that the overall systolic function and that of the segments of the left ventricle can improve.

The majority of studies in which pre- and post-operative ventricular function had been compared in patients with coronary artery disease, the mean ejection fraction increased significantly following the surgical intervention (Table 2) [64-72]. Nevertheless, it needs to be taken into account that these results were obtained in a series of patients in whom the surgical indication was not uniquely for cardiac insufficiency but included angina as well. Milano et al. [70] reported the surgical results from a series of 118 patients with ejection fraction <25%. About 58% of the patients were in class III-IV heart failure. Surgical mortality was 11% and the actuarial survival rates were 77% in the first year and 57% at 5 years. Clinical improvement in heart failure class (p<0.0001) of angina (p<0.0001) and of ejection fraction (p<0.005) were highly significant.

TABLE 2. Ejection fraction changes post-revascularisation.

	n	Angina (%)	Follow up (months)	EF pre. (%)	EF post. (%)	Hospital mortality (%)
Kron et al.[64]	39	56	21	19	26	2.6
Louie et al.[65]	22	23	12	23	36	13.6
Luciani et al.[66]	49	67	26	23	41	14
Van Trigt et al.[67]	118	100	27	21	27	11
Elefteriades et al.[68]	83	49	22	25	33	8.4
Lansman et al.[69]	42	100	34	16	23	4.8
Milano et al.[70]	118	100	27	21	27	11
Olsen et al.[71]	31	100	-	23	35	9.7
Hausmann et al.[72]	265	100	24	24	38	7.6

When changes in ejection fraction following revascularisation are evaluated, it should be taken into account that during the first weeks following surgery there can still be stunned myocardium and, as such, the full recovery of systolic function should be evaluated much later. Isotopic ventriculography has been used to evaluate post-operative changes in ejection fraction after coronary surgery. Ghods et al. [73]

determined the ejection fraction early-on (6 ± 4 days) and later (62 ± 24 days) after the surgery in 12 patients with normal pre-operative ejection fraction and in 15 patients with depressed ejection fraction. While in the first few patients studied there were no significant changes, subsequently the ejection fraction increased from 26% ± 8% to 30% ± 10% in the early-evaluation study and to 34% ± 8% in the late-evaluation study (p<0.05). Of the 11 patients that in the late-evaluation study had increased ejection fraction >5%, only 4 had had an increased in the early-evaluation study. Hence, a premature post-operative measurement of the ejection fraction can cause an underestimation although it is certain, as well, that later-evaluation results can be influenced by the death of those patients with a more pronounced deterioration of ventricular function [74-81].

Although it is not possible to adopt an extremely rigid attitude regarding indications for surgery in these patients, the criteria for the revascularisation of patients with ischaemic heart disease include the presence of an ejection fraction >20%, a left ventricular end-diastolic diameter of <70-75 mm (index >40-44 mm/m^2), good distal coronary vessels and reversible ischaemia in at least two regions of the left ventricle [75].

In the Spanish multicentre study evaluating myocardial viability using isotopic techniques [76-78] in which 116 patients had been studied (78 with ^{99m}Tc-MIBI and 38 with ^{201}Tl), the assessment of ventricular function was performed using blood pool gated radionuclide ventriculography before and after 3 to 6 months of the revascularisation. No significant differences were observed between the pre-revascularisation EF (41.1 ± 14.5%) and the post-revascularisation EF (41.8 ± 15.7%). In 50% of the patients the pre- and post-operative EF did not differ by more than 5 points. In 28% of patients the post-revascularisation EF was >5 points and in 22% a decrease >5 points in the EF was observed. The EF changes in each of these three groups of patients are presented in Figure 3. It can be seen that there were no differences in the mean EF values pre-revascularisation nor was there a significant variation in the EF between patients with severely and those with moderately depressed systolic function.

Christian et al. [79] of the Mayo Clinic reported similar results recently in a series of 86 patients not specifically studied for viability and with pre-operative EF <50%. These authors did not observe statistically significant differences between the mean pre-operative EF (39 ±8%) and the post-operative EF (39 ±8%). In 21% of the patients the EF increased >8 points and in 12% >4 points. As such, only about a third of the patients had an improvement in the contractility.

Apart from the presence of non-viable tissue, other factors can explain this modest rate of functional recovery and among which (Table 3) the outstanding ones are the skill of the surgeon, the possibility of peri-operative necrosis and an insufficient restoration of coronary flow due to poor distal vascular beds.

Conversely, in our series of patients [76-78], of a total of 1044 segments analysed, 464 (44.4%) counted as severe contractile dysfunction (grades 3, 4 and 5) and 413 (39% of the 1044 and 89% of the 464) were revascularised. Contractility improved in 34.4% (142 of 413) of the revascularised dysfunctional segments. As such, the percentage of patients with overall function improvement was 28% and, in relation to the revascularised segments, the improved contractility was 34.4%. These results are similar to those obtained by other authors. In the series of patients studied by Tamaki et al. [80] improvement was in only 51 of the 130 asynergic segments revascularised (39%) and in the Borges-Neto et al. study [81] this was 46 out of 109 segments (42%).

TABLE 3. Factors that can affect the outcome of myocardial revascularisation.

Extent of viable myocardium
Method and timing of the assessment of revascularisation outcome
Incomplete revascularisation
Peri-operative myocardiual protection
Suitability of the coronary vessels to be revascularised
Experience of the surgeon
Peri-operative myocardial injury
Restenosis or occlusion of the graft
Posibility of primary cardiomyopathy
Left ventricular dilation

4. Prognostic implications of viable myocardium detection

Some studies with echo-dobutamine and with isotopes [82-91] suggest that patients with severe impairment of contractility and with criteria of viability progress unfavourably when not revascularised. Eitzman et al. [83] studied the role of viable myocardium in the subsequent appearance of complication in 82 patients, 40 of whom had been revascularised. The patients with a pattern of discordant perfusion-metabolism who had been revascularised had an improvement in functional class but, of the 18 patients not revascularised, 6 died and 3 suffered a myocardial infarction. For Yoshida and Gould [84], the size of the necrotic myocardium and of the viable myocardium in the jeopardised arterial regions were the predictors of mortality in a follow-up of 3 years, especially in patients with low ejection fraction.

DiCarli et al. [85] using PET with ^{13}N-ammonium and ^{18}F-fluorodesoxiglucose, found that the presence of a mismatch pattern of perfusion-metabolism predicted a low survival in a series containing 93 patients with a mean ejection fraction of 25% and a follow-up for one year. Paolini et al. [86] in patients with multivessel disease without angina, with ejection fraction <30% and with evidence of viability in a significant number of myocardial segments observed that, at the end of two years, all the revascularised patients were alive and had improvement in functional class while more than half of those who were not revascularised had worsened heart failure or had died while awaiting transplant. Lee et al. [87] studied a series containing 129 patients with prior infarction and left ventricular dysfunction. The evaluation was with PET images with ^{82}Rb following the administration of dipyridamole and metabolic images with FDG. Of the patients with positive FDG treated with drugs, 48% had non-fatal ischaemic complications compared with 8% of the patients who were FDG negative. Using multivariate analysis, it was observed that, uniquely, the presence of FDG positive was an independent predictor of the appearance of ischaemic events. Although all these studies indicate a better prognosis for patient revascularisation, none of them have an appropriate study design with sufficient sample size and sufficient long-term follow-up for the proposal of improved prognosis to be unambiguous.

We believe that appropriate studies are still necessary to demonstrate that the presence of viable myocardium, of itself, is an independent prognostic variable, as has been demonstrated for systolic function and the presence of jeopardised myocardium. It must be remembered, also, that the hibernating myocardium is a chronic insufficiently-irrigated myocardium and, as such, should be included in the category of jeopardised myocardium. For this reason, the diagnosis of viable myocardium should be an established part of the studies directed towards evaluating the jeopardised myocardium. Only after an extensive infarction or in coronary artery disease, when the detection of viable myocardium is necessary for the better management of the patient, are studies directed towards its detection and quantification clinically indicated.

References

1. Rahimtoola SH. Hibernating myocardium has reduced blood flow at rest that increases with low-dose dobutamine. Circulation 1996; 94: 3055-3061.
2. Iskandrian AS. Myocardial viability: Unresolved issues. J Nucl Med 1996; 37: 794-797.
3. Kaul S. Response of dysfunctional myocardium to dobutamine. "The eyes see what the mind knows!". J Am Coll Cardiol 1996; 27: 1608-1611.
4. Wackers FJT. Radionuclide detection of myocardial ischemia and myocardial viability: Is the glass half empty or half full?. J Am Coll Cardiol 1996; 27: 1598-1600.
5. Dilsizian V. Myocardial viability: Contractile reserve or cell membrane integrity. J Am Coll Cardiol 1996; 28: 443-446.
6. Beller GA. Comparison of ^{201}Tl scintigraphy and low-dose dobutamine echocardiography for the noninvasive assessment of myocardial viability. Circulation 1996; 94: 2681-2684.
7. McGhie AI, Weyman A. Searching for hibernating myocardium. Time to reevaluate investigative strategies?. Circulation 1996; 94: 2685-2688.
8. Armstrong WF. "Hibernating" myocardium: Asleep or part dead?. J Am Coll Cardiol 1996; 28: 530-535.
9. Vanoverschelde JLJ, Wijns W, Borgers M et al. Chronic myocardial hibernation in humans. From bedside to bench. Circulation 1997; 95: 1961-1971.
10. Lewis SJ, Sawada SG, Ryan T, Segar DS, Armstrong WF, Feigenbaum H. Segmental wall motion abnormalities in the absence of clinically documented myocardial infarction: Clinical significance and evidence of hibernating myocardium. Am Heart J 1991; 121: 1088-1093.
11. Candell-Riera J, Santana-Boado C, Castell-Conesa J, et al. Simultaneous dipyridamole/maximal subjective exercise with 99mTc-MIBI SPECT: improved diagnostic yield in coronary arterty disease. J Am Coll Cardiol 1997; 29: 531-536.
12. Lemlek J, Heo J, Iskandrian AS. The clinical relevance of myocardial viability in patient management. Am Heart J 1992; 124: 1327-1331.
13. Candell-Riera J, Permanyer-Miralda G, Castell J et al. Uncomplicated first myocardial infarction: Strategy for comprehensive prognostic studies. J Am Coll Cardiol 1991; 18: 1207-1219.
14. Olona M, Candell-Riera J, Permanyer-Miralda G et al. Strategies for prognostic assessment of uncomplicated first myocardial infarction: A 5-years follow up study. J Am Coll Cardiol 1995; 25: 815-822.
15. Santana C, Candell-Riera J, Aguadé S et al. Extensión del territorio no viable en el infarto anterior, inferior y no Q. Estudio con ^{99m}Tc-MIBI SPET de reposo. Rev Esp Cardiol 1997; 50 (Supl. 6): 79 (Abstr.).
16. Candell-Riera J, González JM, Castell J et al. Cuantificación de la extensión de miocardio viable mediante 99mTc-MIBI SPET de reposo. Rev Esp Cardiol 1997; 50 (Supl. 6): 57 (Abstr.).

17. Margonato A, Ballarotto C, Bonetti F et al. Assessment of residual tissue viability by exercise testing in recent myocardial infarction: Comparison of the electrocardiogram and myocardial perfusion scintigraphy. J Am Coll Cardiol 1992;19: 948-952.

18. Margonato A, Chierchia SL, Xuereb RG et al. Specificity and sensitivity of exercise-induced ST segment elevation for detection of residual viability: Comparison with fluorodeoxyglucose and positron emission tomography. J Am Coll Cardiol 1995; 25: 1032-1038.

19. Candell-Riera J, Santana-Boado C, Armadans-Gil L et al. Comparison of patients with anterior wall healed myocardial infarction with and without exercise induced ST segment elevation. Am J Cardiol 1998; 81: 12-16.

20. Piérard LA, De Landsheere CM, Berthe C, Rigo P, Kulbertus HE. Identification of viable myocardium by echocardiography during dobutamine infusion in patients with myocardial infarction after thrombolytic therapy: comparison with positron emission tomography. J Am Coll Cardiol 1990; 15: 1021-1031.

21. Barilla F, Gheorgiade M, Alam M, Khaja F, Goldstein S. Low-dose dobutamine in patients with acute myocardial infarction identifies viable but not contractile myocardium and predicts the magnitude of improvement in wall motion abnormalities in response to coronary revascularization. Am Heart J 1991; 122: 1522-1531.

22. Cigarroa CG, deFilippi CR, Brickner ME, Alvarez LG, Wait MA, Grayburn PA. Dobutamine stress echocardiography identifies hibernating myocardium and predicts recovery of left ventricular function after coronary revascularization. Circulation 1993; 88: 430-436.

23. La Canna G, Alfieri O, Giubbini R, Gargano M, Ferrari R, Visioli O. Echocardiography during infusion of dobutamine for identification of reversible dysfunction in patients with chronic coronary artery disease. J Am Coll Cardiol 1994; 23: 617-626.

24. Afridi I, Kleiman NS, Raizner AE, Zoghbi WA. Dobutamine echocardiography in myocardial hibernation. Optimal dose and accuracy in predicting recovery of ventricular function after coronary angioplasty. Circulation 1995; 91: 663-670.

25. Perrone-Filardi P, Pace L, Prastaro M et al. Dobutamine echocardiography predicts improvement of hypoperfused dysfunctional myocardium after revascularization in patients with coronary artery disease. Circulation 1995; 91: 2556-2565.

26. Arnese M, Cornel JH, Salustri A et al. Prediction of improvement of regional left ventricular function after surgical revascularization. A comparison of low-dose dobutamine echocardiography with 201Tl single-photon emission computed tomography. Circulation 1995; 91: 2748-2752.

27. De Filippi CR, Willett DL, Irani WN, Eichhorn EJ, Velasco CE, Grayburn PA. Comparison of myocardial contrast echocardiography and low-dose dobutamine stress echocardiography in predicting recovery of left ventricular function after coronary revascularization in chronic ischemic heart disease. Circulation 1995; 92; 92: 2863-2868.

28. Smart SC, Sawada S, Ryan T et al. Low-dose dobutamine echocardiography detects reversible dysfunction after thrombolytic therapy of acute myocardial infarction. Circulation 1993; 88: 408-415.

29. Chen C, Chen LL, Prada JV et al. Incremental doses of dobutamine induce a biphasic response in dysfunctional left ventricular regions subtending coronary stenoses. Circulation 1995; 92: 756-766.

30. Hoffman R, Lethen H, Marwick T et al. Analysis of interinstitutional observer agreement in interpretation of dobutamine stress echocardiogramas. J Am Coll Cardiol 1996; 27: 330-336.

31. Panza JA, Dilsizian V, Laurienzo JM, Curiel RV, Katsiyiannis PT. Relation between thallium uptake and contractile response to dobutamine. Implications regarding myocardial viability in patients with chronic coronary artery disease and left ventricular dysfunction. Circulation 1995; 91: 990-998

32. Kaul S, Jayaweera AR, Glasheen WP, Villanueva FS, Gutgesel HP, Spotnitz WD. Myocardial contrast echocardiography and the transmural distribution of flow: a critical apraisal during myocardial ischemia not associated with infarction. J Am Coll Cardiol 1992; 20: 1005-1006.

33. De la Torre JM, Martín Durán R. Ecocardiografía de contraste. Rev Esp Cardiol 1997; 50 (Supl. 5): 15-25.

34. Bax JJ, Wijns W, Cornel JH, Visser FC, Boersma E, Fioretti PM. Accuracy of currently available techniques for prediction of functional recovery after revascularization in patients with left ventricular dysfunction due to chronic coronary artery disease: comparison to pooled data. J Am Coll Cardiol 1997; 30: 1451-1460.

35. Scognamiglio R, Fasoli G, Casarotto D et al. Postextrasystolic potentiation and dobutamine echocardiography in predicting recovery of myocardial function after coronary bypass revascularization. Circulation 1997; 96: 816-820.

36. Hoffer EP, Dewé W, Celentano C, Piérard LA. Low-level exercise echocardiography detects contractile reserve and predicts reversible dysfunction after acute myocardial infarction. Comparison with low-dose dobutamine echocardiography. J Am Coll Cardiol 1999; 34: 989-997.

37. Amanullah AM, Chaudhry FA, Heo J et al. Comparison of dobutamine echocardiography, dobutamine sestamibi, and rest-redistribution thallium-201 single-photon emission computed tomography for determining contractile reserve and myocardial ischemia in ischemic cardiomyopathy. Am J Cardiol 1999; 84: 626-631.

38. Spinelli L, Petretta M, Cuocolo A et al. Prediction of recovery of left ventricular dysfunction after acute myocardial infarction: comparison between ^{99m}Tc-sestamibi cardiac tomography and low-dose dobutamine echocardiography. J Nucl Med 1999; 1683-1692.

39. Panza JA, Dilsizian V, Curiel RV, Unger EF, Laurienzo JM, Kitsiou AN. Myocardial blood flow at rest and contractile reserve in patients with chronic coronary artery disease and left ventricular dysfunction. J Nucl Cardiol 1999; 6: 487-494.

40. Bax JJ, Poldermans D, Visser FC et al. Delayed recovery of hibernating myocardium after surgical revascularization: implications for discrepancy between metabolic imaging and dobutamine echocardiography for assessment of myocardial viability. J Nucl Cardiol 1999; 6: 685-687.

41. Everaert H, Vanhove C, Franken PR. Low-dose dobutamine gated single-photon emission tomography: comparison with stress echocardiography. Eur J Nucl Med 2000; 27: 413-418.

42. Lu C, Carlino M, Fragasso G et al. Enoximone echocardiography for predicting recovery of left ventricular dysfunction after revascularization. A novel test for detecting myocardial viability. Circulation 2000; 101: 1255-1260.

43. Iwakura K, Ito H, Nishikawa N et al. Use of echocardiography for predicting myocardial vviability in patients with reperfused anterior wall infarction Am J Cardiol 2000; 85: 744-748.

44. Cwajg JM, Cwajg E, Nagueh SF et al. End-diastolic wall thickness as a predictor of recovery of function in myocardial hibernation. Relation to rest-redistribution Tl-201 tomography and dobutamine stress echocardiography. J Am Coll Cardiol 2000; 35: 1152-1161.

45. Rozanski A, Berman D, Gray R et al. Preoperative prediction of reversible myocardial asynergy by postexercise radionuclide ventriculography. N Engl J Med 1982; 307: 212-216.

46. Borer JS, Bacharach SL, Green MV, Kent KM, Johnston GS, Epstein SE. Effect of nitroglycerin on exercise-induced abnormalities of left ventricular regional function and ejection fraction in coronary artery disease. Assessment by radionuclide cineangiography in symptomatic and asymptomatic patients. Circulation 1978; 57: 314-320.

47. Ritchie JL, Sorensen SG, Kennedy JW, Hamilton GW. Radionuclide angiography: Noninvasive assessment of hemodynamic changes after administration of nitroglycerin. Am J Cardiol 1979; 43: 278-284.

48. Satler LF, Kent KM, Fox LM et al. The assessment of contractile reserve after thrombolytic therapy for acute myocardial infarction. Am Heart J 1986; 111; 821-825.

49. Pérez-Baliño NA, Masoli OH, Meretta AH et al. Amrinone stimulation test: Ability to predict improvement in left ventricular ejection fraction after coronary bypass surgery in patients with poor baseline left ventricular function. J Am Coll Cardiol 1996; 28: 1488-1492.

50. Dove JT, Shah PM, Schreiner BF. Effects of nitroglycerin on left ventricular wall motion in coronary artery disease. Circulation 1974; 49: 682-687.

51. Fujita M, Yamanishi K, Hirai T et al. Significance of collateral circulation in reversible left ventricular asynergy by nitroglycerin in patients with relatively recent myocardial infarction. Am Heart J 1990; 120: 521-528.

52. Baer FM, Voth E, Schneider CA, Theissen P, Schicha H, Sechtem U. Comparison of low-dose dobutamine-gradient-echo magnetic resonance imaging and positron emission tomography with (^{18}F)fluorodeoxyglucose in patients with chronic coronary artery disease: a functional and morphological approach to the detection of residual myocardial viability. Circulation 1995; 91: 1006-1015.

53. Yabe T, Mitsunami K, Inubushi T, Kinoshita M. Quantitative measurements of cardiac phosphorus metabolites in coronary artery disease by phosphorus-31 magnetic resonance spectroscopy. Circulation 1995; 92: 15-23.

54. Baer FM, Theissen P, Crnac J et al. Head to head comparison of dobutamine-transoesophageal echocartdiography and dobutamine-magnetic resonance imaging for the prediction of left ventricular functional recovery in patients with chronic coronary artery disease. Eur Heart J 2000; 21: 981-991.

55. Sechtem U, Baer FM, Theissen P, Voth E, Schicha H (1998) Assessment of myocardial viability by magnetic resonance techniques, in Higgins CB, Ingwall JS and Pohost GM (eds.), Futura Publishing Company, Inc., Armonk, NY, pp. 267-282.

56. Haines DE, Beller GA, Watson DD, Kaiser DL, Sayre SL, Gibson RS. Exercise-induced ST segment elevation 2 weeks after uncomplicated myocardial infarction: Contributing factors and prognostic significance. J Am Coll Cardiol 1987; 9: 996-1003.

57. Gewirtz H, Sullivan M, O'Reilly G, Winter S, Most AS. Role of myocardial ischemia in the genesis of stress-induced S-T segment elevation in previous anterior myocardial infarction. Am J Cardiol 1983; 51: 1289-1293.

58. Mazzotta G, Camerini A, Scopinaro G et al. Predicting cardiac mortality after uncomplicated myocardial infarction by exercise radionuclide ventriculography and exercise-induced ST segment elevation. Eur Heart J 1992; 13: 330-337.

59. Weiner DA, McCabe C, Klein MD, Ryan TJ. ST segment changes post-infarction: Predictive value for multivessel coronary disease and left ventricular aneurysm. J Am Coll Cardiol 1987; 9: 996-1003.

60. Cahine RA, Raizner AE, Ishimori T. The clinical significance of exercise-induced ST-segment elevation. Circulation 1976; 54: 209-213.

61. Coma-Canella I, del Val Gómez M, Terol I, Rodrigo F, Castro JM. Radionuclide studies in patients with stress-induced ST-segment elevation after acute myocardial infarction. J Am Coll Cardiol 1994; 128: 459-465.

62. Elhendy A, Geleijnse ML, Roelandt JRTC et al. Evaluation by quantitative 99m-technetium MIBI SPECT and echocardiography of myocardial perfusion and wall motion abnormalities in patients with dobutamine-induced ST-segment elevation. Am J Cardiol 1995; 76: 441-448.

63. Cinca J, Bardají A, Carreño A et al. ST elevation at the surface of a healed transmural myocardial infarction in pigs. Conditions for passive transmission from the ischemic peri-infarction zone. Circulation 1995; 91: 1552-1559.

64. Kron IL, Flanagan TL, Blackbourne LH et al. Coronary revascularization rather than cardiac transplantation for chronic ischemic cardiomyopathy. Ann Surg 1989; 210: 348-352.

65. Louie HW, Laks H, Milgalter E et al. Ischemic cardiomyopathy. Criteria for coronary revascularization and cardiac transplantation. Circulation , suppl. III 1991; 84: 290-295.

66. Luciani GB, Faggian G, Razzolini R et al. Severe ischemic left ventricular failure. Coronary operation or heart transplantation? Ann Thorac Surg 1993; 55: 719-723.

67. Van Trigt P. Ischemic cardiomyopathy. The role of coronary artery bypass. Coron Artery Dis 1993; 4: 707-712.

68. Elefteriades JA, Tolis G, Jr, Levi E et al. Coronary artery bypass grafting in severe left ventricular dysfunction. Excellent survival with improved ejection fraction and functional state. J Am Coll Cardiol 1993; 22: 1411-1117.

69. Lansman SL, Cohen M, Galla JD et al. Coronary bypass wih ejection fraction of 0.20 or less using centigrade cardioplegia. Long-term follow-up. Ann Thorac Surg 1993; 56: 480-485.

70. Milano CA, White WD, Smith LR et al. Coronary artery bypass in patients with severely depressed ventricular function. Ann Thorac Surg 1993; 56: 487-493.

71. Olsen P, Kassis E, Niebuhr-Jorgensen U. Coronary artery bypass surgery in patients with severe left ventricular dysfunction. Thorac Cardiovasc Surg 1993; 41: 118-120.

72. Hausmann H, Ennker J, Topp H et al. Coronary artery bypass grafting and heart transplantation in end-stage coronary artery disease. A comparison of hemodynamic improvement and ventricular function. J Card Surg 1994; 9: 77-84.

73. Ghods M, Pancholy S, Cave V, Cassell D, Heo J, Iskandrian AS. Serial changes in left ventricular function after coronary artery bypass: implications in viability assessment. Am Heart J 1995; 129: 20-23.

74. Louie HW, Laks H, Milgalter E et al. Ischemic cardiomyopathy: criteria for coronary revascularization and cardiac transplantation. Circulation 1991; 84 (Supl 5): 290-295.

75. Blitz A, Laks H. The role of coronary revascularization in the management of heart failure: identification of candidates and review of results. Curr Opin Cardiol 1996; 11: 276-290.

76. Castell J, Candell-Riera J, Roselló-Urgell J et al. Valoración de la viabilidad miocárdica mediante tecnecio-99m isonitrilo y talio-201. Resultados del protocolo multicéntrico español. Rev Esp Cardiol 1997; 50: 320-330.

77. Candell-Riera J. ^{99m}Tc-MIBI SPET de reposo y esfuerzo-reposo en el diagnóstico de la hibernación miocárdica. Estudio multicéntrico español. Rev Esp Cardiol 1997; 50 (Supl. 6): 57.

78. Candell Riera J, Castell Conesa J, González González J, Rosselló J. Grupo de trabajo de Cardiología Nuclear. Eficacia de la tomogammagrafía miocárdica con ^{99m}Tc-MIBI en la predicción de la recuperabilidad de la función contráctil post-revascularización. Resultados del protocolo multicéntrico español. Rev Esp Cardiol 2000; 53: 903-910.

79. Christian TF, Miller TD, Hodge DO, Orszulak TA, Gibbons RJ. An estimate of the prevalence of reversible left ventricular dysfunction in patients referred for coronary artery bypass surgery. J Nucl Cardiol 1997; 4: 140-146.

80. Tamaki N, Kawamoto M, Tadamura E et al. Prediction of reversible ischemia after revascularization. Perfusion and metabolic studies w2ith positron emission tomography. Circulation 1995; 91: 1697-1705.

81. Borges-Neto S, Shaw LJ, Kesler K et al. Usefulness of serial radionuclide angiography in predicting cardiac death after coronary artery bypass grafting and comparison with clinical and cardiac catheterization data. Am J Cardiol 1997; 79: 851-855.

82. Sicari R, Picano E, Landi P et al. Prognostic value of dobutamine-atropine stress echocardiography early after acute myocardial infarction. J Am Coll Cardiol 1997; 29: 254-260.

83. Eitzman D, Al-Aouar Z, Kanter HL et al. Clinical outcome of patients with advanced coronary artery disease after viability studies with positron emission tomography. J Am Coll Cardiol 1992; 20: 559-565.

84. Yoshida K, Gould KL. Quantitative relation of myocardial infarct size and myocardial viability by positron emission tomography to left ventricular ejection fraction and 3-year mortality with and without revascularization. J Am Coll Cardiol 1993; 22: 984-997.

85. Di Carli MF, Davidson M, Little R et al. Value of metabolic imaging with positron emission tomography for evaluating prognosis in patients with coronary artery disease and left ventricular dysfunction. Am J Cardiol 1994; 73: 527-533.

86. Paolini G, Lucignani G, Zuccari M et al. Identification and revascularization of hibernating myocardium in angina free patients with left ventricular dysfunction. Eur J Cardiothorac Surg 1994; 8: 139-144.

87. Lee KS, Marwick TH, Cook SA et al. Prognosis of patients with left ventricular dysfunction, with and without viable myocardium after myocardial infarction. Relative efficacy of medical therapy and revascularization. Circulation 1994; 90: 2687-2694.

88. Gioia G, Powwers J, Heo J, Iskandrian AS. Prognostic value of rest-redistribution tomographic thallium-201 imaging in ischemic cardiomyopathy. Am J Cardiol 1995; 75: 759-762.

89. Pasquet A, Robert A, D'Hondt AM et al. Prognostic value of myocardial ischemia and viability in patients with chronic left ventricular ischemic dysfunction. Circulation 1999; 100: 141-148.

90. Samady H, Elefteriades JA, Abbott BG, Mattera JA, McPherson CA, Wackers FJT. Failure to improve left ventricular function after coronary revascularization for ischemic cardiomyopathy is not associated with worse outcome. Circulation 1999; 100: 1298-1304.

91. Sharir T, Berman DS, Lewin HC et al. Incremental prognostic value of rest-redistribution 201Tl single-photon emission tomography. Circulation 1999; 100: 1964-1970.

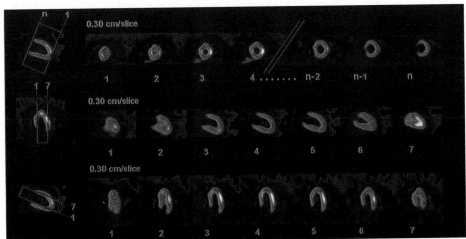

Plate 2.1: Presentation and numeration of the three series of slices. Above: the slices of the short axis with the vertical long axis as reference and with consecutive sections numbered from the apex to the left ventricle valvular plane. Centre: the vertical long axis slices with the horizontal long axis as reference and numbering from the septum up to the lateral wall. Below: the slices of the horizontal long axis with the vertical long axis as reference and with the numbering from the inferior wall up to the anterior wall.

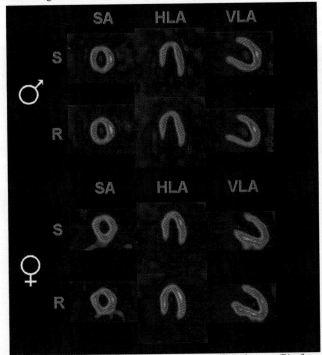

Plate 2.2: Normal images of the three ventricular axes in stress (S) and at rest (R) of a male and a female with a probability of <5% of coronary disease. Of note, particularly in the sections of the short axis, is the accentuated hypo-activity in the inferior region in the male and in the anterior region in the female.
HLA : horizontal long axis, SA : short axis, VLA : vertical long axis

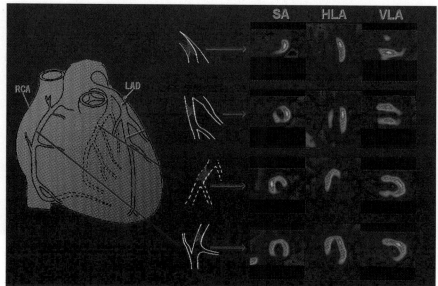

Plate 2.3: Localisation of the perfusion defects corresponding to the occlusion by balloon angioplasty of the principal epicardial arteries. From top to bottom: left anterior descending artery (LAD), middle anterior descending artery (below the first septal branch), proximal circumflex artery (Cx) and right coronary artery (RCA). HLA: horizontal long axis, SA: short axis, VLA: vertical long axis

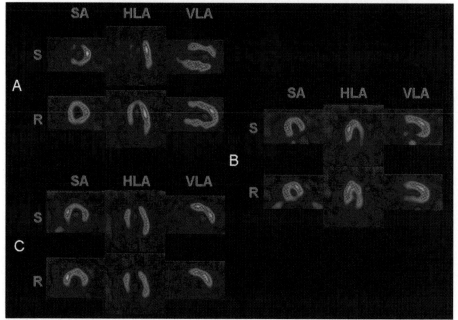

Plate 2.4: Perfusion SPET with tetrofosmin in stress (S) and at rest (R) in the three ventricular axes. Post-stress perfusion defects with total (A), partial (B), and no (C) reversibility. HLA: horizontal long axis, SA: short axis, VLA: vertical long axis

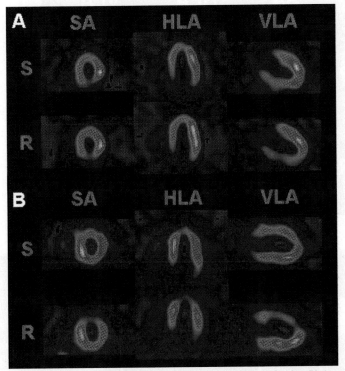

Plate 2.5: A) Inferior reverse pattern in patient without previous myocardial infarction. B) Anterior reverse pattern in patient with previous anterior myocardial infarction..
HLA : horitzontal long axis, SA : short axis, VLA : vertical long axis.

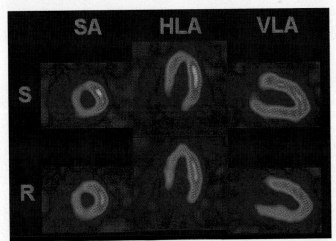

Plate 2.6: Perfusion SPET with tetrofosmin in stress (S) and at rest (R) in patient with left bundle branch block, normal coronary arteries, and abnormal septal movement in the echocardiogram. A light hypo-uptake can be observed limited to the septal zone with minimal variations between the images of stress and rest.
HLA : horitzontal long axis, SA : short axis, VLA : vertical long axis.

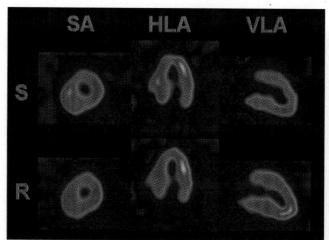

Plate 2.7: Myocardial SPET images of patient with hypertrophic cardiomyopathy with predominant thickening of infero-septal wall. HLA: horizontal long axis, SA: short axis, VLA: vertical long axis.

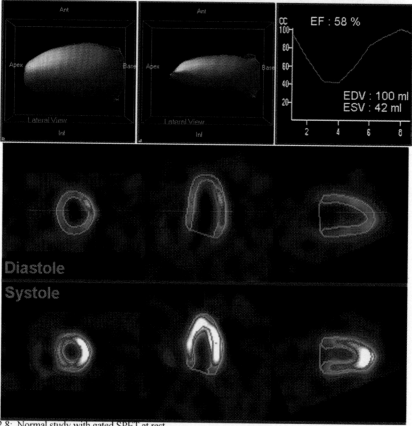

Plate 2.8: Normal study with gated SPET at rest.
EDV: end diastolic volume, EF: ejection fraction, ESV: end systolic volume.

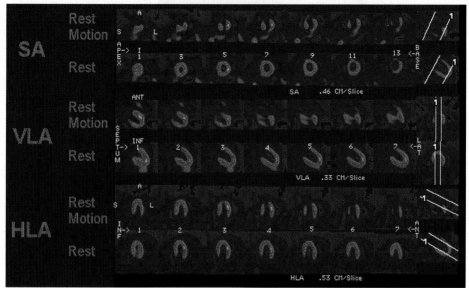

Figure 2.9: Artefacts produced by the patient having moved during the rest SPET image acquisition (rest motion) compared to correct acquisition (rest).
HLA: horitzontal long axis, SA: short axis, VLA: vertical long axis.

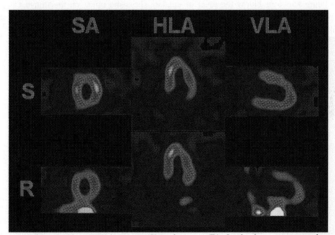

Figure 2.10: Myocardial perfusion SPET in stress (S) and at rest (R). In the images at rest there appears intense extra-cardiac activity in the inferior-basal region corresponding to the biliary-gastric reflux in the stomach and behind the valvular plane due to gastro-oesophageal reflux.
HLA: horizontal long axis, SA: short axis, VLA: vertical long axis.

230

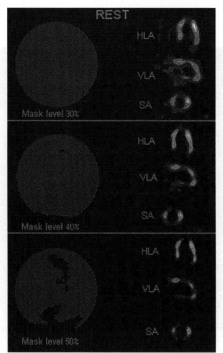

Plate 3.1: Analysis of level of uptake method: Conducted on a normalised polar map on which a mask is maintained for a pre-established level of uptake, a binary effect is achieved in which the zones of the myocardium are expressed as being above or below the level of uptake. The same effect on the image can be achieved by performing a subtraction of background activity of a similar magnitude.

HLA : horizontal long axis, SA : short axis, VLA : vertical long axis

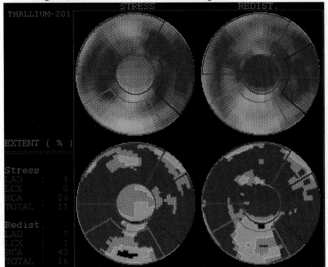

Plate 3.2: Cedars method of polar maps of stress and redistribution of Thallium-201 (above) and visualisation of the comparison with the database of normality in four colours (below), in terms of standard deviations. On the left are expressed the percentages of extent for each of the coronary vessels (LAD: left anterior descending, LCX: left circumflex and RCA: right coronary artery) of the segments of the map with a standard deviation >10% of normal.

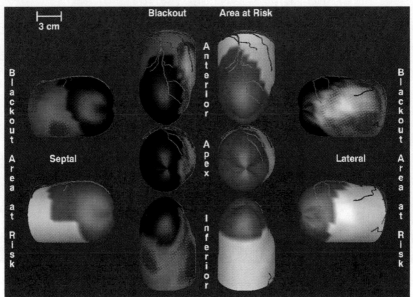

Plate 3.3: Five different views of the unified LV and coronary arteries. Blackout regions on the epicardial surface serve as the gold standard, purple regions on the corresponding views (called "areas-at-risk" in this figure) are those portions of the LV that are predicted to be at-risk, based on coronary artery anatomy and it's unification with the epicardial surface. Note the overlap between blackout and purple (area-at-risk) regions, indicating excellent unification accuracy.

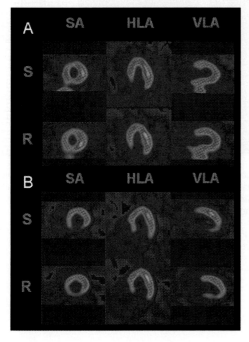

Plate 4.1. Myocardial stress SPET with ^{99m}Tc-tetrofosmin. A) a patient with left branch block and angiographically-normal coronary arteries. No reversible perfusion can be seen. B) a patient with left branch block, inferior infarct and critical stenosis in the right coronary artery. A severe partially-reversible defect in the inferior region can be observed. In no case was there evidence of false image of ischaemia in the septal region that could be attibutable to left branch block.
HLA : Horizontal long axis, R : rest, S : stress, SA : short axis, VLA : vertical long axis.

232

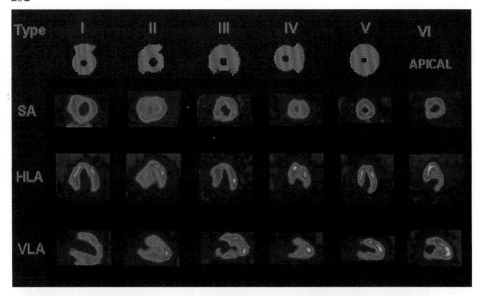

Plate 4.2. Myocardial SPET with ^{99m}Tc-tetrofosmin in different types of hypertrophic cardiomyopathy [168]. HLA: horitzontal long axis, SA: short axis, VLA: vertical long axis.

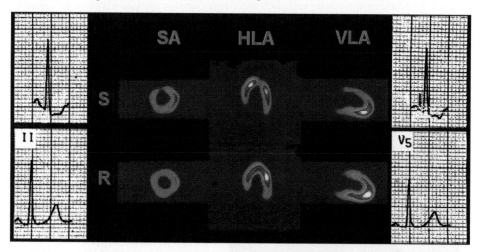

Plate 4.3. Myocardial SPET with ^{99m}Tc-tetrofosmin in a patient with syndrome X, with angina, ST segment depression during stress and angiographically-normal coronary arteries. A slight thinning can be observed and defect of the anterior region which normalised on resting.
HLA : horizontal long axis, R : rest, S: stress, SA : short axis, VLA : vertical long axis.

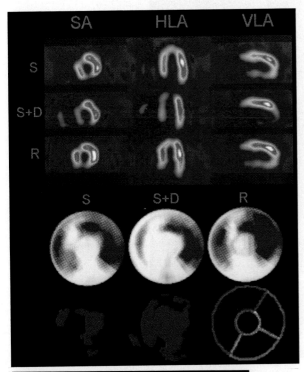

Plate 5.1. SPET sections of the short axis (SA), horizontal long axis (HLA), and verical long axis (VLA) following an insufficient exercise test (S); following the same test together with the administration of dipyridamole (S+D); and at rest (R) in a patient without previous infarction and disease of the right anterior descending coronary artery and of the right coronary artery. The severity of the inferior defect and of the extent of the antero-septal defect is more evident in the S+D. Similarly, the extent of ischaemia (in red) of the polar map in the same patient is higher in S+D.

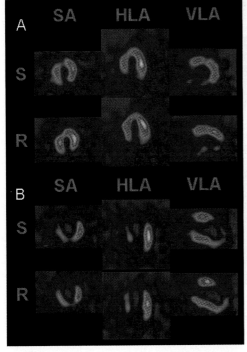

Plate 5.2. A: Patient with inferior infarct and stenosis of 70% of the first diagonal. Apart from the inferior reversible defect (large arrows), a slight reversible defect (ischaemia at distance) in the middle anterior region (small arrows). B: Patient with anterior infarct and stenosis of 90% of the proximal anterior descending. Severe and extensive antero-apical defects and partially reversible septal (residual ischaemia) in the apical and septal regions (arrows) are observed.
HLA : horizontal long axis, R : rest, S : stress, SA : short axis, VLA : vertical long axis.

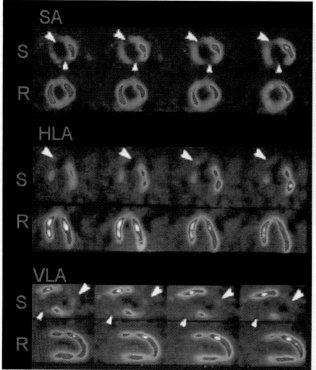

Plate 6.1. ^{99m}Tc-MIBI perfusion SPET in a patient with multivessel disease in which are seen reversible perfusion defects in the anterior-septal and apical regions (large arrows) dependent on the left descending anterior coronary artery and in the inferior region (small arrows) dependent on the right coronary artery. HLA: horizontal long axis, SA: short axis, VLA: vertical long axis.

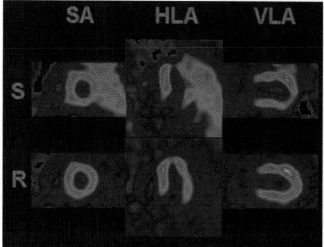

Plate 6.2. Example of abnormal pulmonary uptake corresponding to a ^{99m}Tc-tetrofosmin scintigraphy in a patient with triple vessel disease.
HLA: horizontal long axis, SA: short axis, VLA: vertical long axis.

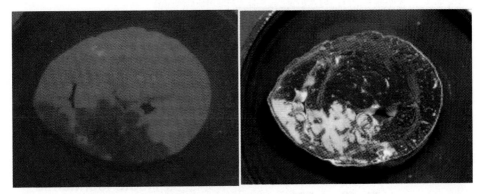

Plate 7.1. Spatial distribution of the salvaged myocardium and of the necrosed myocardium in the reperfused zone in a pig heart subjected to 48 minutes of coronary occlusion and 6 hours of reperfusion. A) The jeopardised area (distribution territory of the occluded artery) appears non-fluorescent under ultraviolet illumination following the injection of fluoresceine during the occlusion. B) Incubation with triphenyltetrazolium reveals the zones of necrosis that appear as areas free of the dye. Note: the intricate distribution of these areas within the jeopardised area.

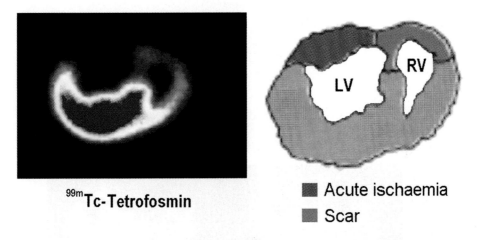

Plate 8.1. Scintigraphic activity of ^{99m}Tc-tetrofosmin in a transverse section of 5mm thickness of the left ventricle of a pig with an infarct of the anterior face of one month's duration subjected to a second occlusion of the anterior descending coronary artery in its proximal portion. The diagrams show the normal myocardium (yelow), the acute ischaemia and the infarct scar. The scar of the infarct shows a greater scintigraphic activity than the regions subjected to acute ischaemia.

236

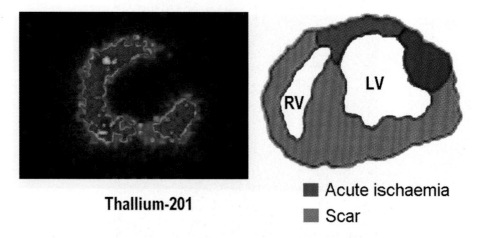

Thallium-201

■ Acute ischaemia
■ Scar

Plate 8.2. Scintigraphic activity of the ^{201}Tl chloride in a transversal section of 5mm thickness of the heart of a pig with an anterior infarct of one month's duration subjected to a second occlusion of the anterior descending coronary artery in its proximal portion. The diagram shows the normal myocardium (yelow), the acute ischaemia and the scar of the infarction. The scintigraphic activity is greater in the infarcted zone than in that of the acute ischaemia.

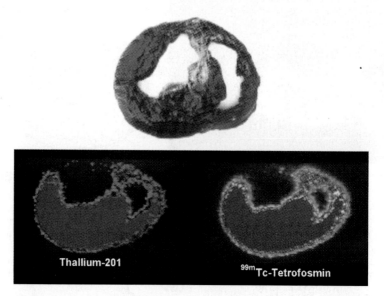

Thallium-201

^{99m}**Tc-Tetrofosmin**

Plate 8.3. Image of a transversal section of 5mm thickness of a porcine heart with its corresponding scintigraphic images using ^{99m}Tc-tetrofosmin and ^{201}Tl. The right ventricular cavity appears to the right and the left ventricular cavity to the left. The area of necrosis is located in the inter-ventricular septum and in a part of the right ventricle. There is greater uptake of both radiotracers in the necrotic than the ischaemic region of the anterior territory of the left ventricle that shows the same level of activity as the background. As can be seen, the distributions of both tracers are identical.

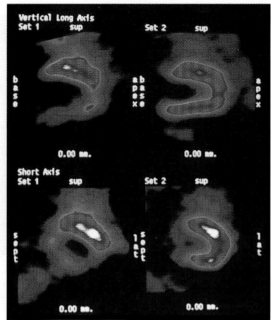

Plate 9.1. Positron emission tomography (PET). Pattern of flow-metabolism mismatch indicative of viability in a region that is severely hypoperfused at rest. To the left, the flow image with ^{13}N-ammonium shows a severe defect in the inferior wall. To the right, intense ^{18}F-Fluordeoxyglucose uptake in the same region is observed. (Courtesy of Dr. J.L Carreras)

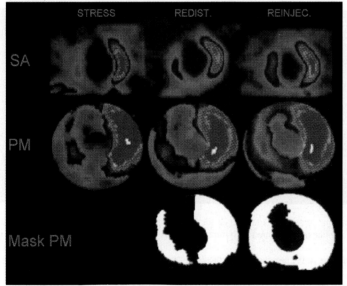

Plate 9.2. From left to right, images of the short axis (SA) post-stress, redistribution and reinjection (with detection at 15 minutes) of a study with ^{201}Tl in a patient with an antero-septal infarction. Polar maps (PM) of stress, redistribution and reinjection, and 50% polar map uptake mask. Severe hypoperfusion in the antero-septal, inferior and apical regions, in stress with minimum redistribution and higher reversibility following reinjection is evident.

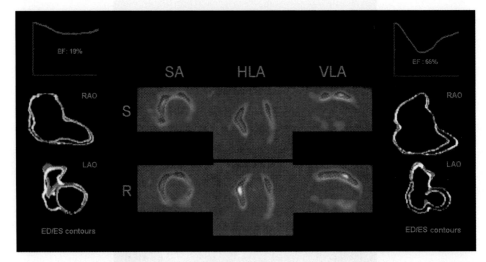

Plate 9.3. On the left, pre-operative study in a patient with severe depression of systolic function (EF 19%) and left ventricular dilation (left panel). The post-stress (S) perfusion study with MIBI showed severe and extensive defects in the apical and inferior regions and moderate anterior and lateral hypoperfusion, partially reversible at rest (R)(central panel). In the right,, the recovery of contractility (EF 55%) 3 months after a triple coronary artery bypass grafft is evident. ED: end-diastolic, EF: ejection fraction, ES: end-systolic, HLA: horitzontal long axis,LAO: left anterior oblique,RAO: right anterior oblique,SA: short axis,VLA: vertical long axis.

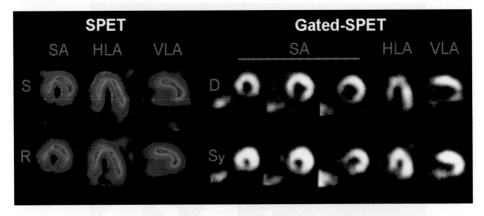

Plate 9.4. Conventional tomographic images on the left (in colour). On the right, images in diastole (D) and systole (Sy) that facilitate the evaluation of systolic thickening and wall motion using a ^{99m}Tc-tetrofosmin rest gated-SPET. The end-diastolic images show an intense inferior defect with a significant increment of activity in end-systole indicative of the presence of contractile myocardium.
S : stress, R : rest, SA : Short axis, HLA : Horitzontal long axis, VLA : Vertical long axis.

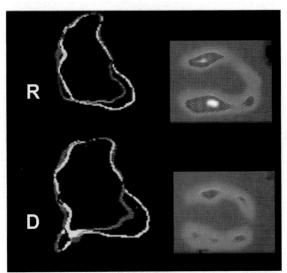

Plate 9.5. Patient with non-extensive anterior infarction. On the left, the ventricular contours obtained in anterior right oblique projection using gated blood pool radionuclide ventriculography. On the right, a section in the long vertical axis of a SPET with MIBI. At rest (R) there appears moderate hypokinesia and hypo-perfusion in the antero-septal region. The administration of 10 ug/kg/min of dobutamine (D) produces an intense increase in the regional contractility (EF-R = 46%, EF-D = 63%) which indicates a preserved contractile reserve, with a slight increase in the antero-apical uptake in the perfusion study.

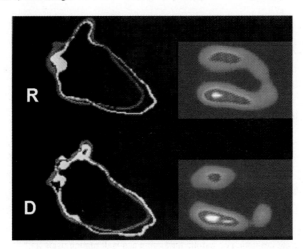

Plate 9.6. Patient with extensive anterior infarction and depressed ventricular function (EF = 32%). On the left, the ventricular contours obtained in right anterior oblique projections using gated blood pool radionuclide ventriculography. On the right, sections of the long vertical axis of a SPET with MIBI. At rest (R) is seen an anterior severe hypokinesia and moderate hypoperfusion in the same territory is seen. The administration of dobutamine (D) at low dose (10 ug/kg/min) worsens the contractility with deterioration of the systolic function (EF = 23%) and induces defects that are more intense and extensive in the anterior and in the apical regions.

Index